The Essentials of Respiratory Therapy

The Essentials of Respiratory Therapy

Second Edition

ROBERT M. KACMAREK, Ph.D., R.R.T.

Director, Respiratory Care Department
Massachusetts General Hospital
Boston, Massachusetts

CRAIG W. MACK, R.R.T.

Director, Department of Respiratory Therapy
Gottlieb Memorial Hospital
Melrose Park, Illinois

STEVEN DIMAS, R.R.T.

Regional Director, Respiratory Therapy Program
Foster Medical Corporation
Home Health Care Division
Berkeley, Illinois

YEAR BOOK MEDICAL PUBLISHERS, INC.
CHICAGO ● LONDON ● BOCA RATON

34567890K898887

Library of Congress Cataloging in Publication Data
Kacmarek, Robert M.
     Essentials of respiratory therapy.

     Includes bibliographies and index.
     1. Respiratory therapy.   2. Respiration.   I. Dimas,
Steven.   II. Mack, Craig W.   III. Title.   [DNLM:
1. Respiratory Therapy.   WB 342 K113e]
RC735.I5K32   1985   615.8'36   84-26945
ISBN 0-8151-4955-7

Sponsoring Editor: Diana L. McAninch
Editing Supervisor: Frances M. Perveiler
Production Project Manager: R. Allen Reedtz
Proofroom Supervisor: Shirley E. Taylor

With love to
KAREN *and* DARLA;
KAREN, BRIAN *and* JUSTIN;
and
CAROL, ERIC, CASSANDRA *and* JAMES

Contributors

MICHAEL F. ALJETS, R.R.T.

Instructor, Respiratory Therapy Program
Northwestern University Medical School
Chicago, Illinois

JOHN CRONIN, R.R.T.

Instructor, Respiratory Therapy Program
Northwestern University Medical School
Chicago, Illinois

DAVID J. HAUPTMAN, R.R.T.

Instructor, Respiratory Therapy Program
Northwestern University Medical School
Chicago, Illinois

ROBERT F. MOLINA, M.A., R.R.T.

Director, Respiratory Therapy Program
Northwestern University Medical School
Chicago, Illinois

DURINDA MULLINS, R.R.T.

Clinical Specialist
Department of Respiratory Therapy
Northwestern Memorial Hospital
Chicago, Illinois

JANE F. REYNOLDS, M.S., R.N., R.R.T.

Clinical Coordinator, Respiratory Therapy Program
Northwestern University Medical School
Chicago, Illinois

CHARLES B. SPEARMAN, R.R.T.

Instructor, Department of Respiratory Therapy
School of Allied Health Professions
Loma Linda University
Loma Linda, California

STEPHEN L. THOMPSON, M.S., R.R.T

Instructor, Department of Respiratory Therapy
Northwestern University Medical School
Chicago, Illinois

PAUL YINGER, R.R.T.

Supervisor, Department of Respiratory Therapy
Northwestern University Medical School
Chicago, Illinois

Preface to the First Edition

Over the years the field of respiratory therapy has expanded significantly and become increasingly complex. Along with this maturing of the profession has come an increase in the level and diversity of knowledge required of the respiratory care practitioner. In order to keep abreast of the educational needs of the field, many texts have been developed by a myriad of authors, each highlighting various aspects of the field.

The purpose of this text, *The Essentials of Respiratory Therapy,* is to unite in a simple and logical presentation areas in which the respiratory care practitioner must develop expertise. In format the text is an extensive presentation of the essential aspects of respiratory therapy; the basic sciences, anatomy and physiology, and the therapeutic aspects of the field are organized in an easily followed outline. As this format indicates, the text is intended as a secondary rather than a primary text; that is, a certain level of overall understanding of respiratory therapy is assumed. The individual requiring in-depth, detailed discussion on a topic should refer to texts of a primary nature.

The text begins with a presentation of the chemistry and gas physics related to respiratory therapy, followed by an extensive, detailed outline of the anatomy and physiology of the respiratory, cardiovascular and nervous systems. Pharmacology, pulmonary functions, neonatal comparative anatomy and obstructive and restrictive pulmonary diseases are then presented. A description of specific therapeutic methods, ventilators, analyzers, microbiology and sterilization techniques completes the text.

At the end of each chapter, references are provided for those interested in pursuing the topic in greater detail.

The general organization of the text makes it an excellent tool for the individual preparing for the registry or certification examinations.

ROBERT M. KACMAREK

STEVEN DIMAS

CRAIG W. MACK

Preface to the Second Edition

THE PROFESSION OF RESPIRATORY CARE is presently undergoing significant changes. The responsibilities of respiratory care practitioners seem to differ from institution to institution. In spite of these variations and alterations in focus, there is still a basic body of knowledge essential to the practice of respiratory care.

The purpose of this text, *The Essentials of Respiratory Therapy*, is to present this required common knowledge base in a logical, well organized manner for quick reference and review. This text is presented as an outline, highlighting all essential aspects of a topic and detailing those more difficult areas. In addition, each chapter is followed by an extensive bibliography including primary texts for additional explanation and periodical literature identifying original research in given areas.

The text begins with chapters on gas physics and chemistry. Following these are a number of chapters detailing pulmonary anatomy and physiology, as well as cardiovascular, neurological, and renal anatomy and physiology. Shunting and deadspace, blood gas interpretation, and fluid and electrolytes are addressed in independent chapters. Chapters addressing all therapeutic aspects of respiratory therapy follow with extensive chapters on mechanical ventilation and PEEP. The text ends with chapters addressing pharmacology, microbiology, sterilization and cleaning.

Those using this text to prepare for both registry and certification examinations will find the book a necessary aid in organizing their study plans and identifying topics requiring additional emphasis.

ROBERT M. KACMAREK

CRAIG W. MACK

STEVEN DIMAS

Acknowledgments

A very sincere and special thank you to all those respected colleagues whose guidance, assistance, and critique over the years has made this text possible: Terry L. Alfredson, R.R.T., David Assmann, R.R.T., Michael Callahan, R.R.T., Ronald Harrison, M.D., Fred Helmholz, M.D., Sally Hixon, R.R.T., Norman Pucilo, R.R.T., Barry Shapiro, M.D., Charles (Bud) Spearman, R.R.T., John Walton, R.R.T., Roger Wilson, M.D., and Camille Woodward, R.N., R.R.T.

In addition, the deepest of thanks to all of our past students who have continually provided the enthusiasm and the dedication to inspire us to grow and continually question, and to the staff at Northwestern University Medical School, Respiratory Therapy Program, whose tolerance was monumental and whose assistance made this text a reality: Michael Aljets, R.R.T., Glenna Bonnin-Fukuda, John Cronin, R.R.T., David Hauptman, R.R.T., Robert Molina, M.A., R.R.T., Steve Thompson, M.A., R.R.T., Jane Reynold, M.A., R.R.T., and Paul Yinger, R.R.T.

A very special thank you to Durinda Mullins, R.R.T., for her fine graphs.

Finally, we are eternally indebted to Pat Prange for her understanding, skill, and everlasting patience in the preparation of the manuscript.

ROBERT M. KACMAREK

CRAIG W. MACK

STEVEN DIMAS

Contents

1 / Basic Chemistry

1. Atomic Structure
   A. Atom: The smallest subdivision of a substance that still maintains the properties of that substance. An atom is composed of the following:
      1. Nucleus: Central portion of an atom, which contains protons and neutrons.
         a. Proton: Positively charged particle with a mass of one atomic mass unit.
         b. Neutron: Neutral particle with a mass of one atomic mass unit.
      2. Electron: Negatively charged particle that revolves around the nucleus of the atom with a mass of about 1/1,000 of an atomic mass unit.
      3. Normally, in its nonreactive state, an atom contains the same number of protons and electrons. The number of neutrons of the same substance may vary from one atom to another.
   B. Element: General term applied to each of the 106 different types of atoms.
   C. Isotope: Atom of a substance with the same number of protons but with a varying number of neutrons. All elements have at least two isotopes.
   D. Atomic weight: Average weight of an atom of a particular substance based on the atomic weight of the carbon 12 isotope. The atomic weight is about equal to the sum of the weights of protons and neutrons in the nucleus of an atom and is not a whole number because of the presence of isotopes (Table 1–1).
   E. Gram atomic weight: Mass in grams of an element equal to its atomic weight (see Table 1–1).
   F. Atomic number: Number equal to the number of protons in the nucleus of an atom (see Table 1–1).
   G. Ion: Charged species of a particular atom.
II. Molecular Structure
   A. Molecule: Particle that results from chemical combination of two or more atoms and normally having a neutral charge.
   B. Compound: Molecule formed from two or more elements.

1

TABLE 1–1.—ATOMIC WEIGHTS AND VALENCES OF 13
COMMON ELEMENTS

ELEMENT	SYMBOL	ATOMIC NUMBER	ATOMIC WEIGHT	VALENCE
Calcium	Ca	20	40.08	+2
Carbon	C	6	12.0	±4
Chlorine	Cl	17	35.5	−1
Fluorine	F	9	18.99	−1
Hydrogen	H	1	1.00	+1
Iron	Fe	26	55.84	+1 or +2
Lithium	Li	3	6.94	+1
Magnesium	Mg	12	24.31	+2
Oxygen	O	8	15.99	−2
Phosphorus	P	15	30.97	−3
Potassium	K	19	39.09	+1
Sodium	Na	11	22.98	+1
Sulfur	S	16	32.06	−2

C. Free radical: Charged compound, reacting as any other ion reacts.
D. Molecular formula: Expression indicating the types of atoms and their numbers in the molecule. The particle that is positively charged is usually listed first.
   Examples:
   $NaCl$ = 1 sodium atom and 1 chloride atom contained in the molecule.
   H_2SO_4 = 2 hydrogen atoms, 1 sulfur atom, and 4 oxygen atoms contained in the molecule
E. Molecular weight: Sum total of all individual atomic weights of atoms that make up a molecule.
   Example (H_2SO_4):

Atom	No. of Atoms		Atomic Wt.	Total Contributing Wt.
H	2	×	1	2
S	1	×	32	32
O	4	×	16	64
			Molecular wt.	98

   Example (CO_2):

Atom	No. of Atoms		Atomic Wt.	Total Contributing Wt.
C	1	×	12	12
O	2	×	16	32
			Molecular wt.	44

F. Gram molecular weight: Mass in grams of a molecule equal to its molecular weight.

III. Valence
  A. Valence: Number given to an atom that indicates its tendency to gain or lose electrons in a chemical reaction.
  Examples (see Table 1–1):
    Na (sodium): Valence of $+1$ indicates that it will react so as to lose one electron.
    Ca (calcium): Valence of $+2$ indicates that it will react so as to lose two electrons.
    F (fluorine): Valence of -1 indicates that it will react so as to gain one electron.
  B. Generally, valences of elements allow predictions of their reactivity with each other.
IV. Chemical Compounds
  A. Ionic compound: Compound formed as a result of the atoms in the compound gaining and losing electrons.
  Examples:
    NaCl: Na has a valence of $+1$, and Cl has a valence of -1. Thus the Na atom has lost an electron and the Cl atom has gained an electron.
    CaF_2: Ca has a valence of $+2$, and each F atom has a valence of -1. Thus the Ca atom has lost 2 electrons and each F atom has gained an electron.
    1. Properties of ionic compounds:
      a. High boiling points.
      b. High melting points.
      c. Dissolve readily in polar solvents.
      d. Strong electrolytes: Dissociate readily in polar solvents.

$$NaCl + H_2O \rightarrow Na^+ + Cl^- + H_2O$$
$$CaF_2 + H_2O \rightarrow Ca^{+2} + 2F^- + H_2O$$

  B. Covalent compound: Compound formed by the sharing of electrons between the various atoms in the compound.

$$O^{-2} + O^{-2} \rightarrow O_2$$
$$N^{-3} + N^{-3} \rightarrow N_2$$
$$Cl^- + Cl^- \rightarrow Cl_2$$

    1. Properties of covalent compounds:
      a. Exist only between atoms of the same element.
      b. Low melting points.
      c. Low boiling points.
      d. Dissolve poorly in polar solvents.
  C. Polar covalent compound: Intermediate compound between a

pure covalent compound and an ionic compound characterized by incomplete sharing of electrons.
Examples:

$$H_2O + CO_2 \rightleftharpoons H_2CO_3$$

1. Properties of polar covalent compounds:
   a. Vary according to the particular compound.
   b. These compounds normally are weak electrolytes. Only a small percentage of ionization takes place when polar covalent compounds are added to a polar solution.

V. Volume Percent and Gram Percent
   A. Volume percent (vol%): Method of indicating the number of milliliters of a substance in 100 ml of solution.
   B. Gram percent (gm%): Method of indicating the number of grams of a substance in 100 ml of solution.

VI. Chemical Solutions
   A. Solution: Homogeneous mixture of two substances.
   B. Solute: Substance dissolved in a solution.
   C. Solvent: Substance that is the dissolving agent.
   D. Effects of a solute on the physical characteristics of water:
      1. Solutes cause an increase in the boiling point of water.
      2. Solutes cause a decrease in the freezing point of water.
      3. Osmotic pressure of a solution containing a solute is higher than that of pure water.
   E. As the temperature of the solvent increases, the volume of solute that can be dissolved in the solvent also increases.
   F. Dilute solution: A small amount of solute dissolved in each unit of solvent at a particular temperature.
   G. Saturated solution: Maximum amount of solute dissolved in each unit of solvent at a particular temperature. In a saturated solution a precipitate is seen at the bottom of the solution.
   H. Supersaturated solution: A greater amount of solute than the solvent would normally hold, dissolved at a particular temperature. However, physical disturbance of this solution causes the excess solute to precipitate.

VII. Solution Concentrations
   A. Ratio solution: Solution concentration represented as a ratio between solute and solvent in number of grams to number of milliliters.
      Examples:
         2:500 means 2 gm to 500 ml: 2 indicates the number of grams of solute and 500 indicates the number of milliliters of solvent.

1:1,000 means 1 gm to 1,000 ml: 1 indicates the number of grams of solute and 1,000 indicates the number of milliliters of solvent.

Problems:

1. How many milligrams of solute are there in 1 ml of a 1:200 solution?

$$1:200 \text{ means } 1 \text{ gm to } 200 \text{ ml}$$
$$1 \text{ gm equals } 1,000 \text{ mg, thus}$$
$$\frac{1,000 \text{ mg}}{200 \text{ ml}} = \frac{x}{1 \text{ ml}}$$
$$x = 5 \text{ mg}$$

2. How many milligrams are there in 5 ml of a 1:500 solution?

$$1:500 \text{ means } 1 \text{ gm to } 500 \text{ ml}$$
$$1 \text{ gm equals } 1,000 \text{ mg, thus}$$
$$\frac{1,000 \text{ mg}}{500 \text{ ml}} = \frac{x}{5 \text{ ml}}$$
$$x = 10 \text{ mg}$$

B. Percent W/V: Solution concentration where the actual percentage indicates the number of grams of solute per 100 ml of solution.

Example:

1% W/V solution means 1 gm of solute contained in 100 ml of solution.

Problems:

1. How many milligrams are there in 10 ml of a 3% W/V solution?

$$3\% \text{ W/V means } 3 \text{ gm per } 100 \text{ ml}$$
$$1 \text{ gm equals } 1,000 \text{ mg, thus}$$
$$3 \text{ gm equals } 3,000 \text{ mg}$$
$$\frac{3,000 \text{ mg}}{100 \text{ ml}} = \frac{x}{10 \text{ ml}}$$
$$x = 300 \text{ mg}$$

2. How many milligrams are there in 3 ml of a 0.5% W/V solution?

$$0.5\% \text{ W/V means } 0.5 \text{ gm per } 100 \text{ ml}$$
$$1 \text{ gm equals } 1,000 \text{ mg, thus}$$

$$0.5 \text{ gm equals } 500 \text{ mg}$$

$$\frac{500 \text{ mg}}{100 \text{ ml}} = \frac{x}{3 \text{ ml}}$$

$$x = 15 \text{ mg}$$

C. True percent solution: Solution concentration where *both* solute and solvent are expressed in either weight or volume. The solute is expressed as a true percentage of the solution.

Examples:

10% solution with a total solution of 100 gm means 10 gm of solute and 90 gm of solvent.

3% solution with a total solution volume of 500 ml means 15 ml of solute and 485 ml of solvent.

Problems:

1. How many grams of solute are there in 250 gm of a 5% solution (5% indicates the percent by weight that the solute is of the total solution)?

$$\underset{\text{solution}}{(250)(0.05)} = \underset{\text{solute}}{12.5 \text{ gm}}$$

$$(250 - 12.5) = \underset{\text{solvent}}{237.5 \text{ gm}}$$

2. How many milliliters of solute are there in 500 ml of a 10% solution (10% indicates the percent by volume that the solute is of the total solution)?

$$\underset{\text{solution}}{(500)(0.10)} = \underset{\text{solute}}{50 \text{ ml}}$$

$$(500 - 50) = \underset{\text{solvent}}{450 \text{ ml}}$$

VIII. Dilution Calculations

A. The following formula is used to determine the concentration that will result when a solution is diluted:

$$V_1 \times C_1 = V_2 \times C_2 \qquad\qquad (1)$$

where

V_1 is the volume before dilution
C_1 is the concentration before dilution
V_2 is the volume after dilution
C_2 is the concentration after dilution

B. In order to use equation 1, three of the four variables must be known.

Problems:

1. What volume of water should be added to 50 ml of a 40% W/V solution of alcohol to dilute it to a 20% W/V solution?

$$V_1 \times C_1 = V_2 \times C_2$$
$$(50)(40) = (x)(20)$$
$$x = 100 \text{ ml}$$
$$100 \text{ ml} = V_2$$
$$V_2 - V_1 = \text{added volume}$$
$$100 \text{ ml} - 50 \text{ ml} = 50 \text{ ml of water to be added.}$$

2. If 4 ml is added to 0.5 ml of a 15% W/V solution, what is the solution's final concentration?

$$V_1 \times C_1 = V_2 \times C_2$$
$$(0.5)(15\%) = (4.5)(x)$$
$$x = 1.67\% \text{ W/V}$$

IX. Gram Equivalent Weights

A. Gram equivalent weight (GEW): Amount of a substance that will react completely with 1 mole of H^+ or OH^- or 1 mole of any monovalent substance.

B. The gram equivalent weight of an element is determined by dividing the gram atomic weight of the substance by its valence. The charge of the valence is disregarded.

Examples:

Na^+ atomic weight 23 gm

$$\frac{23 \text{ gm}}{1} = 23 \text{ gm/GEW}$$

Al^{+3} atomic weight 27 gm

$$\frac{27 \text{ gm}}{3} = 9 \text{ gm/GEW}$$

S^{-2} atomic weight 32 gm

$$\frac{32 \text{ gm}}{2} = 16 \text{ gm/GEW}$$

C. The gram equivalent weight of an acid is determined by dividing its gram molecular weight by the number of replaceable hydrogen ions in the molecular formula. Normally all H^+ are replaceable. However, H_2CO_3 is an exception: only one H^+ is replaceable.

Examples:

H_2SO_4 GMW = 98 gm, 2 replaceable H^+

$$\frac{98 \text{ gm}}{2} = 49 \text{ gm/GEW}$$

H_3PO_4 GMW = 98 gm, 3 replaceable H^+

$$\frac{98 \text{ gm}}{3} = 32.66 \text{ gm/GEW}$$

H_2CO_3 GMW = 62 gm, 1 replaceable H^+

$$\frac{62 \text{ gm}}{1} = 62 \text{ gm/GEW}$$

D. The gram equivalent weight of a base is determined by dividing its gram molecular weight by the number of replaceable hydroxyl ions (OH^-) in the molecular formula. Normally all OH^- are replaceable.
   Examples:

NaOH GMW = 40 gm, 1 replaceable OH^-

$$\frac{40 \text{ gm}}{1} = 40 \text{ gm/GEW}$$

$Ca(OH)_2$ GMW = 74 gm, 2 replaceable OH^-

$$\frac{74 \text{ gm}}{2} = 37 \text{ gm/GEW}$$

$Al(OH)_3$ GMW = 78 gm, 3 replaceable OH^-

$$\frac{78 \text{ gm}}{3} = 26 \text{ gm/GEW}$$

E. The gram equivalent weight of a salt is determined by dividing its gram molecular weight by the total valence of the positive ions or free radicals in the molecule.
   Examples:

NaCl GMW = 58.5 gm, 1 Na^+ with a total valence of $+1$

$$\frac{58.5 \text{ gm}}{1} = 58.5 \text{ gm/GEW}$$

CaF_2 GMW = 78 gm, 1 Ca^{+2} with a total valence of $+2$

$$\frac{78 \text{ gm}}{2} = 39 \text{ gm/GEW}$$

$Al_2(CO_3)_3$ GMW = 234 gm, 2 Al^{+3} with a total valence of +6

$$\frac{234 \text{ gm}}{6} = 39 \text{ gm/GEW}$$

F. The gram equivalent weight of a free radical is determined by dividing its gram molecular weight by its valence, disregarding the charge of the valence.
Examples:

HCO_3^{-} GMW = 61 gm, valence 1

$$\frac{61 \text{ gm}}{1} = 61 \text{ gm/GEW}$$

PO_4^{-3} GMW = 95 gm, valence 3

$$\frac{95 \text{ gm}}{3} = 31.67 \text{ gm/GEW}$$

CO_3^{-2} GMW = 60 gm, valence 2

$$\frac{60 \text{ gm}}{2} = 30 \text{ gm/GEW}$$

G. Milliequivalent weight (mEq): Weight of a substance that will react with one millimole (mmole) of H^+, OH^-, or any monovalent substance. Numerically, the mEq of a substance is equal to its GEW.
Examples:

NaCl 58.5 gm/GEW, 58.5 mg/mEq
H_2CO_3 62 gm/GEW, 62 mg/mEq
Na^+ 23 gm/GEW, 23 mg/mEq

H. Equivalent weights are used to determine the precise quantity of a substance that reacts completely with a given quantity of another substance.
X. Temperature Scales
  A. Temperature scales (in degrees) in general use:
    1. Fahrenheit (F)
    2. Celsius or Centigrade (C)
    3. Rankine (R)
    4. Kelvin (K)
  B. The Rankine and Kelvin scales are absolute zero scales, i.e., zero on their scales represents the point where all molecular activity stops.
  C. Conversion formulas for temperature scales

     1. $C = 5/9 \, (F - 32)$
     2. $F = (9/5 \, C) + 32$
     3. $K = C + 273$
     4. $R = F + 460$

XI. Osmosis

   A. The movement of water from an area of high concentration of water to an area of low concentration of water.

   B. Osmosis occurs when two compartments of fluid are separated by a membrane that is selectively permeable.

   C. Osmosis will proceed in a system until the concentration of water in the involved compartments is equal. When concentrations are equal, no net movement of fluid occurs; however, molecules still move back and forth across the system.

   D. Osmosis occurs between two solutions as a result of osmotic pressure differences in the solutions.

     1. The potential pressure of the molecules of pure H_2O is about 1,073,000 mm Hg.

     2. When a solute is dissolved in H_2O, the potential pressure of the H_2O is decreased.

     3. The osmotic pressure of a solution is equal to the potential pressure of pure water minus the potential pressure of the solution.

     Example:

Pure H_2O	1,073,000 mm Hg
Solution	1,000,000 mm Hg
Osmotic pressure	73,000 mm Hg

     4. Osmotic pressure is a force *drawing* water into the solution.

     5. Osmosis can be stopped by exerting a force on a solution equal to the osmotic pressure of the solution.

XII. Hydrostatic Pressure

   A. This is the amount of force exerted by the weight of a column of water (cm H_2O).

XIII. Expressions of H^+ Ion Concentration

   A. pH: Negative log of the H^+ concentration per liter (L) of solution, [ ] is used to symbolize molar concentration.

     1. $pH = -\log_{10} [H^+]$ or $\log_{10} \dfrac{1}{[H^+]}$

     2. pH of 7.0: Neutral

     3. pH greater than 7.0: Basic or alkalotic

     4. pH less than 7.0: Acidic or acidotic

5. pH scale: 1 to 14, equivalent to an $[H^+]$ of 10^{-1} to 10^{-14} moles/L

B. Nanomoles per liter (nmoles/L): H^+ concentration in number of billionths of a mole of H^+ per liter.
1. The $[H^+]$ is expressed as a number multiplied by 10^{-9}.
2. A pH of 7.0 = 3.98×10^{-8} moles/L or 39.8×10^{-9} moles/L or 39.8 nmoles/L.
3. Nanomole expressions normally are used for $[H^+]$ in the physiologic range.
   a. pH of 6.90 = 126 nmoles/L
   b. pH of 7.70 = 20.1 nmoles/L

XIV. Acids and Bases
A. Acid: A compound that donates H^+ ions when placed into solution.
1. The active compound responsible for the properties of acids is the hydronium ion (H_3O^+).
2. In solution the liberated H^+ reacts with H_2O to form the H_3O^+ ion.

$$H^+ + H_2O \rightarrow H_3O^+$$

B. Base: A compound that accepts H^+ ions when placed into solution. The active compound responsible for the properties of most bases is the OH^- (hydroxyl ion).
C. Neutralization reaction: The reaction between an acid and a base, where the results are a salt plus water.

$$NaOH + HCl \rightarrow NaCl + H_2O$$

XV. Oxidation and Reduction
A. Oxidation: Process in a chemical reaction whereby a substance loses electrons.
B. Reduction: Process in a chemical reaction whereby a substance gains electrons.
XVI. Metric System
A. Length
1. The basic unit of length is the meter (m). One meter is equal to 39.37 inches (in.).
2. One meter is equal to all of the following, and they are thus equal to each other:
   a. 100 centimeters (10^2 cm)
   b. 1,000 millimeters (10^3 mm)
   c. 1,000,000 microns (10^6 μ)

d. 10,000,000,000 angstroms (10^{10} Å)
3. Basic factors used in converting from the metric to the British system or British to the metric system:
a. 1 m = 39.37 in.
b. 1 in. = 2.54 cm
B. Weight
1. The basic unit of weight in the metric system is the kilogram (kg). One kilogram is equal to 2.2 pounds (lb).
2. One kilogram is equal to all of the following, and they are thus equal to each other:
a. 1,000 gm (10^3 gm)
b. 1,000,000 mg (10^6 mg)
3. Basic factors used in converting from metric to British system or from British to metric system:
a. 1 kg = 2.2 lb
b. 1 lb = 454 gm
C. Volume
1. The basic unit of volume in the metric system is the liter (L), which is equal to 1.057 quarts (qt).
2. One liter is equal to 1,000 ml (10^3 ml) and also to 1,000 cc (10^3 cc).
a. The volume of 1 cc is 1 ml.
b. 1 ml of water weighs 1 gm.
3. One cubic meter contains 10^3 L.
4. Basic factors used in converting from the metric to British system or from British to metric system:
a. 1 L = 1.057 qt
b. 1 cu ft = 28.3 L

BIBLIOGRAPHY
Beckenback E.F., Drooyar I., Wooton W.: *College Algebra*, ed. 4. Belmont, Calif., Wadsworth Publishing Co., Inc., 1966.
Brooks S.M.: *Integrated Basic Sciences*, ed. 3. St. Louis, C.V. Mosby Co., 1970.
Epstein L.I., Kuzava B.A.: *Basic Physics in Anesthesiology: A Programmed Approach*. Chicago, Year Book Medical Publishers, Inc., 1976.
Johnson R.H., Grunwald E.: *Atoms, Molecules, and Chemical Change*, ed. 2. Englewood Cliffs, N.J., Prentice-Hall, Inc., 1965.
Masterton W.L., Slowinski E.: *Chemical Principles*, ed. 4. Philadelphia, W.B. Saunders Co., 1977.
Sackheim G.I.: *Chemical Calculations*, Series B, ed. 8. Champaign, Ill., Stipes Publishing Co., 1962.
Sackheim G.I., Schultz R.M.: *Chemistry for the Health Sciences*, ed. 2. New York, Macmillan Publishing Co., Inc., 1973.

Shapiro B.A., Harrison R.A., Walton J.R.: *Clinical Application of Blood Gases*, ed. 3. Chicago, Year Book Medical Publishers, Inc., 1982.

Spearman C.B., Sheldon R.L., Egan D.F.: *Egan's Fundamentals of Respiratory Therapy*, ed. 4. St. Louis, C.V. Mosby Co., 1982.

Young J.A., Crocker D.: *Principles and Practice of Respiratory Therapy*, ed. 2. Chicago, Year Book Medical Publishers, Inc., 1976.

2 / General Principles of Gas Physics

I. Basic Units and Relationships
   A. Mass: The property of matter defined as its ability to occupy space, and if in motion to stay in motion, and if at rest to stay at rest.
   B. Weight: A method of quantifying the mass of an object. The effect of gravitational attraction on the object.
   C. Velocity: The speed with which movement between two points occurs. Expressed in miles per hour or centimeters per second.
   D. Acceleration: The rate at which the velocity of an object increases. The units of acceleration are cm/sec^2 or $miles/hr^2$.
   E. Work is equal to the product of force and distance:

$$\text{Work} = \text{Force} \times \text{Distance} \qquad (1)$$

   1. Force is defined as mass $\times$ acceleration. The units of force are:
      a. Dyne $=$ gm $\cdot$ cm/sec
      b. Newton $=$ kg $\cdot$ m/sec
   2. Work is not performed unless the applied force causes movement.
   3. The units of work are:
      a. ERG $=$ dyne-centimeter
      b. Joule $=$ Newton-meter
   F. Energy is defined as the ability to do work.
   1. Potential and kinetic energy are the two types of mechanical energy.
   2. Potential energy is the energy of position.
   3. Kinetic energy is the energy of motion.
   4. Kinetic energy (KE) is equal to:

$$KE = 0.5\ MV^2 \qquad (2)$$

   where M $=$ mass and V $=$ velocity.
   5. Kinetic energy of gases is normally expressed as:

$$KE = 0.5\ DV^2 \qquad (3)$$

   where D $=$ density.

14

G. Pressure is the force applied per unit area. The units of pressure are:
   1. Pounds per square inch (lb/in.^{2}, or PSI)
   2. Grams per square centimeter (gm/cm^2)

II. States of Matter
   A. All matter exists in one of three basic states:
      1. Solid
      2. Liquid
      3. Gas
   B. The state of a substance is determined by the relationship of two forces.
      1. Kinetic energy of the molecules.
      2. Intermolecular attractive forces among the molecules.
   C. The kinetic energy of a substance is directly related to temperature.
      1. The greater the kinetic energy of a substance, the greater is its tendency to exist as a liquid or gas.
      2. Molecules of every substance are in constant motion as a result of kinetic energy.
      3. At absolute zero the kinetic activity of a substance is theoretically zero.
   D. Intermolecular attractive forces oppose the kinetic energy of molecules and tend to force them to exist in less free (solid, or liquid) states. Basically there are three types of intermolecular attractive forces: dipole, hydrogen bonding, and dispersion.
      1. Dipole forces: Forces that exist between molecules that have electrostatic polarity; the negative aspect of one molecule is lined up and attracted to the positive aspect of another molecule, as seen with NaCl. These substances frequently form crystals.
      2. Hydrogen bonding: A force that exists between molecules formed by hydrogen reacting with fluorine, oxygen, or nitrogen.
         a. As a result of the electronegative difference between hydrogen and fluorine, oxygen or nitrogen, the hydrogen atom in the molecule appears as a pure proton.
         b. The hydrogen of one molecule is thus attracted to the negative aspect of another molecule of the substance.
         c. Hydrogen bonding occurs only with compounds of fluorine, oxygen, and nitrogen because of their:
            (1) Strong electronegativity
            (2) Small atomic diameter

3. Dispersion forces (London or van der Waals forces): Forces between molecules of relatively nonpolar substances.
   a. In nonpolar substances the electron cloud normally is distributed equally among all of the atoms in the molecule.
   b. However, at some point in time the electron cloud may be instantaneously concentrated at one end of the molecule. When this occurs, a polarity is set up on the molecule.
   c. This instantaneous polarity allows attraction between adjacent molecules.
   d. Dispersion forces are the weakest of all intermolecular forces.
E. Units of heat
   1. Calorie: Unit of heat in metric system. Essentially it is the amount of heat necessary to cause a 1° C increase in the temperature of 1 gm of water.
   2. British thermal unit (BTU): Unit of heat in the British system. Essentially it is the amount of heat necessary to cause a 1° F increase in the temperature of 1 lb of water.
   3. One BTU is equal to 252 calories of heat.
   4. Heat capacity: Number of calories needed to raise the temperature of 1 gm of a substance 1° C.
   5. Specific heat: Ratio of heat capacity of a substance compared to heat capacity of water.
F. Change of state
   1. A specific amount of heat is needed to cause the molecules of a substance to change their state.
   2. Latent heat of fusion is the amount of heat necessary to change 1 gm of a substance at its melting point from a solid to a liquid without causing a change in temperature.
      a. The melting point is the temperature (at 1 atm of pressure) at which a substance will change from a solid to a liquid.
      b. The total volume of a substance must change from a solid to a liquid before its temperature will change.
      c. Latent heats of fusion and melting points for various substances:

SUBSTANCE	HEAT OF FUSION (CALORIES/GM)	MELTING POINT (C)
Water	80	0
Hydrogen	13.8	−259.25
Carbon dioxide	43.2	−57.6
Nitrogen	6.15	−210
Oxygen	3.3	−218.8

3. The latent heat of vaporization is the amount of heat necessary to change 1 gm of a substance at its boiling point from a liquid to a gas without causing a change in temperature.
   a. Boiling point is the temperature at 1 atm pressure at which a substance will change from a liquid to a gas.
   b. The total volume of a substance must change from a liquid to a gas before its temperature will change.
      (1) In order for a substance to boil, its vapor pressure must equal the pressure of the atmosphere above it.
      (2) Evaporation is a surface phenomenon whereby individual molecules of a substance gain enough heat to change their state. Boiling, on the other hand, occurs throughout the entire volume of the substance.
   c. Latent heats of vaporization and boiling points for various substances:

SUBSTANCE	HEAT OF VAPORIZATION (CALORIES/GM)	BOILING POINT (C)
Water	540	100
Hydrogen	40	− 252.5
Carbon dioxide	83	− 78.5
Nitrogen	. . .	− 196
Oxygen	50	− 183

G. Effects of pressure on melting and boiling points
   1. In general, the greater the pressure over a substance, the higher the temperature necessary to cause the substance to change its state. Pressure has a greater effect on the boiling point of a substance than on its melting point.
   2. Critical temperature: The highest temperature at which a substance can exist as a liquid, regardless of the amount of pressure applied to it (O_2 = − 118.8° C).
   3. Critical pressure: The lowest pressure necessary at the critical temperature of a substance to maintain it in its liquid state (O_2 = 49.7 atm pressure).
   4. Critical point: Combination of critical temperature and critical pressure of a substance.
H. Triple point: Specific combination of temperature and pressure in which a substance can exist in all three states of matter in dynamic equilibrium.
I. Sublimation: Transition of a substance from a solid directly to a gas without existence in a liquid state. The heat of sublimation equals the heat of fusion plus the heat of vaporization.

III. Kinetic Theory of Gases
  A. The kinetic theory normally is applied to relatively dilute gas volumes.
  B. Principles of kinetic theory
    1. Gases are composed of molecules that are in rapid continuous random motion.
    2. The molecules undergo near collisions with each other and collide with the walls of their container.
    3. All molecular collisions are elastic, and as long as the container is properly insulated, the temperature of the gas remains constant.
    4. The kinetic energy of molecules of a gas is directly proportional to the absolute temperature.
      a. An increase in temperature will cause an increase in kinetic energy of the gas.
      b. The increased kinetic energy will cause an increase in the velocity of the gas molecules.
      c. The increased velocity will cause an increase in the frequency of collisions.
      d. The increased frequency of collisions will cause an increase in the pressure in the system.
      e. With an increase in temperature, the degree of increase in the velocity of gas molecules is indirectly related to their molecular weight.
IV. Avogadro's Law
  A. One gram molecular weight, 1 gm atomic weight, 1 gm ionic weight, etc., of a substance contains 6.02×10^{23} particles of that substance.
  B. The above mass of any substance is referred to as a mole.
  C. One mole of a gas at 0° C and 760 mm Hg (standard temperature and pressure; STP) occupies a volume of about 22.4 L. (There is a small percent variation in this number for individual gases, i.e., CO_2 = 22.3 L.)
  D. An equal number or fractions of moles of different gases at a specific temperature and pressure occupy the same volume and contain the same number of particles.
V. Density
  A. Density is the mass of an object per unit volume and usually is expressed as grams per liter:

$$D = \frac{M}{V} \qquad (4)$$

B. On the surface of the earth, mass in equation 4 may be replaced by weight.

C. Calculation of densities of solids and liquids is straightforward since their volumes are relatively stable at various temperatures and pressures.

D. The volumes of gases, on the other hand, are severely affected by temperature and pressure.

E. For this reason, the standard density of all gases is determined at STP conditions where the volume used is 22.4 L and the weight used is the gram molecular weight (GMW) of the particular gas:

$$\text{Density of gas } = \frac{\text{GMW}}{22.4 \text{ L}} = x \text{ gm/L} \tag{5}$$

$$\text{Density of oxygen } = \frac{32 \text{ gm (GMW)}}{22.4 \text{ L}} = 1.43 \text{ gm/L}$$

F. Standard densities of various substances:
   1. Oxygen: 1.43 gm/L
   2. Nitrogen: 1.25 gm/L
   3. Carbon dioxide: 1.965 gm/L

G. The density of a mixture of gases is determined by the following equation:

$$D = \frac{(\%_A)(\text{GMW}_A) + (\%_B)(\text{GMW}_B) + (\%_C)(\text{GMW}_C)}{22.4 \text{ L}} \tag{6}$$

Example: The density of a gas containing 40% oxygen, 55% nitrogen, and 5% carbon dioxide would be computed as follows:

$$D = \frac{(0.4)(32) + (0.55)(28) + (0.05)(44)\text{gm}}{22.4 \text{ L}}$$

$$D = \frac{(12.8) + (15.4) + (2.2)\text{gm}}{22.4 \text{ L}}$$

$$D = \frac{30.4 \text{ gm}}{22.4 \text{ L}}$$

$$D = 1.36 \text{ gm/L}$$

H. Specific gravity: Ratio of the density of a substance to the density of a standard. The specific gravity of solids and liquids is determined using water as the standard; for gases, oxygen is used as the standard. Specific gravity is expressed purely as a ratio.

VI. Gas Pressure
  A. Pressure (P) in any sense is equal to force per unit area:

$$P = \frac{gm}{sq\ cm}; \qquad P = \frac{lb}{sq\ in.} \tag{7}$$

  B. The pressure of a gas is directly related to the kinetic energy of the gas (see Section II) and to the gravitational attraction of the earth.
  C. With an increase in altitude, the gravitational attraction of the earth on molecules of gas in the atmosphere decreases.
    1. This causes a decrease in density of the atmospheric gases.
    2. Decreased density results in fewer molecular collisions.
    3. Thus, with increasing altitude there is a nonlinear decrease in the pressure of the total atmosphere and of individual gases.
    4. Even though there is a steady decrease in the pressure of the atmosphere with altitude, the concentration of gases in the atmosphere remains stable to an elevation of about 50 miles.
    5. Concentration of atmospheric gases:
      a. Oxygen: 20.95%
      b. Nitrogen: 78.08%
      c. Argon: 0.93%
      d. Carbon dioxide: 0.03%
      e. Trace elements: 0.01%
  D. The barometric pressure (PB) of the atmosphere is equal to the height of a column of fluid times the fluid's density:

$$PB = (height\ of\ column\ of\ fluid)(fluid's\ density) \tag{8}$$

If the fluid used is mercury (psi = pounds per square inch):

14.7 psi = (29.9 in. Hg)(0.491 lb/cu in.)

  E. Mercury's density in the metric system is 13.6 gm/cc; in the British system it is 0.491 lb/cu in.
  F. Gas pressure is frequently expressed as the height of a substance, i.e., mm Hg, cm H_2O. These are not true pressure expressions but they may be easily converted to the proper pressure notation by use of equation 8 if necessary.
  G. Atmospheric pressure normally is determined by a mercury or an aneroid barometer.
  H. Equivalent expressions of normal atmospheric pressure:
    1. 14.7 psi

    2. 760 mm Hg

    3. 1,034 gm/sq cm

    4. 33 ft of salt H_2O

    5. 33.9 ft of fresh H_2O

    6. 29.9 in. Hg

    7. 76 cm Hg

    8. 1,034 cm H_2O

VII. Humidity

    A. Water vapor content of the air under atmospheric conditions is variable. Temperature is the factor that most significantly affects water vapor content in the atmosphere.

    B. At a particular temperature, there is a maximum amount of water that a gas can hold.

    C. Since the boiling point of water (100° C) is considerably higher than the normal temperature of the atmosphere, the maximum water vapor content of the atmosphere varies with temperature.

        1. As the temperature increases, the rate of evaporation of water accelerates and the capacity of the atmosphere to hold water increases.

        2. All other standard gases in the atmosphere have boiling points much lower than atmospheric temperature. This causes stability in their concentrations.

        3. Water is the only standard atmospheric gas that responds to temperature changes in this manner.

    D. Expressions of water vapor content

        1. Partial pressure of water vapor (P_{H_2O}), maximum P_{H_2O} at 37° C, is equal to 47 mm Hg.

        2. Absolute humidity is defined as the actual weight of water vapor contained in a given volume of gas.

            a. Absolute humidity may be expressed as grams per cubic meter or milligrams per liter.

            b. The maximum absolute humidity at 37° C is 43.8 gm/cu m or 43.8 mg/L.

        3. Relative humidity (RH) is defined as a relationship between the actual weight or pressure (content) of water in air at a specific temperature and the maximum weight or pressure (capacity) of water that air can hold at that specific temperature. Relative humidity is expressed as a percentage.

            a. Expressions of actual and maximum amounts of water:

                (1) mm Hg

                (2) gm/cu m

                (3) mg/L

b. Formula for calculating relative humidity:

$$RH = \frac{content}{capacity} \times 100 \qquad (9)$$

Example: At 37° C, if the actual water vapor pressure is 20 mm Hg, what is the relative humidity?

$$RH = \frac{20 \text{ mm Hg}}{47 \text{ mm Hg}} \times 100 = 43\%$$

c. If water content is kept constant and temperature is increased, relative humidity decreases because capacity of air for water increases. As temperature decreases, the opposite effect is seen.

VIII. Dalton's Law of Partial Pressure

A. Dalton's law states that the sum of the individual partial pressures of the gases in a mixture is equal to the total barometric pressure of the system.

B. The partial pressure (PP) of a gas is equal to the barometric pressure (PB) times the concentration of gas in the mixture:

$$(PP) = (PB)(conc.) \qquad (10)$$

Example: If the PB is 760 mm Hg and the concentration of O_2 is 21%, what is the PO_2?

$$PO_2 = (760)(0.21) = 159.6 \text{ mm Hg}$$

C. The concentration of a gas is equal to the partial pressure of the gas divided by the barometric pressure:

$$Conc. = \frac{PP}{PB} \times 100 \qquad (11)$$

Example: If the PB is 750 mm Hg and the PO_2 is 200 mm Hg, what is the concentration of O_2?

$$O_2 \text{ conc.} = \frac{200 \text{ mm Hg}}{750 \text{ mm Hg}} \times 100 = 26.7\%$$

IX. Effect of Humidity on Dalton's Law

A. Water vapor pressure does not follow Dalton's law because under normal atmospheric conditions, PH_2O is dependent primarily on temperature.

B. When calculating the partial pressure of a gas where water vapor is present, the total barometric pressure of the system must be corrected before the partial pressure of any other gas can be calculated.

C. Following is a modification of Dalton's law to account for the presence of water vapor:

$$(\text{PP}) = (\text{PB} - \text{P}_{\text{H}_2\text{O}})(\text{conc.}) \qquad (12)$$

Example: If PB is 770 mm Hg, $\text{P}_{\text{H}_2\text{O}}$ is 30 mm Hg, and the concentration of O_2 is 50%, what is the Po_2?

$$\text{Po}_2 = (770 \text{ mm Hg} - 30 \text{ mm Hg})(0.50)$$
$$\text{Po}_2 = 370 \text{ mm Hg}$$

D. When the temperature is 37°C with barometric pressure at 760 mm Hg, the gas saturated with water vapor, and the oxygen concentration 21%, the Po_2 is 149.7 mm Hg:

$$\text{Po}_2 = (760 \text{ mm Hg} - 47 \text{ mm Hg})(0.21) = 149.7 \text{ mm Hg}$$

X. Ideal Gas Laws
  A. The ideal gas laws apply to dilute gases at temperatures above the gases' boiling point.
  B. The closer the temperature to the boiling point of a gas, the greater the error involved in using the gas laws.
  C. The *ideal gas law* demonstrates the interrelationships among volume, pressure, temperature, and amount of gas.
     1. According to the ideal gas law, multiplying the pressure of the system by the volume of the system and dividing this by the product of the temperature (absolute) and amount of gas in any gas system yields a result that is a constant. This is referred to as Boltzmann's constant, which is a constant that can be applied to all gas systems.
     2. The ideal gas law is normally expressed as

$$PV = nRT$$

$$\text{or} \qquad (13)$$

$$R = \frac{PV}{nT}$$

     where P = pressure, V = volume, and n = amount of gas (expressed normally in moles), R = Boltzmann's constant, and T = temperature (expressed in degrees Kelvin).
     3. Boltzmann's constant is equal to
        a. 82.1 ml · atm/mole · degree K when pressure is expressed in atmospheres and volume in milliliters.

      b. 62.3 L · mm Hg/mole · degree K when pressure is expressed in mm Hg and volume in liters.

D. *Boyle's law* states that pressure and volume of a gas system vary inversely if the temperature and amount of gas in the system are constant.

    1. Boyle's law mathematically is

$$PV = nRT \qquad (14)$$

where nRT is equal to a constant, thus

$$PV = K \qquad (15)$$

    2. In a system where temperature and amount of gas are constant, the original pressure and volume equal the final pressure and volume:

$$P_1 V_1 = P_2 V_2 \qquad (16)$$

E. *Charles' law* states that the temperature and volume of a gas system vary directly if the pressure and amount of gas in the system are constant.

    1. Charles' law mathematically is

$$\frac{V}{T} = \frac{nR}{P} \qquad (17)$$

where nR/P is equal to a constant, thus

$$\frac{V}{T} = K \qquad (18)$$

    2. In a system where the pressure and amount of gas are constant, the original temperature and volume equal the final temperature and volume:

$$\frac{V_1}{T_1} = \frac{V_2}{T_2} \qquad (19)$$

F. *Gay-Lussac's law* states that the pressure and temperature of a gas system vary directly if the volume and amount of gas in the system are constant.

    1. Gay-Lussac's law mathematically is

$$\frac{P}{T} = \frac{nR}{V} \qquad (20)$$

where $\dfrac{nR}{V}$ is equal to a constant, thus

$$\frac{P}{T} = K \tag{21}$$

2. In a system where the volume and amount of gas are constant, the original pressure and temperature equal the final pressure and temperature:

$$\frac{P_1}{T_1} = \frac{P_2}{T_2} \tag{22}$$

G. The *combined gas law* states that pressure, temperature, and volume of gas are specifically related if the amount of gas remains constant.
   1. The combined gas law mathematically is

$$\frac{PV}{T} = nR \tag{23}$$

where nR is equal to a constant, thus

$$\frac{PV}{T} = K \tag{24}$$

   2. In a system where the amount of gas in a system is constant, the original pressure, temperature, and volume are equal to the final pressure, temperature, and volume:

$$\frac{P_1 V_1}{T_1} = \frac{P_2 V_2}{T_2} \tag{25}$$

H. All gas law calculations must use temperature on the Kelvin scale for accurate results.
I. Water vapor does not react as an ideal gas; therefore, in a system where water vapor is present, water vapor pressure must be subtracted from total pressure before calculations are made.
J. When precision is needed, the barometric pressure reading should be corrected for expansion of mercury as affected by temperature.

XI. Diffusion
   A. Diffusion is movement of gas from an area of high concentration of a gas to an area of low concentration.

B. As diffusion occurs, a gas will occupy the total container as if it were the only gas present; i.e., a gas in a container will distribute itself *with time* equally throughout the whole container.
C. The rate of diffusion of a gas through another gas is affected by the following factors:
  1. The concentration gradient, which is directly related to the rate of diffusion.
  2. The temperature, which is directly related to the rate of diffusion.
  3. The cross-sectional area available for diffusion, which is directly related to the rate of diffusion.
  4. The molecular weight, which is indirectly related to the rate of diffusion.
  5. The distance the gas has to diffuse, which is indirectly related to the rate of diffusion:

$$\text{Rate of diffusion of a gas through a gas} = \frac{(\text{press.})(\text{temp.})(\text{cross-sectional area})}{(\text{MW})(\text{distance})} \qquad (26)$$

D. *Henry's law* states that the amount of a gas that can dissolve in a liquid is directly related to the partial pressure of the gas over the liquid and indirectly related to the temperature of the system.
  1. Henry's law expresses the solubility coefficients of gases in liquids.
  2. Solubility coefficients of oxygen and carbon dioxide in plasma at 37° C:
    a. 0.023 ml of O_2/ml of blood/760 mm Hg P_{O_2}
    b. 0.510 ml of CO_2/ml of blood/760 mm Hg P_{CO_2}
E. *Graham's law* states that the rate of diffusion of a gas through a liquid is indirectly related to the square root of the gram molecular weight (GMW) of the gas.
F. If Henry's and Graham's laws are combined, the rates of diffusion of carbon dioxide to oxygen can be compared under conditions of equal pressure gradients, distances, cross-sectional areas, and temperatures.
  1. When the above variables are equal, the only factors affecting the comparison would be the GMW of the gases and their solubility coefficients.
  2. The comparison may be mathematically represented as follows:

Rate of diffusion of

$$\frac{CO_2}{O_2} = \frac{(\text{sol. coef. } CO_2)(\sqrt{GMW\ O_2})}{(\text{sol. coef. } O_2)(\sqrt{GMW\ CO_2})}$$

$$= \frac{(0.510)(5.66)}{(0.023)(6.66)}$$

$$\approx \frac{19}{1} \tag{27}$$

3. Thus, under the above-mentioned conditions, carbon dioxide would diffuse about 19 times faster than would oxygen.
4. However, *at the alveolar capillary membrane, pressure gradients for oxygen and carbon dioxide are not equal.*
   a. Diffusion gradient for oxygen is 60 mm Hg.
   b. Diffusion gradient for carbon dioxide is 6 mm Hg.
   c. As a result of the above pressure gradients, oxygen equilibrates across the alveolar-capillary membrane slightly faster than does carbon dioxide.
   d. Oxygen equilibrates in about 0.23 second, while carbon dioxide equilibrates in about 0.25 second.

XII. Elastance and Compliance
   A. Elastance (E) is the ability of a distorted object to return to its original shape.
   B. Compliance (C) is the ease with which an object can be distorted.
   C. Compliance and elastance are inversely related:

$$C = \frac{1}{E} \tag{28}$$

   D. If the compliance of a system increases, the elastance of the system decreases.
   E. If the compliance of a system decreases, the elastance of the system increases.
   F. *Hook's law* defines the response of elastic bodies to distorting forces.
      1. It states that an elastic body stretches equal units of length or volume for each unit of weight or force applied to it.
      2. This relationship holds until the elastic limit of the system is reached.
      3. Beyond the elastic limit, each unit of weight or force produces smaller and smaller changes in length or volume.

    4. With a true spring, exceeding the elastic limit results in permanent distortion.

G. Elastance can be mathematically defined as:

$$E = \frac{\Delta P}{\Delta V} \qquad (29)$$

where ΔP = change in pressure and ΔV = change in volume.

H. Compliance can be mathematically defined as:

$$C = \frac{\Delta V}{\Delta P} \qquad (30)$$

XIII. Surface Tension
  A. Surface tension is a force that exists at the interface between a liquid and a gas or between two liquids.
  B. The surface tension of a liquid is the result of like molecules being attracted to each other and thus moving away from the interface. This causes the liquid to occupy the smallest volume possible.
  C. As a result of surface tension, a force is necessary to cause a tear in the surface of the liquid.
  D. The surface tension of a liquid is expressed in dynes per linear centimeter.
  E. Surface tension is indirectly related to temperature.
  F. *LaPlace's law* is used to determine the amount of pressure generated inside a system as a result of surface tension.
    1. The law states that the pressure (P) in dynes/sq cm as a result of surface tension (ST) in dynes/cm is equal to the surface tension of the liquid multiplied by 1 over the radii (r) in centimeters of curvature:

$$P = ST\left(\frac{1}{r_1} + \frac{1}{r_2} + \frac{1}{r_3} + \ldots \frac{1}{r_n}\right) \qquad (31)$$

    2. LaPlace's law as applied to a drop is:

$$P = \frac{2\ ST}{r} \qquad (32)$$

Here reference is made to a perfect sphere that has only two radii of curvature, one in the vertical plane and one in the horizontal plane.

3. LaPlace's law as applied to a bubble is:

$$P = \frac{4\ ST}{r} \tag{33}$$

There are two interfaces in a bubble, one on the inside of the bubble and one on the outside; thus, there is a total of four radii. All are considered equal because the film of the bubble is only angstroms in diameter.

4. LaPlace's law as applied to a blood vessel is:

$$P = \frac{ST}{r} \tag{34}$$

When the radii of curvature of a blood vessel are considered, the only radius used in the calculation is that of the vessel's width, because the radius of length is so great. When the inverse of the radii of length is calculated, the number essentially goes to infinity and is meaningless in calculating the pressure as a result of surface tension.

5. It is important to remember that the pressure as a result of surface tension is indirectly related to the radius. *The smaller the sphere, the greater the pressure as a result of surface tension* (Fig 2–1).

G. *Critical volume* is a volume below which the effects of surface tension are so great that the structure collapses. Once the critical volume is reached, collapse is always imminent.

H. The force necessary to inflate a deflated object increases significantly as the critical volume is reached but rapidly decreases once the critical volume is exceeded (Fig 2–2).

I. The surface tension of a fluid is reduced by chemicals referred to as surfactants. Surfactants are surface-active agents that interfere with the molecules of the fluid at the surface, causing a reduction in the force (ST) that draws the fluid centrally. Soaps and detergents are common surfactants.

XIV. Fluid Dynamics

A. Law of continuity

1. The product of the cross-sectional area of a system times the velocity for a given flow rate is constant.

2. Thus, if the flow of gas is constant, the cross-sectional area and velocity of gas are inversely related.

3. In any system with varying radii, the velocity of gas movement must change as the radius changes.

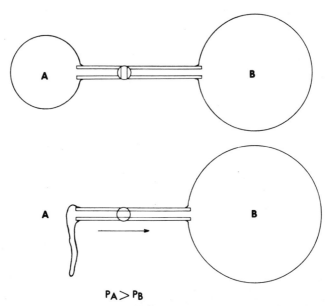

$$P_A > P_B$$

Fig 2–1.—When two bubbles of different sizes *(A and B)* but with the same surface tension are allowed to communicate, the greater pressure as a result of surface tension in the smaller bubble causes it to empty into the larger. (From Spearman C.B., Sheldon R.L., Egan D.F.: *Egan's Fundamentals of Respiratory Therapy,* ed. 4. St. Louis, C.V. Mosby Co., 1982. Reproduced by permission.)

B. Velocity vs. flow
   1. Velocity is the speed with which movement between two points occurs (miles/hour, cm/second).
   2. Flow is the volume passing a single point per unit of time (L/min).
   3. The two are related and may change directly or indirectly with each other, depending on the specific changes that occur in the structure of the system.
C. Resistance to gas flow
   1. In general, resistance is defined as the force (pressure) necessary to maintain a specific flow in a particular system.
   2. In order for gas movement to occur, there must be a pressure gradient. The magnitude of the pressure gradient is determined by the overall resistance of the system. In gas physics, airway resistance is equal to the change in pressure divided by flow:

$$R = \frac{\Delta P}{\dot{V}} \qquad (35)$$

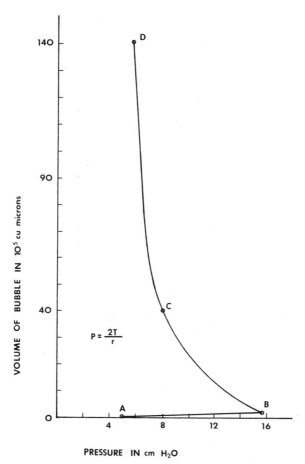

Fig 2–2.—Pressure-volume curve of a bubble as it is inflated. *A*, minimal volume providing shape. *B*, critical volume. *C* and *D*, decreased pressure is necessary to maintain a given volume as the radius of the sphere increases. See text for details.

where R = airway resistance, ΔP = change in pressure, and $\dot{V}$ = flow.

4. Airway resistance is a physical property of the system.
5. The change in pressure reflects the amount of pressure necessary to maintain a *specific flow* in the system.
6. The resistance of a system is increased under the following situations:
   a. Decreased lumen of the system.
   b. Directional changes in the system.
   c. Branching of the system.

7. If the resistance of a system is constant, an increase in pressure gradient results in an increase in system flow.
8. An increase in resistance with a constant pressure gradient results in a decrease in flow.
9. In general, if resistance is constant, pressure gradient and system flow are directly related.

D. Conductance
   1. Conductance is the capability of a system to maintain flow.
   2. Conductance is the inverse of resistance.
   3. Mathematically, conductance is equal to:

$$\text{Conductance} = \frac{\dot{V}}{\Delta P} \tag{36}$$

E. Types of flow
   1. *Laminar flow* is a smooth, even, nontumbling flow.
      a. Laminar flow proceeds with a cone front. The molecules of gas in the center of the system encounter the least frictional resistance and move at a greater velocity than those at the sides of the system (Fig 2–3).
      b. In all laminar flow situations, the pressure necessary to overcome airway resistance is directly related to flow:

$$R = \frac{\Delta P}{\dot{V}} \tag{37}$$

   2. *Turbulent flow* is a rough, tumbling, uneven flow pattern.
      a. Turbulent flow proceeds with a blunt front. Due to a tumbling effect, all of the molecules in the system encounter the walls of the vessel (see Fig 2–3).
      b. In a turbulent flow system, the pressure necessary to overcome airway resistance is directly related to the *square* of the flow:

$$R = \frac{P}{\dot{V}^2} \tag{38}$$

      c. *The pressure gradient necessary to maintain turbulent flow is much higher than that necessary to maintain laminar flow.*
   3. *Tracheobronchial flow* is a combination of areas of laminar and turbulent flow. Tracheobronchial flow is believed to be the type of flow maintained throughout the respiratory system.

LAMINAR

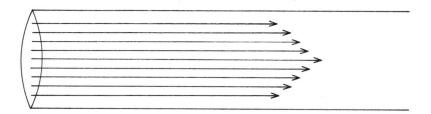

TURBULENT

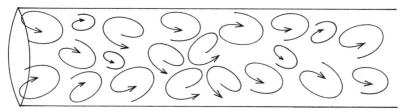

Fig 2–3.—Laminar and turbulent flow.

F. *Reynold's number*
  1. Reynold's number (RN) is a dimensionless number that indicates whether flow through a system is laminar or turbulent.
  2. Reynold's number is calculated as follows:

$$\text{RN} = \frac{(\text{diameter})(\text{velocity})(\text{density})}{(\text{viscosity})} \qquad (39)$$

  where the diameter refers to the diameter of the system and velocity, density, and viscosity refer to the gas that is flowing in the system.
  3. If Reynold's number is 2,000 or greater, the flow in the system will be turbulent. If it is less than 2,000, the flow will be laminar.
G. *Bernoulli effect*
  1. Bernoulli effect: As a gas moves through a free-flowing system, transmural pressure is inversely related to velocity of the gas; i.e., as the velocity of the gas increases, the transmural pressure decreases (Fig 2–4).
  2. The above statement holds true because the total energy in a free-flowing system is equal at all points.

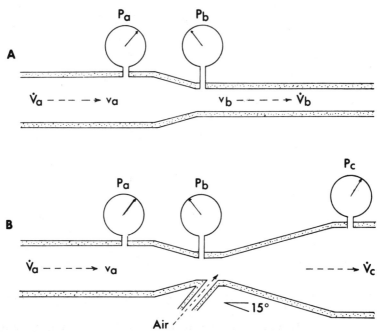

Fig 2–4.—A, the Bernoulli effect demonstrates that the *pressure* exerted by a steady flow of gas or liquid in a conducting tube varies *inversely* as the *velocity* of the fluid. With an abrupt narrowing of the passage since the volume of fluid per unit of time leaving $(\dot{V_b})$ must equal the time-volume entering the tube $(\dot{V_a})$, the linear motion of the fluid per unit of time (velocity, v) must increase as it traverses the structure $(v_b > v_a)$. Thus there is a pressure drop distal to the restriction $(P_b < P_a)$. **B,** according to the Venturi principle, the pressure drop distal to a restriction can be closely restored to the prerestriction pressure if there is a dilation of the passage immediately distal to the stenosis, with an angle of divergence not exceeding 15 degrees. Thus P_c approximately equals P_a. The Venturi is a widely used device to entrain a second gas to mix with the main-flow gas. The subambient pressure distal to the restriction draws in the second gas just past the restriction, and the increased outflow $(\dot{V_c} > \dot{V_a})$ is accomodated by the widened distal passage. (From Spearman C.B., Sheldon R.L., Egan D.F.: *Egan's Fundamentals of Respiratory Therapy,* ed. 4. St. Louis, C.V. Mosby Co., 1982. Reproduced by permission.)

      3. In a free-flowing system of limited size functioning essentially as a non-gravity-dependent system, the total energy is equal to the sum of the kinetic energy and the transmural pressure energy.

      4. Transmural pressure energy is purely a measure of the force that the gas flow exerts on the walls of the system.

5. Kinetic energy in this sense is equal to 0.5 times the gas density times the gas velocity squared:

$$\text{Kinetic energy} = 0.5\ (D)(V^2) \qquad (40)$$

6. Thus, in a free-flowing system

$$\text{Total energy} = 0.5\ (D)(V^2) + P_{transmural} \qquad (41)$$

This illustrates the fact that velocity and transmural pressure are inversely related.

7. As the radius of the system decreases and velocity of the gas moving through the system increases, transmural pressure decreases, per equation 41.
8. The lower the density of a gas, the smaller the decrease in transmural pressure as the gas moves through a stenosis. This relationship demonstrates the effect of density on maintaining a more laminar flow.
9. *Venturi principle*
   a. The Venturi principle is an extension of the Bernoulli effect (see Fig 2–4).
   b. It states that distal to a stenosis in a free-flowing system, prestenotic pressure can be restored if the angle of divergence of the system from the midline does not exceed 15 degrees.
   c. Also, if the stenosis in the system is small enough, subatmospheric transmural pressure can be developed and used to entrain a second gas or liquid.
   d. Venturi systems can be designed to deliver specific oxygen concentrations.
   e. The concentration of oxygen delivered by a venturi system can be varied by:
      (1) Altering the size of the venturi's stenosis.
      (2) Altering the size of the entrainment ports.
   f. Backpressure on a venturi system decreases the volume of fluid or gas entrained. This causes the oxygen concentration delivered by the system to increase.
H. Jet mixing
   1. The use of a constant pressure flow of gas (jet) to entrain a second gas.
   2. No pressure gradient exists between the jet flow and the ambient environment.
   3. Air entrainment is a result of the viscous shearing force be-

tween a dynamic fluid and a stationary fluid resulting in a change in velocities.
   a. The dynamic fluid's velocity decreases.
   b. The stationary fluid's velocity increases.
   4. Provided free access is allowed for the entrained gas, mixing at specific ratios can be maintained.
   5. Altering the *flow* of the gas from the jet alters the total volume exiting the system but does not alter entrainment ratios or FI_{O_2}.
   6. Entrainment ratios are the same as those commonly listed for Venturi systems (see Chap. 24).
   7. Backpressure on the system decreases entrainment and increases FI_{O_2}.
   8. Jet mixing is responsible for the function of air entrainment masks and most other systems in respiratory care commonly attributed to the Venturi effect.
I. *Poiseuille's Law*
   1. Poiseuille's law is used in the determination of the viscosity of a fluid.
   2. Viscosity is defined as a fluid's resistance to deformity and, for gases, increases with increased temperature.
   3. Poiseuille's law states that viscosity (μ) is equal to the change in pressure (ΔP) times pi (π) times the radius to the fourth power (r^4) divided by eight times the length of the system ($8l$) times flow ($\dot{V}$):

$$n = \frac{\Delta P \pi r^4}{8l\dot{V}} \tag{42}$$

   4. Rearranging equation 42 and placing on the left side of the equation those factors that would be constant when ventilating a patient and on the right side of the equation those factors that would vary, the result is

$$\frac{n8l}{\pi} = \frac{\Delta P r^4}{\dot{V}} \tag{43}$$

   5. The right side of equation 43 indicates the relationship between pressure, flow, and radius of a gas flow system.
   6. If the radius were to decrease by one half, there would be a 16-fold change in the right side of the equation.
   7. In order to maintain the left side of the equation constant, a 16-fold change in pressure or flow or a combination of both

would be necessary to minimize the effects of the decrease in radius.

8. Thus, in order to minimize the effects of an airway diameter decrease, it would be necessary to increase the pressure gradient and/or decrease the flow in the system.

9. Theoretically, Poiseuille's law can only be applied to homogeneous fluid flow systems that are nonpulsatile and laminar through a single cylinder.

10. Thus, Poiseuille's law cannot be directly applied to the respiratory and cardiovascular systems, but it does provide insights into the interrelationships between pressure, flow, and system radius.

BIBLIOGRAPHY

Carr H.Y., Weidner R.T.: *Physics from the Ground Up.* New York, McGraw-Hill Book Co., 1971.

Cherniack R.M., Cherniack L.: *Respiration in Health and Disease,* ed. 3. Philadelphia, W.B. Saunders Co., 1983.

Comroe J.H.: *Physiology of Respiration,* ed. 2. Chicago, Year Book Medical Publishers, Inc., 1974.

Dejours P.: *Respiration.* New York, Oxford University Press, 1966.

Epstein L.I., Kuzava B.A.: *Basic Physics in Anesthesiology.* Chicago, Year Book Medical Publishers, Inc., 1976.

Guyton A.C.: *Textbook of Medical Physiology,* ed. 6. Philadelphia, W.B. Saunders Co., 1981.

Murray J.F.: *The Normal Lung.* Philadelphia, W.B. Saunders Co., 1976.

Nunn J.F.: *Applied Respiratory Physiology With Special Reference to Anesthesia,* ed. 2. London, Butterworth & Co., Ltd., 1977.

Sacheim G.I., Schultz R.M.: *Chemistry for the Health Sciences,* ed. 2. New York, Macmillan Publishing Co., Inc., 1973.

Scacci R.: Air entrainment masks: Jet mixing is how they work; the Bernoulli and Venturi principles is how they don't. *Respir. Care* 24:928–934, 1979.

Schaim U.R., et al.: *College Physics.* New York, Raytheon Education Co., Physical Science Study Committee, 1968.

Shapiro B.A., Harrison R.A., Kacmarek R.M., et al.: *Clinical Application of Respiratory Care,* ed. 3. Chicago, Year Book Medical Publishers, Inc., 1985.

Shapiro B.A., Harrison R.A., Walton J.R.: *Clinical Application of Blood Gases,* ed. 3. Chicago, Year Book Medical Publishers, Inc., 1982.

Young J.A., Crocker D.: *Principles and Practice of Respiratory Therapy,* ed. 2. Chicago, Year Book Medical Publishers, Inc., 1976.

3 / Anatomy of the Respiratory System

I. Boundaries and Functions of the Upper Airway
- Boundaries: From the anterior nares to the true vocal cords.
- Functions:
  1. Heating or cooling inspired gases to body temperature (37° C).
  2. Filtering inspired gases.
  3. Humidifying inspired gases to a relative humidity of about 100% at body temperature.
  4. Olfaction: Act of smelling.
  5. Phonation: Production of sound.
  6. Conduction passageway for ventilating gases.

A. The nose
  1. The nose is a rigid structure of cartilage and bone, the superior one third made up of the nasal and maxilla bones, the inferior two thirds made up of five large pieces of cartilage.
  2. The two external openings are called the nostrils, external nares, or anterior nares. Their lateral borders are termed the alae.
  3. The nasal cavity is divided into two nasal fossae by the septal cartilage.
  4. Each nasal fossa is divided into three regions: vestibular, olfactory, and respiratory (Fig 3–1).
     a. *Vestibular* region: An area of slight dilation inside the nostril, bordered laterally by the alae and medially by the nasal septal cartilage.
        (1) Contained are coarse nasal hairs (vibrissae) that project anteriorly and inferiorly.
        (2) Sebaceous glands secrete sebum, a greasy substance that keeps the nasal hairs soft and pliable.
        (3) The nasal hairs are the first line of defense for the upper airway, acting as very gross filters of inspired air.
        (4) The vestibular region is lined with stratified squamous epithelium (Table 3–1).
     b. *Olfactory* region: An area in each nasal cavity defined by

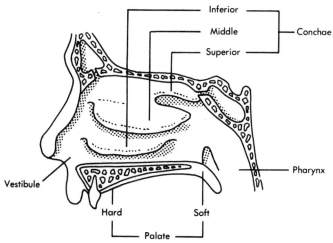

Fig 3–1.—Lateral view of the nasal cavity, representing one complete nasal fossa. (From Dail D.H.: Anatomy of the respiratory system, in Moser K.M., Spragg R.G. (eds.): *Respiratory Emergencies,* ed. 2. St. Louis, C.V. Mosby Co., 1982. Reproduced by permission.)

the superior concha laterally, nasal septal cartilage medially, and roof of the nasal cavity superiorly.

(1) Contained is the olfactory epithelium responsible for the sense of smell.

(2) The olfactory epithelium is yellowish brown and appears as pseudostratified columnar epithelial cells. These cells are interspersed with more deeply placed olfactory cells whose sensory filament, the olfactory hairs, protrude to the epithelial surface.

(3) Due largely to the architecture of the nasal cavity, sniffing causes inspired gases to be drawn to the olfactory

TABLE 3–1.—ANATOMICAL COMPARISON
OF EPITHELIUM IN UPPER RESPIRATORY TRACT

STRUCTURE	EPITHELIUM
Vestibular region/nose	Stratified squamous
Olfactory region/nose	Pseudostratified columnar
Respiratory region/nose	Pseudostratified ciliated columnar
Paranasal sinuses	Pseudostratified ciliated columnar
Nasopharynx	Pseudostratified ciliated columnar
Oropharynx	Stratified squamous
Laryngopharynx	Stratified squamous
Larynx/above true cords	Stratified squamous

region and not much farther into the respiratory tract. This provides a protective mechanism for sampling potentially noxious environmental gases.

c. *Respiratory* region: An area in each nasal cavity inferior to the olfactory region and posterior to the vestibular region. The respiratory region comprises most of the surface area of the nasal fossa.

(1) Contained in the respiratory region of each nasal fossa are three bony plates called turbinates or conchae. The turbinates extend in a medial and inferior direction from the lateral walls of the nasal fossa.

(2) The three turbinates (superior, middle, and inferior) overhang and define the three corresponding passageways through each nasal cavity, respectively the superior, middle, and inferior meati.

(3) Because of the arrangement of the turbinates and folded mucous membrane covering the turbinates in the nose, it has a volume of about 20 cc and a remarkably large surface area of about 160 sq cm.

(4) Turbulent flow is created through the respective meati, which serve the three primary functions of the nose: heating, humidifying, and filtering inspired gases.

(5) Heating, humidifying, and filtering of inspired gases are accomplished by the turbulent flow, which provides a greater probability that each gas molecule will come in contact with the very large surface area of the vascular nasal mucous membrane. This large gas to nasal surface interface allows the following:

(a) The abundant underlying vasculature to heat inspired gases to body temperature.

(b) The moist nasal mucous membrane to give up 650–1,000 ml of H_2O per day in bringing inspired gases to a relative humidity of 80% on leaving the nose and entering the nasopharynx.

(c) Particles suspended in the inspired gas to contact the sticky mucous membrane, thus filtering out particles greater than 5 μ by inertial impaction to an efficiency of about 100%.

(6) The epithelial lining of the respiratory region of the nasal cavity is pseudostratified ciliated columnar epithelium (Fig 3–2).

(a) The cells are cylindrical and appear to be two cell

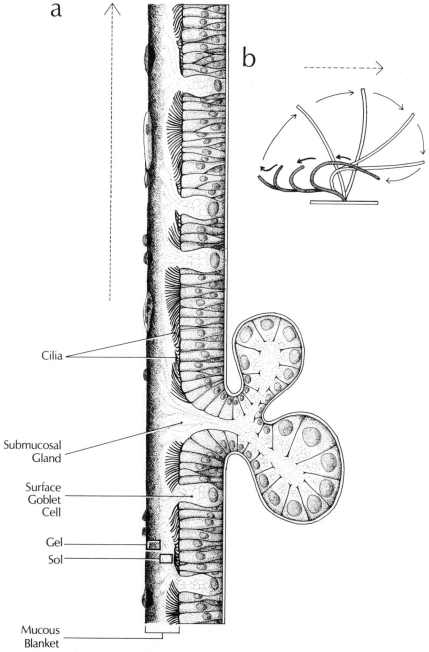

a

b

Cilia

Submucosal
Gland

Surface
Goblet
Cell

Gel

Sol

Mucous
Blanket

Fig 3–2.—Conceptual depiction of the respiratory epithelium (pseudostratified ciliated columnar epithelium). (From Shapiro B.A., Harrison R.A., Kacmarek R.M., et al.: *Clinical Application of Respiratory Care,* ed. 3. Chicago, Year Book Medical Publishers, Inc., 1985. Reproduced by permission.)

layers thick due to the high lateral pressures compressing the cells. Actually the epithelium is only
one cell layer thick, each columnar cell making contact with the basement membrane.
  (b) Each columnar cell has 200–250 cilia on its luminal
surface. Each of the cilia contains two central and
nine paired peripheral fibrils. It is the sliding interaction of these fibrils that is thought to cause the
beating of the cilia.
  (c) Goblet cells and submucosal glands are interspersed
throughout the epithelium and, along with capillary
seepage, are responsible for production of mucus
(100 ml/day in health).
  (d) Mucus exists in two layers:
    (i) Sol layer: Fluid bottom layer housing the cilia.
    (ii) Gel layer: A viscous layer overlying the cilia.
  (e) On the forward stroke, the cilia become rigid. Their
tips touch the undersurface of the gel layer and pro-
pel it toward the oropharynx. On the backward
stroke, the cilia become flaccid, fold upon themselves, and slide entirely through the sol layer to
their resting position without producing a retrograde motion of the gel layer.
  (f) The cilia of a particular cell and adjacent cells beat
in a coordinated and sequential fashion that produces a motion very similar to a wave. This allows a
unidirectional flow of mucus. The cilia beat about
1,000–1,500 times per minute and move the mucous layer at a rate of 2 cm/minute.
  (g) Functions of the mucus and pseudostratified ciliated
columnar epithelium (mucociliary blanket):
    (i) To entrap inspired particles.
    (ii) To humidify inspired gas.
    (iii) To transport debris-laden mucus out of the re-
spiratory tract.
5. The nose is responsible for one half to two thirds of the total
airway resistance during nasal breathing. It therefore is not
surprising that during stress (e.g., exercise or disease) a switch
is made to mouth breathing.
6. The nose ends with the outlet of the nasal cavity into the nasopharynx through the internal nares (posterior nares or
choanae).

B. Paranasal sinuses (Fig 3–3)
1. Sinuses are cavities of air in the bones of the cranium.
2. The function of the sinuses is not clearly understood, but it may be twofold:
    a. To give the voice resonance (prolongation and intensification of sound).
    b. To lighten the head to some extent, the space occupied by the sinuses being filled with air rather than bone.
3. The sinuses are absent or rudimentary at birth and grow almost simultaneously with the development of the permanent teeth. Formation of the sinuses is responsible for the alteration in facial shape that occurs at this time.
4. All of the air sinuses are lined with pseudostratified ciliated columnar epithelium and produce mucus, which drains into the nasal meati.
5. If sinus drainage is blocked by nasogastric tubes or nasotracheal intubation, sinusitis and sinus infection often result.
6. Groups of paranasal sinuses: Frontal, maxillary, sphenoidal, and ethmoidal.
    a. The *frontal sinuses* appear as paired sinuses medial to the orbits of the eye and superior to the roof of the nasal cavity between the external and internal surfaces of the frontal bone. They drain into the anterior portion of the middle meati.
    b. The *maxillary sinuses* appear as paired sinuses lateral to each nasal cavity and inferior to the orbits of the eye in the body of the maxilla. These sinuses, the largest of all the air sinuses, drain into the middle meati.
    c. The *sphenoidal sinuses* appear as paired sinuses posterior and inferior to the roof of the nasal cavity and superior to the internal nares (choanae) in the body of the sphenoid bone. They drain into the superior meati.
    d. The *ethmoidal sinuses* are paired sinuses that exist in three groups: anterior, medial, and posterior ethmoidal. They exist just lateral to the superior and middle conchae, medial to the orbits of the eyes, inferior to the frontal sinuses, and superior to the maxillary sinuses in the ethmoid bone. The ethmoidal sinuses drain into the superior and middle meati.
C. Pharynx
1. The pharynx is a hollow muscular structure lined with epithelium (Fig 3–4).
2. Major functions

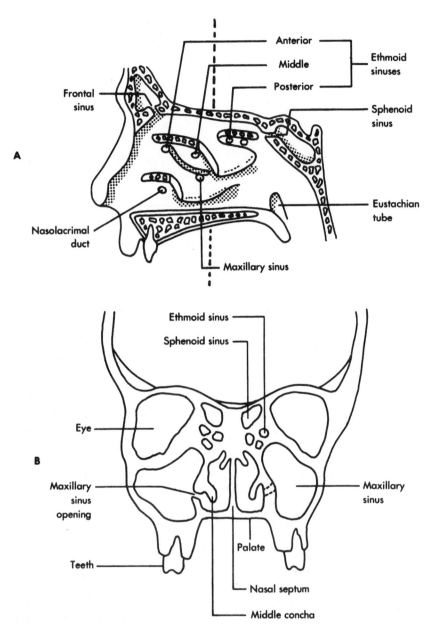

Fig 3–3.—A, lateral view of the nasal cavity, representing one complete nasal fossa with sites of sinus drainage. **B,** frontal section of the nasal cavity taken through the dotted line in **A.** (From Dail D.H.: Anatomy of the respiratory system, in Moser K.M., Spragg R.G. (eds.): *Respiratory Emergencies,* ed. 2. St. Louis, C.V. Mosby Co., 1982. Reproduced by permission.)

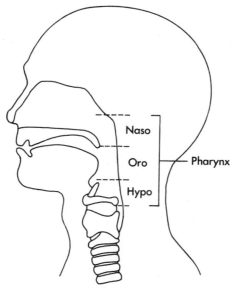

Fig 3–4.—Lateral view of the upper airway indicating the three sections of the pharynx. (From Dail D.H.: Anatomy of the respiratory system, in Moser K.M., Spragg R.G. (eds.): *Respiratory Emergencies,* ed. 2. St. Louis, C.V. Mosby Co., 1982. Reproduced by permission.)

      a. To produce the vowel sounds (phonation) by changing its shape.

      b. To serve as a common passageway for ventilatory gases, food, and liquid.

  3. The pharynx is about 5 in. long and extends from the internal nares (choanae) inferiorly to the esophagus.

  4. Sections of the pharynx: Nasopharynx, oropharynx, and laryngopharynx.

      a. The *nasopharynx* is located behind the nasal cavity and extends from the internal nares superiorly to the tip of the uvula inferiorly.

        (1) The epithelium is continuous with the epithelium of the nasal cavity and is pseudostratified ciliated columnar epithelium.

        (2) The eustachian or auditory tubes open into the nasopharynx on each of its lateral walls and communicate with the tympanic cavity or middle ear (see Fig 3–3).

          (a) This allows equilibration of pressure on each side of the tympanic membrane (eardrum) with environmental pressure changes.

(b) Nasal intubation may block the eustachian tube openings and may cause otitis media.

(3) The pharyngeal tonsil or adenoid is located in the superior and posterior wall of the nasopharynx.

   (a) The pharyngeal tonsil consists of a large concentration of lymphoid tissue comprising the superior portion of Waldeyer's ring. This ring of lymphoid tissue surrounds and guards the entrance to the respiratory and gastrointestinal tracts.

(4) During the process of swallowing, the uvula and soft palate move in a posterior and superior direction to protect the nasopharynx and nasal cavity from the entrance of food and/or liquid.

(5) Major functions of the nasopharynx:

   (a) Gas conduction

   (b) Filtration of gases

   (c) Defense mechanism of the body (tonsils)

b. The *oropharynx* is located behind the oral or buccal cavity and extends from the tip of the uvula superiorly to the tip of the epiglottis inferiorly.

(1) The epithelial lining is stratified squamous epithelium.

(2) The palatine tonsils are located lateral to the uvula on the lateral and anterior aspects of the oropharynx.

(3) The lingual tonsil is located at the base of the tongue, superior and anterior to the vallecula (the space between the epiglottis and base of the tongue).

(4) The two palatine tonsils, one lingual and one pharyngeal (adenoid), are the major components of Waldeyer's ring.

(5) Major functions of the oropharynx:

   (a) Gas conduction

   (b) Food and fluid conduction

   (c) Filtration of inspired gases

   (d) Defense mechanism of the body (Waldeyer's ring)

c. The laryngopharynx or hypopharynx extends superiorly from the tip of the epiglottis to a point inferiorly where it bifurcates into larynx and esophagus.

(1) The epithelial lining is stratified squamous epithelium.

(2) Major functions of the laryngopharynx:

   (a) Gas conduction

   (b) Food and fluid conduction

(3) The laryngopharynx leads anteriorly into the larynx and posteriorly into the esophagus.

(4) The larynx* is considered the connection between the upper and lower airways, the exact division being the true vocal cords.

II. Boundaries and Functions of the Lower Airway
- Boundaries: From the true vocal cords to the terminal air spaces (alveoli).
- Functions:
  1. Ventilation: To and fro movement of gas (gas conduction).
  2. External respiration: Actual gas exchange between body (pulmonary capillary blood) and external environment (alveolar gas).
  3. Sphincter or glottic mechanisms.
     a. Valsalva maneuver: Forced expiration against closed glottis.
     b. Müller maneuver: Forced inspiration against closed glottis.
     c. Cough mechanism.
     d. Protection of laryngeal inlet.
  4. Phonation: Production of sound.

A. The larynx (Fig 3–5)
  1. The larynx is a boxlike structure made of cartilage connected by extrinsic and intrinsic muscles and ligaments. It is lined internally by a mucous membrane.
  2. Functions
     a. Gas conduction: Ventilation.
     b. Phonation: Production of sound.
     c. Sphincter or glottic mechanism.
  3. The larynx extends from the third to sixth cervical vertebrae in the anterior portion of the neck.
  4. Unpaired cartilages of the larynx: Epiglottis, thyroid, and cricoid.
     a. *Epiglottic cartilage*
        (1) Leaf-shaped piece of fibrocartilage.
        (2) Anteriorly attached to thyroid cartilage just inferior to the thyroid notch.
        (3) Laterally attached to folds of mucous membrane called aryepiglottic folds.
        (4) On swallowing, the epiglottis is squeezed between the base of the tongue and thyroid cartilage, causing the epiglottis to pivot in a posterior and inferior direction to cover the laryngeal inlet.

*For discussion and organizational purposes, a complete description of the larynx will follow after Section II on the lower airway (please note that the superior portion of the larynx is part of the upper airway and the inferior portion of the larynx is part of the lower airway).

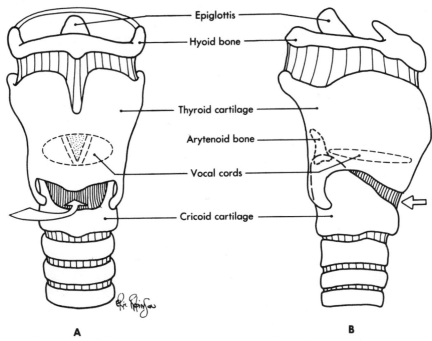

Fig 3–5.—Frontal and lateral view of the larynx. (From Dail D.H.: Anatomy of the respiratory system, in Moser K.M., Spragg R.G. (eds.): *Respiratory Emergencies,* ed. 2. St. Louis, C.V. Mosby Co., 1982. Reproduced by permission.)

    b. *Thyroid cartilage*
       (1) The largest laryngeal cartilage.
       (2) The anterior aspect is called the laryngeal prominence or Adam's apple.
       (3) Directly superior to the laryngeal prominence is the thyroid notch.
       (4) The posterior and lateral aspects of this cartilage have two superior and two inferior projections, the superior and inferior cornua.
         (a) The superior cornu articulates with the hyoid bone, which serves as a support from which the lower respiratory tract is suspended.
         (b) The inferior cornu articulates with the cricoid cartilage below.
    c. *Cricoid cartilage*
       (1) Shaped like a signet ring.

(2) Forms the entire inferior aspect and most of the posterior aspect of the larynx.

(3) On the posterolateral surface exist articulating surfaces for the inferior cornu of the thyroid cartilage.

(4) On the posterosuperior surface exist articulating surfaces for the paired arytenoid cartilages.

(5) Lies inferior to the thyroid and superior to the trachea, to which it attaches.

(6) Lies anterior to the esophagus. Therefore, external cricoid pressure may facilitate viewing of the glottis during tracheal intubation and prevent reflux from the stomach by compressing the esophagus.

5. Paired cartilages of the larynx: Arytenoid, corniculate, and cuneiform.

   a. *Arytenoid cartilages*

     (1) Shaped like upright pyramids.

     (2) The base of each cartilage articulates with the posterosuperior surface of the cricoid cartilage.

     (3) Each arytenoid cartilage has a ventral-medial projection from its base called the vocal process, to which the vocal ligaments attach.

     (4) Arytenoid cartilages, along with the cricoid cartilage, make up the entire posterior surface of the larynx.

   b. *Corniculate cartilages*

     (1) Shaped like cones and are the smallest cartilages of the larynx.

     (2) Articulate with the arytenoid cartilages on their superior surface, to which the corniculate cartilages are sometimes fused.

     (3) When the larynx is viewed from above, the corniculate cartilages appear as two small elevations on the posteromedial aspect of the laryngeal inlet.

     (4) Housed in mucosal folds called the aryepiglottic folds.

   c. *Cuneiform cartilages*

     (1) Shaped like small, elongated clubs.

     (2) Located lateral and anterior to the corniculate cartilages.

     (3) When the larynx is viewed from above, the cuneiform cartilages appear as two small elevations just lateral and anterior to the corniculate cartilages.

     (4) Housed in the aryepiglottic folds.

     (5) The cuneiforms, along with the aryepiglottic folds, form

    the lateral aspect of the laryngeal inlet. The epiglottis forms the anterior aspect, the corniculates the posterior aspect of the laryngeal inlet.

6. Extrinsic ligaments of the larynx
   a. Extrinsic ligaments attach cartilages of the larynx to structures outside the larynx.
   b. The *thyrohyoid membrane* is a broad fibroelastic sheet that attaches the anterior and lateral superior aspects of the thyroid cartilage to the inferior surface of the hyoid bone (the posterior portion of the thyroid cartilage is attached to the hyoid bone by the superior cornu of the thyroid cartilage).
   c. The *hyoepiglottic ligament* is an elastic band that attaches the anterior surface of the epiglottis to the hyoid bone.
   d. The *cricotracheal ligament* connects the lower portion of the cricoid cartilage to the trachea by a very broad fibrous membrane.
7. Intrinsic ligaments of the larynx
   a. Intrinsic ligaments attach cartilages of the larynx to one another.
   b. The *thyroepiglottic ligament* attaches the inferior aspect of the epiglottis to the thyroid cartilage on its internal surface below the thyroid notch.
   c. The *aryepiglottic ligament* attaches the arytenoid cartilages to the epiglottis and acts as a point of attachment for the aryepiglottic folds.
   d. The *cricothyroid ligament* attaches the anterior portion of the thyroid cartilage to the anterior portion of the cricoid cartilage. It is through this ligament that an emergency cricothyroidotomy is performed.
   e. The *vocal ligament* is a thick band that stretches from the vocal process of the arytenoid cartilages across the cavity of the larynx to attach to the thyroid cartilage just inferior to the thyroepiglottic ligament. The lateral borders of the vocal ligament attach to the inverted free borders of the cricothyroid ligament.
   f. The *ventricular ligament* is a thick band that stretches from the arytenoid cartilage across the cavity of the larynx to the thyroid cartilage. It exists superior and lateral to the vocal ligament.
8. Cavity of the larynx (Fig 3–6)
   a. The larynx is divided into three sections by the pair of ventricular folds and vocal folds.

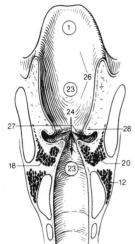

Fig 3–6.—Frontal section of larynx, posterior view, depicting laryngeal cavities. *1*, epiglottis; *18*, true vocal cords; *23*, laryngeal cavity; *24*, entrance to larynx through the rima vestibuli and rima glottidis; *26*, vestibule of larynx; *27*, rima vestibuli; *28*, ventricular folds. (From Feneis H.: *Pocket Atlas of Human Anatomy,* ed. 4. New York, Thieme-Stratton, Inc., 1976. Reproduced by permission.)

b. The *upper section*, the vestibule of the larynx, extends from the laryngeal inlet to the level of the ventricular folds.

  (1) The ventricular folds are called the false vocal cords.

  (2) The space between the ventricular folds is the rima vestibuli.

c. The *middle section*, the ventricle of the larynx, extends from the ventricular folds to the vocal cords.

  (1) The vocal folds are the true vocal cords.

  (2) The space between the vocal folds is the rima glottidis or glottis.

    (a) The glottis is triangular, the base being posterior, the apex anterior.

    (b) It is the smallest opening of the adult airway (important when selecting endotracheal tube size).

    (c) The dimensions of the glottis are smaller in the female than in the male.

      (i) Average female transverse diameter: 7–8 mm.

      (ii) Average male transverse diameter: 9–10 mm.

      (iii) Average anteroposterior diameter in the female: 17 mm.

      (iv) Average anteroposterior diameter in the male: 24 mm.

  (3) The size of the rima glottidis also is variable, depending on the state of the vocal cords (Fig 3–7).

    (a) Adduction is accomplished by medial rotation and

Front

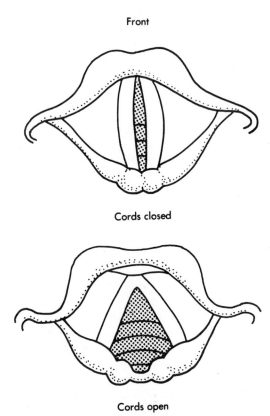

Cords closed

Cords open

Fig 3–7.—View into the larynx with the vocal cords closed (adduction) and opened (abduction). See text for details. (From Dail D.H.: Anatomy of the respiratory system, in Mosen K.M., Spragg R.G. (eds.): *Respiratory Emergencies,* ed. 2. St. Louis, C.V. Mosby Co., 1982. Reproduced by permission.)

approximation of the arytenoids, thus sealing the glottis.
   (b) Abduction is accomplished by lateral rotation of the arytenoids, thus increasing the size of the glottis.
   (4) The glottic or sphincter mechanism requires aryepiglottic folds, epiglottis, ventricular folds, and vocal folds to act in a very coordinated fashion in sealing the laryngeal inlet.
   d. The *lower section,* subglottic cavity of the larynx, extends from vocal folds to cricoid cartilage.
   e. The epithelial lining of the larynx above the true vocal cords

is continuous with the laryngopharynx and is stratified squamous epithelium (see Table 3–1).

  f. The epithelial lining of the larynx below the true vocal cords is pseudostratified ciliated columnar epithelium.

B. Tracheobronchial tree and lung parenchyma

  1. The tracheobronchial tree functions in ventilation (to and fro movement of air) and is sometimes referred to as the conducting airway.

  2. The lung parenchyma functions in external respiration and is the area of the lung where actual gas exchange occurs.

  3. As the lower airway subdivides, it gives way to more and more airways (generations). Each new generation of airways is assigned a number. The numbering system below begins with assigning generation 0 to the trachea. The first branching or division of the trachea constitutes the mainstem bronchi, which are assigned generation 1. Each subsequent branching of the lower airway is assigned the subsequent generation number.

C. Trachea (generation 0)

  1. The trachea is a cartilaginous, membranous tube 10–13 cm in length and 2–2.5 cm in diameter.

  2. The trachea extends from the cricoid cartilage at the sixth cervical vertebra to its point of bifurcation (carina) at the fifth thoracic vertebra.

  3. Sixteen to twenty incomplete cartilaginous rings open posteriorly and are arranged horizontally. The open ends of the cartilage and the area between individual cartilages are joined by a combination of fibrous, elastic, and smooth muscle tissue.

    a. The smooth muscle is arranged longitudinally to shorten and elongate the trachea.

    b. The smooth muscle also is arranged transversely to constrict and dilate the trachea.

  4. The posterior wall of the trachea is separated from the anterior wall of the esophagus by loose connective tissue.

  5. The trachea and following large airways (bronchi) contain three characteristic layers (Fig 3–8):

    a. Cartilaginous layer.

    b. Lamina propria, which contains small blood vessels, lymphatic vessels, nerve tracts, elastic fibers, smooth muscle, and submucosal glands.

    c. Epithelial, or intraluminal, layer, which is separated from the lamina propria by a noncellular basement membrane.

  6. The epithelial lining of the trachea is continuous with the lar-

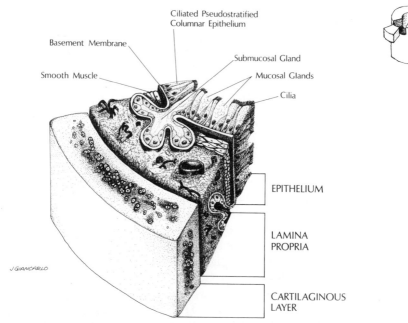

Fig 3–8.—Section of the trachea showing the three layers: epithelium, lamina propria, and cartilaginous layer. (From Shapiro B.A., Harrison R.A., Kacmarek R.M., et al.: *Clinical Application of Respiratory Care,* ed. 3. Chicago, Year Book Medical Publishers, Inc., 1985. Reproduced by permission.)

ynx above and consists of pseudostratified ciliated columnar epithelium (Table 3–2).

   D. Mainstem bronchi (generation 1)
      1. The trachea bifurcates into two airways, the right and left mainstem bronchi, at the carina.
        a. Right mainstem bronchus
          (1) Branches off the trachea at an angle of about 20 to 30 degrees with respect to the midline.
          (2) Diameter: About 1.4 cm.
          (3) Length: About 2.5 cm.
        b. Left mainstem bronchus
          (1) Branches off the trachea at an angle of 40 to 60 degrees with respect to the midline.
          (2) Diameter: About 1.0 cm.
          (3) Length: About 5 cm.
      2. A portion of mainstem bronchi is extrapulmonary (exists outside the lung, in the mediastinum), but the majority of it is intrapulmonary (inside the lung proper).

TABLE 3–2.—ANATOMICAL COMPARISON OF STRUCTURES
IN THE LOWER RESPIRATORY TRACT

STRUCTURE	EPITHELIUM	DIVISION
Larynx/below true cords	Pseudostratified ciliated columnar	X
Trachea	Pseudostratified ciliated columnar	0
Mainstem bronchi	Pseudostratified ciliated columnar	1
Lobar bronchi	Pseudostratified ciliated columnar	2
Segmental bronchi	Pseudostratified ciliated columnar	3
Subsegmental bronchi	Pseudostratified ciliated columnar	4–9
Bronchioles	Pseudostratified ciliated cuboidal	10–15
Terminal bronchioles	Cuboidal to simple squamous	16
Respiratory bronchioles	Simple squamous	17–19
Alveolar ducts	Simple squamous	20–24
Alveolar sacs	Simple squamous	25
Alveoli	Type I; squamous	. . .
	Type II; granular	. . .
	Type III; macrophage	. . .

3. The structural arrangement of the mainstem bronchi is the same as that of the trachea, with C-shaped pieces of cartilage, a lamina propria, and pseudostratified ciliated columnar epithelium.

4. The only structural difference between the mainstem bronchi and the trachea is that the intrapulmonary section of the mainstem bronchi is covered with a sheath of connective tissue, the peribronchiolar connective tissue.

   a. The function of peribronchiolar connective tissue is to encase large nerve, lymphatic, and bronchial blood vessels as they follow the branchings of the subdividing airways.

   b. The peribronchiolar connective tissue continues to follow the branching of the airways until the level of the bronchioles, where it disappears.

5. Mainstem bronchi are sometimes referred to as primary bronchi.

E. Lobar bronchi (generation 2)

1. Five lobar bronchi correspond, respectively, to the five lobes of the lung.

2. The right mainstem bronchus trifurcates into right upper, middle, and lower lobar bronchi.

3. The left mainstem bronchus bifurcates into left upper and lower lobar bronchi.

4. The structural arrangement of lobar bronchi is the same as that of mainstem bronchi.

5. The epithelial lining of lobar bronchi is pseudostratified ciliated columnar epithelium (see Table 3–2).

  6. Lobar bronchi are sometimes referred to as secondary bronchi.
F. Segmental bronchi (generation 3)
  1. There are 18 segmental bronchi, corresponding to the 18 segments of the lung.
  2. The structural arrangement of segmental bronchi is similar to that of lobar and mainstem bronchi except that the C-shaped pieces of cartilage become less regular in shape and volume (see Fig 3–9)
  3. The epithelial lining of segmental bronchi is pseudostratified ciliated columnar epithelium.
  4. Segmental bronchi are sometimes referred to as tertiary bronchi.
G. Subsegmental bronchi (generations 4–9)
  1. The diameter of subsegmental bronchi ranges from 1 mm to 6 mm.
  2. Cartilaginous rings give way to irregularly placed pieces of cartilage circumscribing the airway, the cartilaginous plaques (see Fig 3–9).
  3. By the ninth generation of airways, cartilage is only scantily present.
  4. As volume and regularity of cartilage have decreased from generation 0 to generation 9, so has the number of submucosal glands and goblet cells.
  5. The epithelial lining of subsegmental bronchi is pseudostratified ciliated columnar epithelium.
H. Bronchioles (generations 10–15)
  1. Diameter is characteristically 1 mm.
  2. Cartilage is totally absent (see Fig 3–9).
  3. Peribronchiolar connective tissue is absent, the lamina propria of these airways being directly embedded in surrounding lung parenchyma.
  4. Airway patency is dependent not on the structural rigidity of surrounding cartilage, but on fibrous, elastic, and smooth muscle tissue.
  5. The epithelial lining of bronchioles is pseudostratified ciliated cuboidal epithelium.
    a. This epithelium is functionally the same as pseudostratified ciliated columnar epithelium.
    b. It differs from pseudostratified ciliated columnar epithelium in three ways:
      (1) It is thinner, being constructed of cuboidal cells rather than columnar cells.

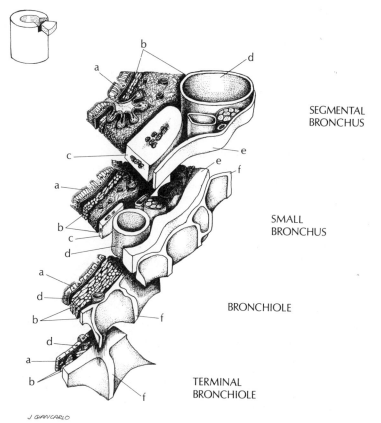

J GIANCARLO

Fig 3–9.—Sections at various levels of the tracheobronchial tree: *a,* pulmonary mucosa; *b,* lamina propria; *c,* cartilage; *d,* blood vessels; *e,* peribronchial connective tissue; *f,* lung parenchyma. (From Shapiro B.A., Harrison R.A., Kacmarek R.M., et al.: *Clinical Application of Respiratory Care,* ed. 3. Chicago, Year Book Medical Publishers, Inc., 1985. Reproduced by permission.)

    (2) The number of goblet cells and submucosal glands gradually decreases, until they are almost nonexistent by generation 15.

    (3) The number of cilia also decreases and cilia are all but gone by the end of generation 15.

I. Terminal bronchioles (generation 16)

  1. Average diameter is 0.5 mm.

  2. Goblet cells and submucosal glands disappear, although mucus is found in these airways (see Fig 3–9).

  3. Cilia are absent from the epithelium of terminal bronchioles.

This epithelium serves as a transition from the cuboidal epithelium of generation 15 to the squamous epithelium of generation 17.

4. Clara cells are located in the terminal bronchioles.
   a. Plump columnar cells that bulge into the lumen of terminal bronchioles.
   b. Probably responsible for mucus and/or surfactant found in terminal bronchioles.
5. Terminal bronchioles mark the end of the conducting airways; all airway generations distal to the terminal bronchioles are considered part of the lung parenchyma.

J. Respiratory bronchioles (generations 17–19) (Fig 3–10)
   1. Average diameter is 0.5 mm.
   2. Alveoli arise from the external surface of the respiratory bronchioles, where a very small portion of external respiration takes place.
   3. The epithelial lining of respiratory bronchioles is a very low cuboidal epithelium interspersed with actual alveoli (simple squamous epithelium).

K. Alveolar ducts (generations 20–24) (see Fig 3–10)
   1. Alveolar ducts arise from respiratory bronchioles.
   2. The only difference between alveolar ducts and respiratory bronchioles is that the walls of the alveolar ducts are totally made up of alveoli.
   3. About one half of the total number of alveoli arise from alveolar ducts.
   4. Alveolar ducts give way to alveolar sacs.

L. Alveolar sacs (generation 25) (see Fig 3–10)
   1. Alveolar sacs are the last generation of airways and are blind passageways.

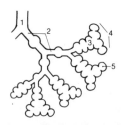

Fig 3–10.—Schematic representation of parenchymal portions of the lung: *1,* terminal bronchiole; *2,* respiratory bronchiole; *3,* alveolar ducts; *4,* alveolar sacs; *5,* alveolus. (From Feneis H.: *Pocket Atlas of Human Anatomy,* ed. 4. New York, Thieme-Stratton, Inc., 1976. Reproduced by permission.)

2. These appear functionally the same as alveolar ducts but differ in that they form grapelike clusters having common walls with other alveoli.

3. The remaining half of alveoli rise from alveolar sacs.

M. Alveoli (Fig 3–11)

1. The alveoli are terminal air spaces that contain numerous capillaries in their septa, which serve as sites for gas exchange.

2. The average number of total alveoli contained in both lungs combined is 300,000,000, but varies directly with the height of the individual and may be as many as 600,000,000.

3. The total cross-sectional area provided by the alveolar surface is about 80 sq m.

4. The total cross-sectional area provided by the pulmonary capillaries is 70 sq m, thus constituting an alveolar gas-pulmonary blood interface of 70 sq m (the size of a tennis court).

N. Alveolar capillary membrane (Fig 3–12)

1. The alveolar capillary membrane has four components: surfactant layer, alveolar epithelium, interstitial space, and capillary endothelium.

a. The surfactant is composed of a phospholipid attached to a lecithin molecule.

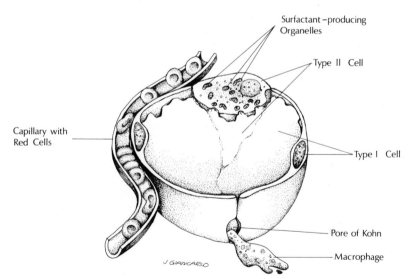

Fig 3–11.—Schematic representation of an alveoli. (From Shapiro B.A., Harrison R.A., Kacmarek R.M., et al.: *Clinical Application of Respiratory Care,* ed. 3. Chicago, Year Book Medical Publishers, Inc., 1985. Reproduced by permission.)

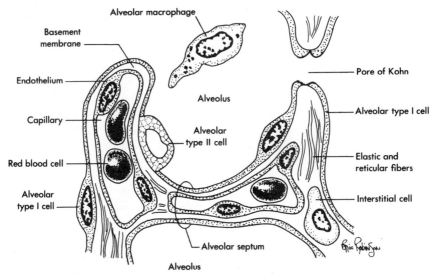

Fig 3–12.—Schematic representation of the alveolar-capillary membrane. (From Dail D.H.: Anatomy of the respiratory system, in Moser K.M., Spragg R.G. (eds.): *Respiratory Emergencies,* ed. 2. St. Louis, C.V. Mosby Co., 1982. Reproduced by permission.)

    (1) Surfactant lines the internal alveolar surface.

    (2) It reduces surface tension, facilitating inspiration and expiration.

  b. Alveolar epithelium (simple squamous epithelium) is a continuous layer of tissue made up of Type I and II cells lying on a basement membrane (see Table 3–2).

    (1) Type I cells, or squamous pneumocytes: Very flat, thin simple squames making up 95% of alveolar surface.

    (2) Type II cells, or granular pneumocytes: Plump, highly metabolic cells credited with surfactant production and alveolar repair.

    (3) Type III cells, or alveolar macrophages: Free, wandering phagocytic cells which ingest foreign material on the alveolar surface.

  c. The interstitial space is the area that separates the basement membrane of alveolar epithelium from the basement membrane of capillary endothelium.

    (1) It contains interstitial fluid.

    (2) This space may be so small, especially where diffusion is to take place, that the basement membranes appear fused.

d. Capillary endothelium is a continuous layer of tissue made up of flat, interlocking squames supported on a basement membrane.

2. Thickness of the alveolar capillary membrane varies from 0.35 μ to 1 μ.

III. The Lung

    A. The lung is situated in the thoracic cavity separated by a structure (mediastinum) containing the heart, great vessels, esophagus, and trachea (Fig 3–13).

        1. Each thoracic cavity is lined with a very fine serous membrane, the parietal pleura, which also covers the dome of each hemi-diaphragm.

        2. The lung and each of its lobes are encased in a similar serous membrane called the visceral pleura.

        3. A potential space (intrapleural space) between the two pleura contains a small amount of fluid called pleural fluid.

           a. Pleural fluid allows cohesion of visceral and parietal pleura.

           b. Pleural fluid allows the two pleura to slide over each other with reduced frictional resistance.

    B. The lung is a conical-shaped organ with four surfaces: apex, base, medial surface, and costal surface (Fig 3–14).

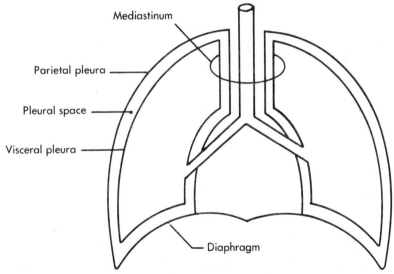

Fig 3–13.—Schematic representation of the lung and thorax. (From Dail D.H.: Anatomy of the respiratory system, in Moser K.M., Spragg R.G. (eds.): *Respiratory Emergencies,* ed. 2. St. Louis, C.V. Mosby Co., 1982. Reproduced by permission.)

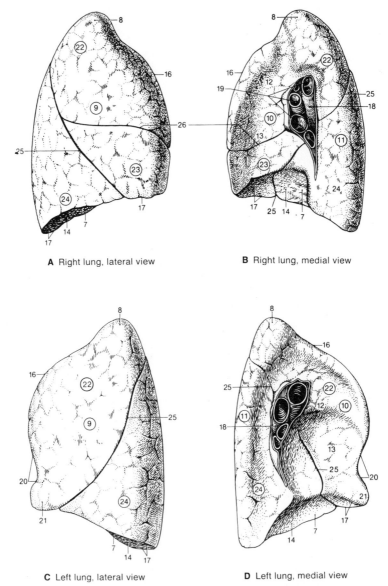

A Right lung, lateral view   **B** Right lung, medial view

C Left lung, lateral view   **D** Left lung, medial view

Fig 3–14.—Lateral and medial view of right and left lungs with fissures and hilar structures depicted. *7,* base of lung; *8,* apex of lung; *9,* costal surface; *10,* medial surface; *13,* cardiac impression; *18,* hilus of lung; *19,* root of lung; *22,* upper lobe; *23,* middle lobe; *24,* lower lobe; *25,* oblique fissure; *26,* horizontal fissure. (From Feneis H.: *Pocket Atlas of Human Anatomy,* ed. 4. New York, Thieme-Straton Inc., 1976. Reproduced by permission.)

1. The apices are rounded superior sections of the lung. They extend 1–2 in. above the clavicles.
2. The bases are concave inferior surfaces of the lung. They rest on the hemidiaphragm. The right base lies higher in the thorax than the left to accommodate the large, underlying liver.
3. The medial surface of each lung exhibits a deep concavity to accept the heart and great vessels. This concavity is called the cardiac impression. The left cardiac impression is deeper than the right because the heart projects to the left of the midline.
4. The costal surface constitutes most of the lung surface in contact with the pleura lining the thoracic cavity.

C. The root of the lung enters the lung proper at the hilum.
1. The root of the lung consists of a mainstem bronchus, a pulmonary artery, two pulmonary veins, major lymph vessels, and nerve tracts.
2. The hilum is the area where the root enters the lung. There the mediastinal and visceral pleura become continuous, forming the pulmonary ligament. This arrangement keeps the pleural cavity sealed and allows the root to enter the sealed lung.

D. The right lung is divided into three lobes by the horizontal and oblique fissures (see Fig 3–14 and Fig 3–15).
1. The oblique fissure isolates the right lower lobe from the right middle and right upper lobe.
2. The horizontal fissure divides the right upper lobe from the right middle lobe.
3. Externally the oblique fissure courses through the following landmarks:
   a. Junction of sixth rib and midclavicular line.
   b. Junction of fifth rib and midaxillary line.
   c. Spinous process of third thoracic vertebra.
4. Externally the horizontal fissure courses through the following landmarks:
   a. Junction of fifth rib and midaxillary line.
   b. Follows the medial course of fourth rib.

E. The left lung is divided into two lobes by the oblique fissure.
1. The oblique fissure divides the left upper lobe from the left lower lobe.
2. Externally the left oblique fissure courses through the same landmarks as does the right oblique fissure.

F. The lobes of the lung are further subdivided into segments (see Fig 3–15).

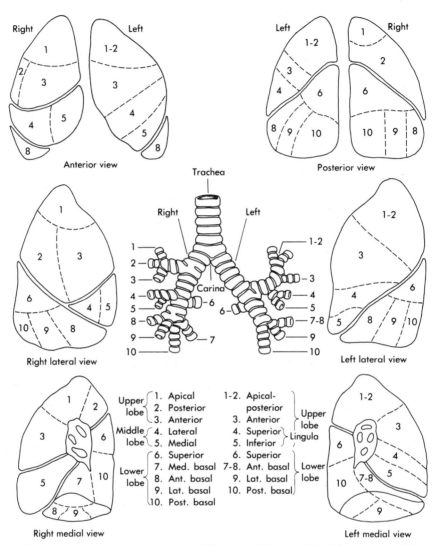

Fig 3–15.—Segmental anatomy of the lung. (From Dail D.H.: Anatomy of the respiratory system, in Moser K.M., Spragg R.G. (eds.): *Respiratory Emergencies,* ed. 2. St. Louis, C.V. Mosby Co., 1982. Reproduced by permission.)

1. Right upper lobe
   a. Anterior segment
   b. Apical segment
   c. Posterior segment
2. Right middle lobe

       a. Lateral segment
       b. Medial segment
    3. Right lower lobe
       a. Superior segment
       b. Anterior basal segment
       c. Lateral basal segment
       d. Medial basal segment
       e. Posterior basal segment
    4. Left upper lobe
       a. Apical-posterior segment
       b. Anterior segment
       c. Superior segment ⎤ Lingula (anatomically corresponds to
       d. Inferior segment ⎦   right middle lobe)
    5. Left lower lobe
       a. Superior segment
       b. Anteromedial basal segment
       c. Lateral basal segment
       d. Posterior basal segment
    6. Knowledge of bronchopulmonary segmentation becomes important when postural drainage, auscultation, x-ray findings, and bronchoscopy are considered.
G. The segments are further subdivided into secondary lobules.
    1. *Secondary lobules* consist of a 15th-order airway (bronchiole) associated with three to five terminal bronchioles and the distal respiratory bronchioles, alveolar ducts, and alveolar sacs.
    2. The secondary lobule is the smallest self-contained unit of the lung that is surrounded by connective tissue.
    3. Secondary lobules appear as polyhedral masses observable on the lung surface and between fissures as dark intersecting lines.
    4. Secondary lobules have their own discrete single pulmonary arteriole, venule, lymphatic, and nerve supply.
    5. Secondary lobules are the building blocks of segments and are discernible on chest x-ray.
    6. Each secondary lobule comprises 30–50 primary lobules and measures 1–2.5 cm in diameter.
       a. Primary lobules consist of a 19th-order respiratory bronchiole and every generation distal to it.
       b. Primary lobules are not self-contained in connective tissue.
       c. There are about 23 million primary lobules in the lung.
    7. Secondary lobules may be important in isolating and maintaining disease entities locally. They also may be responsible for local matching of ventilation to perfusion.

   H. Bronchiolar and alveolar intercommunicating channels.
   1. The canals of Lambert may be important structures implicated in collateral ventilation of bronchioles.
   2. The pores of Kohn are interalveolar pores that allow collateral ventilation of alveoli. Their diameter varies from 3 μ to 13 μ.
IV. Bony Thorax (Fig 3–16)
   A. It is a bony and cartilaginous frame within which lie the principal organs of circulation and respiration.
   B. It is conical, narrow above and broad below.
   C. Posteriorly the thorax includes the 12 thoracic vertebrae and the posterior portion of the ribs.
   D. Laterally the thorax is convex and formed by the ribs.
   E. Anteriorly it is composed of the sternum, anterior ends of the ribs, and the costal cartilage.
   F. The superior opening into the thorax—defined by the manubrium, first rib, and first thoracic vertebra—is called the thoracic inlet or operculum.
   G. The inferior opening out of the thorax—defined by the 12th rib, costal cartilage of ribs 7 through 10, and 12th thoracic vertebra—is called the thoracic outlet.
   H. Functions of the bony thorax are to protect underlying organs, to aid in ventilation, and to provide a point of attachment for various bones and muscles.
   I. Sternum (see Fig 3–16)
   1. The sternum is about 17 cm long.
   2. Divided into three sections
      a. Manubrium: Superior portion
      b. Body: Middle portion
      c. Xiphoid process: Inferior portion
   3. The manubrium articulates with the clavicle and the first and second ribs.
   4. The junction of the manubrium and the body is called the angle of Louis. The trachea bifurcates beneath this junction.
   5. The body of the sternum articulates with ribs 2 through 7.
   6. The xiphoid process articulates with the 7th rib.
   J. Ribs (see Fig 3–16)
   1. Twelve elastic arches of bone, posteriorly connected to vertebral column.
   2. Types of ribs: True, false, and floating.
   3. True ribs
      a. Rib pairs 1 through 7.
      b. Called vertebrosternal ribs because they connect to the

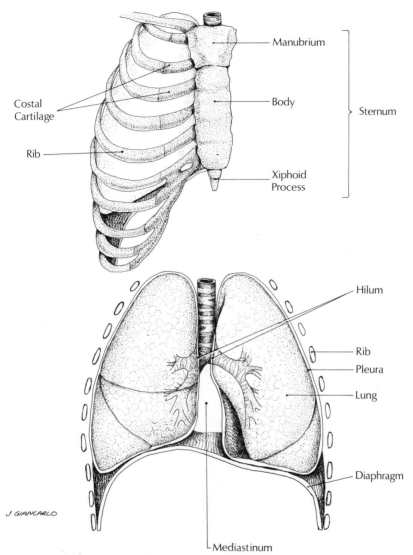

Fig 3–16.—The bony thorax and its relationship to the lung. (From Shapiro B.A., Harrison R.A., Kacmarek R.M., et al.: *Clinical Application of Respiratory Care,* ed. 3. Chicago, Year Book Medical Publishers, Inc., 1985. Reproduced by permission.)

sternum via costal cartilage and the vertebrae of the spinal column.
4. False ribs
   a. Rib pairs 8 through 10.
   b. Called vertebrocostal ribs because they connect to costal cartilage of superior rib and the vertebrae of the spinal column.
5. Floating ribs
   a. Rib pairs 11 and 12.
   b. Have no anterior attachment, lying free in abdominal musculature.
6. The space between the ribs is called the intercostal space.
   a. Wider anteriorly than posteriorly.
   b. Wider superiorly than inferiorly.
7. All 12 pairs of ribs are positioned in an inferior direction. Contraction of the intercostal muscles elevates the ribs from their natural inclined position.
   a. A superoinferior motion of the ribs causes an increase in the transverse diameter of the thorax and is called the bucket handle effect.
   b. An anteroposterior motion of the ribs causes an increase in the anteroposterior diameter of the thorax and is called the pump handle effect.
V. Muscles of Inspiration (Fig 3–17)
   A. The diaphragm and external intercostal muscles are those normally used for resting inspiration.
      1. Diaphragm: Dome-shaped muscle that separates thoracic from abdominal cavity.
         a. It is the major muscle of ventilation.
         b. Origin: Thoracic outlet.
         c. Insertion: Central tendon.
         d. Action: Increases vertical diameter of thorax.
         e. Innervation: Cervical spinal motor nerves 3, 4, and 5 (phrenic nerve).
      2. External intercostals
         a. Origin: Inferior border of superior rib.
         b. Insertion: Superior border of inferior rib.
         c. Action: Elevate ribs, increasing anteroposterior and transverse diameters of thorax (pump and bucket handle effects).
         d. Innervation: Thoracic spinal motor nerves 1 through 11.
         e. Along with internal intercostals, this muscle group prevents the intercostal space from bulging and recessing with normal ventilatory efforts.

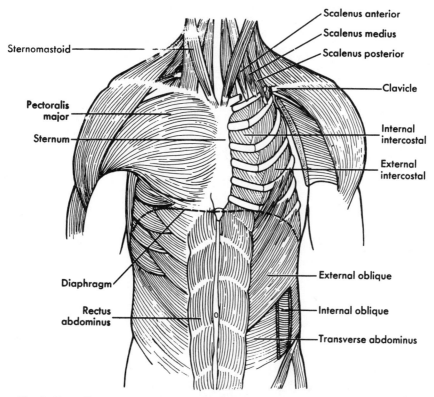

Fig 3–17.—The muscles of ventilation. (From Spearman C.B., Sheldon R.L., Egan D.F.: *Egan's Fundamentals of Respiratory Therapy,* ed. 4. St. Louis, C.V. Mosby Co., 1982. Reproduced by permission.)

    B. Accessory muscles of inspiration
        1. Each tends to perform one of two actions, either raising the thorax or stabilizing the thorax so that other muscles can effectively raise the thorax.
           a. Sternocleidomastoid
           b. Scalenes
               (1) Anterior
               (2) Middle
               (3) Posterior
           c. Pectoralis major
           d. Pectoralis minor
           e. Trapezius
           f. Serratus anterior
           g. Levatores costarum

      h. Serratus posterior

      i. Sacrospinalis

   2. It should be noted that use of accessory muscles for resting inspiration is abnormal and that accessory muscle use should occur only with deep or forced inspiration.

VI. Accessory Muscles of Expiration (see Fig 3–17)

   A. There are no muscles of quiet resting expiration. Expiration is purely a passive process brought about by the normal elastic tendencies of the lung coupled with cessation of inspiratory muscle contraction. Therefore, any muscles used for expiration are termed accessory muscles of expiration.

   B. Any muscle usage for quiet resting expiration is abnormal.

   C. Accessory muscles of expiration are used only for forced expiration, making expiration an active process.

   D. The accessory muscles of expiration are either of the back, thorax, or abdomen and tend either to pull the thorax down or to support the thorax so that other muscle groups can effectively pull down on the thorax.

      1. Latissimus dorsi

      2. Internal intercostals

      3. Rectus abdominis

      4. External oblique

      5. Internal oblique

      6. Transverse abdominis

BIBLIOGRAPHY

Anthony C.P., Kolthoff N.J.: *Textbook of Anatomy and Physiology,* ed. 10. St. Louis: C.V. Mosby Co., 1981.

Comroe J.H.: *Physiology of Respiration,* ed. 2. Chicago, Year Book Medical Publishers, Inc., 1974.

Crowley L.V.: *Introducing Concepts in Anatomy and Physiology.* Chicago, Year Book Medical Publishers, Inc., 1976.

Feneis H.: *Pocket Atlas of Human Anatomy,* ed. 4. Chicago, Year Book Medical Publishers, Inc., 1976.

Fraser R.G., Paré J.A.: *Organ Physiology: Structure and Function of the Lung.* Philadelphia, W.B. Saunders Co., 1977.

Gray H., Goss C.M.: *Gray's Anatomy of the Human Body,* ed. 30. Philadelphia, Lea & Febiger, 1979.

Guyton A.C.: *Textbook of Medical Physiology,* ed. 6. Philadelphia, W.B. Saunders Co., 1981.

Jacob S.W., Francone C.A.: *Structure and Function in Man,* ed. 4. Philadelphia, W.B. Saunders Co., 1979.

McLaughlin A.J.: *Essentials of Physiology for Advanced Respiratory Therapy.* St. Louis, C.V. Mosby Co., 1977.

Murray J.F.: *The Normal Lung.* Philadelphia, W.B. Saunders Co., 1976.

Ruch T.C., Patton H.D.: *Physiology and Biophysics,* ed. 20. Philadelphia, W.B. Saunders Co., 1974.

Shapiro B.A., Harrison R.A., Kacmarek R.M., et al.: *Clinical Application of Respiratory Care,* ed. 3. Chicago, Year Book Medical Publishers, Inc., 1985.

Shibel E.M., Moser K.M.: *Respiratory Emergencies.* St. Louis, C.V. Mosby Co., 1977.

Slonim N.B., Hamilton L.H.: *Respiratory Physiology,* ed. 2. St. Louis, C.V. Mosby Co., 1971.

Spearman C.B., Sheldon R.L., Egan D.F.: *Egan's Fundamentals of Respiratory Therapy,* ed. 4. St. Louis, C.V. Mosby Co., 1982.

4 / Mechanics of Ventilation

I. The Lung-Thorax System
   A. As described in Chapter 3, the lung and the thorax are both lined by thin tissues; the parietal pleura on the inside of the thoracic cage and the visceral pleura on the outside of the lung and mediastinum.
   B. These two pleura are in contact with each other, being separated by only a thin film of fluid.
   C. Since the lungs have a tendency to contract inward and the thorax to expand outward, during normal breathing a negative (subatmospheric) pressure is maintained between the pleura (Fig 4–1).
   D. A convenient way of viewing the lung-thorax system is to consider it as a two-springed system held together by the pleura (Fig 4–2). The thorax can be conceptualized as a band spring tending to expand outward and the lung as a coil spring tending to contract inward.
   E. If the sternum is split, the lung and thorax move to their independent resting positions (see Fig 4–1).
      1. The lung collapses.
      2. The thorax expands.
   F. If air is allowed to enter the potential pleural space, a pneumothorax develops.
   G. Any interference with the integrity of the pleura interferes with ventilation.
II. Inspiration
   A. Figures 4–3 and 4–4 depict the intrapleural (intrathoracic) and intrapulmonary pressure curves during normal resting ventilation.
   B. At functional residual capacity level (FRC) or resting exhalation, the intrapleural pressure is about -5 cm H_2O while the intrapulmonary pressure is zero (atmospheric).
      1. This pressure gradient is commonly referred to as the transpulmonary pressure (TPP) gradient.
      2. The TPP gradient is equal to the alveolar pressure minus the intrapleural pressure.

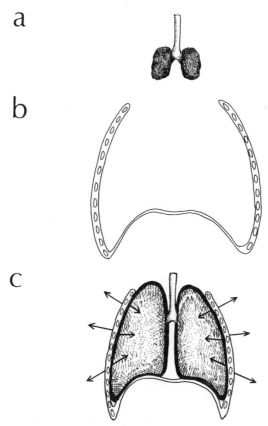

a

b

c

Fig 4–1.—A, resting state of normal lungs when removed from the chest cavity; i.e., elasticity causes total collapse. **B,** resting state of normal chest wall and diaphragm when apex is open to atmosphere and the thoracic contents removed. **C,** end-expiration in the normal, intact thorax. Note that elastic forces of lung and chest wall are in opposite directions. The pleural surfaces link these two opposing forces (see text). (From Shapiro B.A., Harrison R.A., Kacmarek R.M., et al.: *Clinical Application of Respiratory Care,* ed. 3. Chicago, Year Book Medical Publishers, Inc., 1985. Reproduced by permission.)

      3. The TPP is also referred to as the alveolar distending pressure.

  C. Since the lung is a valveless pump, when gas flow stops, intrapulmonary and atmospheric pressures are equal.

  D. In order for inspiration to occur, a pressure gradient with the atmosphere must be established.

      1. Mouth pressure minus alveolar pressure is called transairway pressure.

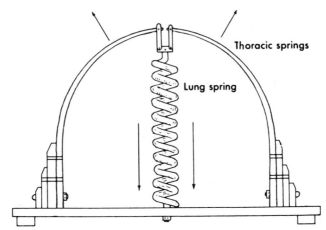

Fig 4–2.—The lung-thorax system may be conceptualized as two springs opposing the movement of each other, the thoracic band spring tending to expand and the lung coil spring tending to contract. (From Spearman C.B., Sheldon R.L., Egan D.L.: *Egan's Fundamentals of Respiratory Therapy,* ed. 4. St. Louis, C.V. Mosby Co., 1982. Reproduced by permission.)

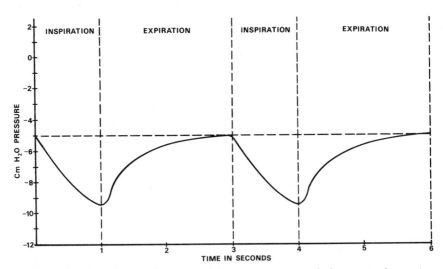

Fig 4–3.—Intrapleural (intrathoracic) pressure curve during normal spontaneous ventilation. Note that normal resting expiratory pressure is about −5 cm H_2O and decreases to −9 cm H_2O during inspiration.

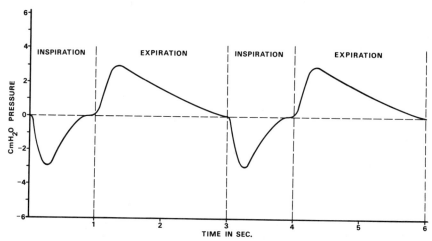

Fig 4–4.—Intrapulmonary pressure during normal spontaneous ventilation has a peak inspiratory pressure of about −3 cm H_2O and peak expiratory pressure of about +3 cm H_2O.

      2. A positive transairway pressure causes gas to enter the lung, while a negative transairway pressure causes exhalation.

  E. This gradient is established by contraction of the diaphragm and the external intercostal muscles.

  F. As a result the thoracic cavity expands, causing the intrapleural pressure to become more negative (about −9 cm H_2O).

  G. This pressure drop increases the volume of the lung. Remember that because of the adherence of the pleura, the lungs must expand as the thorax expands.

  H. The expansion of the lung decreases the intrapulmonary pressure to about −3 cm H_2O.

  I. The decreased intrapulmonary pressure establishes a pressure gradient with the atmosphere, causing gas to enter the lung.

  J. Once the intrapulmonary pressure is returned to normal by gas entering the lung, inspiration stops.

  K. The pressure-volume changes described are all explained by Boyle's law.

III. Exhalation

  A. Exhalation is normally a passive process. The lung-thorax system is returned to its resting state as a result of the elastic recoil of the lung.

  B. Relaxation of the muscles of inspiration allows the intrapleural pressure to return to baseline (−5 cm H_2O); as a result, the intrapulmonary pressure increases to about +3 cm H_2O.

    C. Since the transairway pressure is negative, gas leaves the lung.

    D. Lung volume returns to FRC and transairway pressure returns to zero.

IV. Resistance to Ventilation

    A. Ventilation is opposed by two major factors:

      1. Elastic resistance

      2. Nonelastic resistance

    B. Elastic resistance is a result of distention of pulmonary elastic tissue. The subdivisions of elastic resistance are:

      1. Surface tension

      2. Compliance

    C. Nonelastic resistance is primarily the resistance to gas flow. It is equivalent to the frictional resistance of solids moving across each other. The subdivisions of nonelastic resistance are:

      1. Airway resistance

      2. Tissue viscous resistance

V. Surface Tension

    A. The force occurring at the interface between a liquid and another liquid or a gas that tends to cause the liquid to occupy the smallest volume possible (see Chap. 2).

    B. Surface tension causes alveoli to decrease in size and would cause collapse were it not for the presence of a pulmonary surfactant secreted by Type II alveolar cells.

    C. The volume of surfactant produced by the respiratory tract is relatively constant. The effect the surfactant exerts is indirectly related to the surface area it covers.

    D. At FRC there is a large amount of surfactant applied per unit area. This causes a significant reduction in pressure as a result of surface tension, with the following results:

      1. Prevention of alveolar collapse on exhalation (preventing alveoli from reaching their critical volume).

      2. Reduction in pressure needed to overcome surface tension as inspiration begins.

    E. At maximum inspiration a small volume of surfactant is applied per unit area. Thus, the pressure as a result of surface tension tending to collapse the alveoli is great. This pressure assists in normal passive exhalation.

    F. Pressures as a result of surface tension:

      1. At maximal inspiration: About 40 dynes/sq cm.

      2. At maximal exhalation: About 2–4 dynes/sq cm.

    G. The effect of surface tension cannot be evaluated directly. Changes in surface tension cause a change in compliance.

H. An increase in surface tension increases elastic resistance to ventilation and is reflected in a decrease in compliance, causing an increase in the work of breathing.

VI. Compliance

A. Compliance is the ease of distention of the lung-thorax system and is inversely related to elastance (see Chap. 2).

B. Compliance is normally a static measurement so as to eliminate the effects of nonelastic resistance.

C. Compliance is determined by comparing the change in volume in a system with the pressure necessary to maintain the volume change:

$$C = \frac{\Delta V}{\Delta P} \tag{1}$$

D. In the respiratory system, there are basically three types of compliance:

1. Pulmonary (C_{pul})
2. Thoracic (C_{th})
3. Total (C_{tol})

E. In the lung-thorax system, the tendency of the lung is to collapse to its resting position, whereas the tendency of the thorax is to expand to its resting position.

F. The FRC is that volume maintained in the lung at resting expiratory position as a result of the opposing effects of pulmonary and thoracic compliance.

G. Total compliance of the lung-thorax system is a result of the interaction of pulmonary and thoracic compliance.

H. Compliance is linear only at normal tidal exchange. As the lung volume exceeds or falls below tidal levels, compliance decreases. Thus, the total compliance curve is significantly distorted as lung volume approaches residual volume (RV) or total lung capacity (TLC) (Fig 4–5).

1. As lung volume approaches TLC, the tendency of the lung to collapse far outweighs the tendency of the thorax to expand. Specifically, the thorax reaches its resting position at 70% of TLC. Beyond this level the thorax tends to collapse. Since the lung has been distorted significantly beyond its resting position, continued pulmonary expansion requires significant force. At TLC the organism cannot exert sufficient force to continue expansion (Fig 4–6).

2. As the lung volume approaches RV, the tendency of the thorax to expand far outweighs the tendency of the lung to

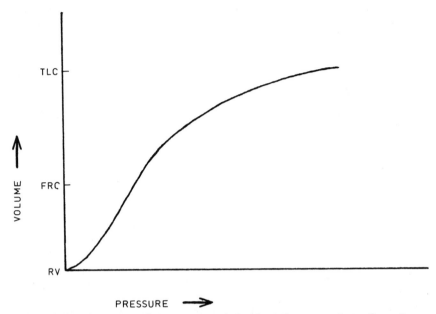

Fig 4–5.—Total compliance curve of the lung-thorax system. Compliance changes linearly about the functional residual capacity *(FRC)*. However, as lung volume nears either residual volume *(RV)* or total lung capacity, *(TLC)*, the pressure needed to cause a volume change increases.

collapse. This occurs because the lung is now near its resting point, whereas the thorax is significantly distorted from its resting point. At RV, the tendency of the thorax to expand is so great that the individual cannot voluntarily exhale a larger volume (see Fig 4–6).

I. Total compliance is determined by dividing the tidal volume (TV) by the static pressure necessary to maintain TV in the lung. *Pressure should be measured at the patient's mouth.* In the average young adult male, total compliance is equal to 0.1 L/cm H_2O.

J. Pulmonary compliance is determined by dividing TV by the static pressure necessary to maintain TV in the lung. *The pressure measured should reflect changes in intrapleural pressures.* A pressure reading taken at the level of the midesophagus reflects pleural pressure changes (the patient swallows a pressure transducer and its level is adjusted to a midesophageal position). In the average young adult male, pulmonary compliance is equal to 0.2 L/cm H_2O.

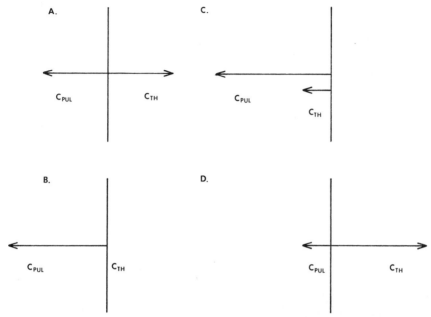

Fig 4–6.—Pulmonary *(C_{pul})* and thoracic *(C_{th})* compliance (elastance) vector forces compared at different lung volumes. **A,** at FRC, the vector forces of C_{pul} and C_{th} are equal and opposite in direction. **B,** at 70% of TLC, the thorax is at its resting position, and C_{pul} tends to cause lung volume to decrease. **C,** at TLC, the vector forces of both C_{pul} and C_{th} tend to decrease lung volume. **D,** at RV, the lung is near its resting level; therefore its vector is decreased, while the vector force of the thorax tends to expand the system.

    K. Thoracic compliance is a calculated value based on the following equation:

$$\frac{1}{C_{total}} = \frac{1}{C_{pulmonary}} + \frac{1}{C_{thoracic}} \tag{2}$$

In the average young adult male, thoracic compliance is equal to 0.2 L/cm H_2O.

    L. Changes in total compliance reflect total elastic resistance to ventilation.

      1. Total compliance reflects surface tension and tissue elastance.

      2. A decrease in total compliance results in a decrease in FRC.

      3. An increase in total compliance results in an increase in FRC.

      4. Alterations in C_{pul} or C_{th} result in an alteration of total compliance.

M. With an increase in total compliance, there is a corresponding decrease in elastance. This tends to increase the ease of inspiration but also increases the difficulty of expiration. In this situation a slow, deep ventilatory pattern may be assumed to minimize the work of breathing (see Chap. 18).

N. With a decrease in total compliance, there is a corresponding increase in elastance. This tends to decrease the ease of inspiration but increases the ease of exhalation. In this situation a rapid, shallow ventilatory pattern may be assumed to minimize the work of breathing (see Chap. 18).

O. Total compliance is decreased by any pathophysiologic change that inhibits lung expansion:
   1. Pneumonitis
   2. Pulmonary consolidation
   3. Pulmonary edema
   4. Pneumothorax
   5. Abdominal distention
   6. Adult respiratory distress syndrome (ARDS)
   7. Pulmonary fibrosis
   8. Thoracic deformities
   9. Complete airway obstruction

P. Total compliance may be increased by any factor that causes a loss of elastic lung tissue.
   1. Alveolar septal destruction
   2. Alveolar distention

Q. *Specific compliance* is a method of comparing the compliance of individuals of different sizes.
   1. The formula for its determination takes into consideration the patient's measured FRC.
   2. Specific compliance (C_s) is equal to pulmonary compliance divided by the patient's FRC and normally is equal to about 0.08 (dimensionless number):

$$C_s = \frac{C_{pul}}{FRC} = 0.08 \qquad (3)$$

   3. C_s can be determined for a lung segment or lobe (Fig 4–7).

VII. Airway Resistance

A. Airway resistance results from the movement of molecules of inspired gas over the surface of the airway.

B. It accounts for about 85% of nonelastic resistance to ventilation.

C. Airway resistance in laminar flow situations is equal to:

$$R = \frac{\Delta P}{\dot{V}} \qquad (3)$$

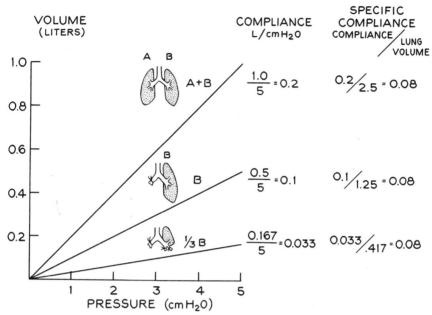

Fig 4–7.—Compliance and specific compliance for both lungs, one lung, and one lobe. Compliance decreases with decreasing lung volume; specific compliance does not. (From Comroe J.R.: *Physiology of Respiration.* Chicago, Year Book Medical Publishers, Inc., 1965. Reproduced by permission.)

whereas in turbulent flow situations the relationship is:

$$R = \frac{\Delta P}{\dot{V}^2} \tag{4}$$

D. More than 60% of normal airway resistance is a result of turbulent gas flow through the nose, pharynx, and larynx.

E. Resistance to gas flow decreases as gas moves into smaller generations of the airway. Since the cross-sectional area of the respiratory tract increases dramatically with increasing generations, flow through any single airway becomes progressively smaller. The pressure necessary to maintain that flow decreases as does total airway resistance.

F. At the level of the respiratory bronchioles, flow is almost absent and gas movement basically is a result of diffusion.

G. Airway resistance is increased when the lumen of the airway is decreased. The airway lumen is primarily decreased as a result of:

1. Bronchospasm

      2. Mucosal edema

      3. Partial airway obstruction (retained secretions)

    H. Normal airway resistance is equal to about 0.6–2.4 cm $H_2O/L/$ second when measured at a standard flow rate of 0.5 L/second.

VIII. Tissue Viscous Resistance

    A. The force necessary to overcome the inertia of the nonelastic structures of the lung-thorax system (i.e., bone, pleurae sliding over each other).

    B. Accounts for about 15% of the nonelastic resistance to ventilation.

IX. Functional Residual Capacity

    A. As stated previously, the thorax tends to expand, whereas the lung tends to collapse. At the FRC level the vector forces of pulmonary and thoracic elastance are equal in magnitude and opposite in direction.

    B. The FRC is the most stable of all lung volumes and capacities because it is the level that is assumed when complete relaxation of ventilatory muscles occurs.

    C. If elastance of thorax and/or lung were to increase or decrease, the volume of FRC would be altered.

X. Ventilation/Perfusion Relationships

    A. Distribution of ventilation is unequal because of:

      1. Variation in compliance and airway resistance within the lung.

        a. If the compliance of part of the lung is multiplied by resistance of that part of the lung, a time constant is determined:

$$\text{Compliance} \times \text{resistance} = \text{time constant} \quad (5)$$

        b. The time constant of a lung unit determines the amount of time it takes for that unit to fill.

      2. Regional variation in transpulmonary pressure throughout the respiratory tract.

        a. In the vertical position, the TPP gradient is greater in the apices than in the bases. The reasons for this variation are:

        (1) Weight of the lung.

        (2) Effect of gravity on the total system, forcing blood flow to dependent areas.

        (3) Support of lung at the hilum.

        b. Transpulmonary pressure differences cause alveoli in the apices to contain a greater volume at FRC level than alveoli in the bases.

      c. Differences in alveolar size decrease as inspiration nears TLC.
3. The results of differing pulmonary time constants and TPP gradients on ventilation from FRC level.
      a. Alveoli in the apices fill slowly and empty slowly (slow alveoli).
      b. Alveoli in the bases fill rapidly and empty rapidly (fast alveoli).
      c. In normal tidal exchange most of the ventilation goes to the bases. Figure 4–8 illustrates the compliance curve of the total lung. The position of the apices on the curve during tidal exchange is on the flatter aspect of the curve, whereas the bases are positioned on the steeper aspect of the curve. Points B to B' indicate the volume change during normal ventilation in the bases; points A to A' indicate the volume change during normal ventilation of the apices. There is a considerably larger volume change in the bases than in the apices per unit pressure change.
B. Distribution of pulmonary blood flow normally is greater in the bases than in the apices.

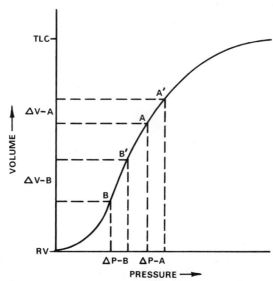

Fig 4–8.—Compliance curve of total lung at functional residual capacity (FRC). *A to A'* indicates volume change in the apices during tidal exchange; *B to B'* indicates volume change in the bases during tidal exchange. The change in volume of B *(ΔV-B)* is greater than the change in volume of A *(ΔV-A)* for the same pressure change *(ΔP-B is equal to P-A).*

1. Perfusion of any aspect of the lung depends on the relationship between pulmonary hydrostatic pressure and the TPP gradient.
2. Since the pulmonary vascular system is a low-pressure system, in the erect individual the apices of the lung receive virtually no blood flow, whereas the bases are engorged with blood because of the effect of gravity.
3. In general, the most gravity-dependent aspect of the lung receives the majority of the blood flow, whereas the least gravity-dependent areas receive little or no blood flow.
4. Basically, in the upright lung, three zones exist (Fig 4–9).
   a. Zone 1: The extreme apex, where there is virtually no blood flow.
   b. Zone 2: The remainder of the apex and middle part of the lung, where blood flow is intermittent.
   c. Zone 3: The bases, where blood flow is constant.
C. Ventilation/perfusion ratios ($\dot{V}/\dot{Q}$ ratios).
   1. The overall $\dot{V}/\dot{Q}$ ratio for the lung is 0.8.
   2. In the apices the $\dot{V}/\dot{Q}$ ratio is about 3.3, in the bases about 0.6.
   3. During normal ventilation and perfusion:
      a. Bases are better perfused than apices.
      b. Bases are better ventilated than apices.
      c. Apices are better ventilated than perfused.
      d. Bases are better perfused than ventilated.
XI. Ideal Alveolar Gas Equation
   A. In addition to the effects of P_{H_2O} on the partial pressure of gases in the alveoli, the carbon dioxide diffusing from the bloodstream into the alveoli will further decrease alveolar P_{O_2}.
   B. Since carbon dioxide is leaving the bloodstream, a closed system, and entering the respiratory tract, an open system, there is an indirect relationship between the alveolar pressures of carbon dioxide and oxygen. Increases in $P_{A_{CO_2}}$ result in decreases in $P_{A_{O_2}}$.
   C. This indirect relationship basically involves only carbon dioxide and oxygen because they are the only metabolically active gases.
   D. In addition, the amount of oxygen and carbon dioxide moving across the alveolar capillary membrane is unequal, 200 ml of carbon dioxide being produced for every 250 ml of oxygen consumed. Thus, the respiratory exchange ratio (R) must be considered when estimating the alveolar P_{O_2}.

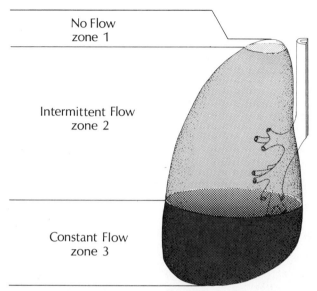

Fig 4–9.—The three-zone pulmonary blood flow model illustrating the effects of gravity on pulmonary perfusion (see text). (From Shapiro B.A., Harrison R.A., Kacmarek R.M., et al.: *Clinical Application of Respiratory Care,* ed. 3. Chicago, Year Book Medical Publishers, Inc., 1985. Reproduced by permission.)

E. The ideal alveolar gas equation is:

$$P_{A_{O_2}} = (P_B - P_{H_2O})(F_{I_{O_2}}) - (Pa_{CO_2})\left(F_{I_{O_2}} + \frac{1 - F_{I_{O_2}}}{R}\right) \quad (6)$$

R normally equals 0.8. Pa_{CO_2} is used instead of $P_{A_{CO_2}}$ because under physiologic conditions compatible with life these are equal, and $P_{A_{CO_2}}$ is impossible to determine clinically.

F. A modification of the above equation may be used for gross estimations of $P_{A_{O_2}}$:

$$P_{A_{O_2}} = (P_B - P_{H_2O})(F_{I_{O_2}}) - \frac{Pa_{CO_2}}{0.8} \quad (7)$$

BIBLIOGRAPHY
Bendixen H.H., et al.: *Respiratory Care.* St. Louis, C.V. Mosby Co., 1965.
Burton G.C., Hodgkin J.E.: *Respiratory Care,* ed. 2. Philadelphia, J.B. Lippincott Co., 1984.
Cherniack R.M., Cherniack L.: *Respiration in Health and Disease,* ed. 3. Philadelphia, W.B. Saunders Co., 1983.

Comroe J.H.: *Phy.   gy of Respiration,* ed. 2. Chicago, Year Book Medical Publishers, Inc., 1974.

Dejours P.: *Respiration.* New York, Oxford University Press, 1966.

Frownfelter D.L.: *Chest Physical Therapy and Pulmonary Rehabilitation.* Chicago, Year Book Medical Publishers, 1979.

Guyton A.C.: *Textbook of Medical Physiology,* ed. 6. Philadelphia, W.B. Saunders Co., 1980.

Hedley-Whyte J., Burgess G.E., Feeley T.W., et al.: *Applied Physiology of Respiratory Care.* Boston, Little, Brown & Co., 1976.

McLaughlin A.J.: *Essentials of Physiology for Advanced Respiratory Therapy.* St. Louis, C.V. Mosby Co., 1977.

Murray J.F.: *The Normal Lung.* Philadelphia, W.B. Saunders Co., 1976.

Nunn J.F.: *Applied Respiratory Physiology With Special Reference to Anaesthesia,* ed. 2. London, Butterworth & Co., Ltd., 1977.

Petty T.L.: *Intensive and Rehabilitative Respiratory Care,* ed. 3. Philadelphia, Lea & Febiger, 1982.

Shapiro B.A., Harrison R.A., Kacmarek R.M., et al.: *Clinical Application of Respiratory Care,* ed. 3. Chicago, Year Book Medical Publishers, Inc., 1985.

Spearman C.B., Sheldon R.L., Egan D.F.: *Egan's Fundamentals of Respiratory Therapy,* ed. 4. St. Louis, C.V. Mosby Co., 1982.

Tisi G.M.: *Pulmonary Physiology in Clinical Medicine,* ed. 2. Baltimore, Williams & Wilkins Co., 1983.

West J.B.: *Respiratory Physiology: The Essentials,* ed. 2. Baltimore, Williams & Wilkins Co., 1979.

West J.B.: *Ventilation/Blood Flow and Gas Exchange,* ed. 3. Oxford, Blackwell Scientific Publications, 1977.

Whitcomb M.E.: *The Lung Normal and Diseased.* St. Louis, C.V. Mosby Co., 1982.

5 / Neurologic Control of Ventilation

I. The following areas located throughout the organism each play specific roles in the neurologic control of ventilation:
   A. Medulla oblongata
   B. Cerebral cortex
   C. Pons
   D. Upper airway reflexes
   E. Vagus (cranial X) nerve
   F. Glossopharyngeal (cranial IX) nerve
   G. Peripheral chemoreceptors
   H. Central chemoreceptors
II. Medulla Oblongata
   A. Located within the medulla oblongata is the respiratory control center, which receives afferent impulses from all other areas in the organism (Fig 5–1).
   B. Afferent impulses are interpreted and efferent impulses are initiated in the medulla oblongata.
   C. The medullary respiratory center maintains the normal rhythmic pattern of ventilation.
   D. Two fairly distinct areas in the medulla contain respiratory neurons.
      1. Dorsal respiratory group
         a. Functions as initial processing center of afferent impulses.
         b. Originates inspiratory efferent impulses, which travel to ventral respiratory neurons and spinal cord.
      2. Ventral respiratory group
         a. Functions primarily by sending efferent impulses to all expiratory motor neurons.
         b. Originates some inspiratory efferent impulses.
   E. Areas from which afferent impulses are sent to the medulla oblongata:
      1. Cerebral cortex
      2. Pons
      3. Upper airway reflexes
      4. Vagus (cranial X) nerve
      5. Peripheral chemoreceptors

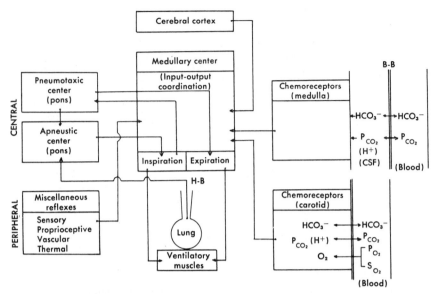

Fig 5–1.—Interrelationships among all areas responsible for ventilatory control (see text). (From Spearman C.B., Sheldon R.L., Egan D.F.: *Egan's Fundamentals of Respiratory Therapy,* ed. 4. St. Louis, C.V. Mosby Co., 1982. Reproduced by permission.)

      6. Glossopharyngeal (cranial IX) nerve

      7. Peripheral chemoreceptors

      8. Central chemoreceptors

III. Cerebral Cortex

    A. Initiates all conscious respiratory control.

    B. Mediates ventilatory changes as a result of pain, anxiety, or other emotional stimuli.

    C. Governs ventilatory control during speech.

IV. Pons

    A. Two distinct centers in the pons contain afferent respiratory neurons.

      1. Pneumotaxic center

        a. Located in upper pons.

        b. Afferent impulses from pneumotaxic center "fine tune" ventilatory rhythmicity by inhibiting length of inspiration.

        c. However, rhythmic ventilation may exist even when the pneumotaxic center is impaired.

        d. If the pneumotaxic center is destroyed, apneustic ventilation (long, sustained inspirations) occurs.

2. Apneustic center
   a. Located in lower pons.
   b. Afferent impulses from apneustic center cause a sustained inspiratory pattern.
   c. However, normal rhythmic ventilation can exist without the apneustic center.
   d. If the apneustic and pneumotaxic centers are destroyed, a rapid, irregular, gasping respiratory pattern develops.

V. Upper Airway Reflexes
   A. Nose
      1. Stimulation of nasal mucosa may cause exhalation.
      2. Exhalation is frequently in the form of a sneeze.
      3. Apnea and bradycardia also may result from nasal stimulation.
   B. Nasopharynx
      1. Stimulation may cause the sniff or aspiration reflex.
      2. A rapid inspiration is initiated to move the irritant from nasopharynx to oropharynx.
      3. Stimulation may also cause bronchodilation and hypertension.
   C. Larynx
      1. Stimulation may result in afferent impulses, causing:
         a. Apnea
         b. Slow, deep breathing
         c. Coughing
         d. Hypertension
         e. Bronchoconstriction
   D. Trachea
      1. Stimulation may result in afferent impulses, causing:
         a. Coughing
         b. Bronchoconstriction
         c. Hypertension

VI. Vagus Nerve
   A. Afferent impulses via the vagus nerve originate from two areas.
      1. Baroreceptors
         a. Located in the aortic arch.
         b. Stimulated by variations in blood pressure.
         c. Afferent impulses from baroreceptors cause alteration of vascular tone in order to maintain normal blood pressure levels.
         d. Ventilatory response is minimal.
            (1) Hyperventilation may be caused by hypotension.
            (2) Hypoventilation may be caused by hypertension.
      2. Pulmonary reflexes

        a. Pulmonary stretch receptors (Hering-Breuer reflex)
            (1) Located in the smooth muscle of conducting airways.
            (2) These receptors are stimulated by lung inflation, deflation, and increased transpulmonary pressures.
            (3) They are slowly adaptive to changes in inflating pressure.
            (4) Stimulation of these receptors may cause:
                (a) Termination of inspiration or expiration
                (b) Bronchodilation
                (c) Tachycardia
                (d) Decreased peripheral vascular resistance
        b. Irritant receptors
            (1) Located in the epithelium of trachea, bronchi, larynx, nose, and pharynx.
            (2) They are rapidly adaptive.
            (3) Stimulation is caused by:
                (a) Inspired irritants
                (b) Mechanical factors
                (c) Anaphylaxis
                (d) Pneumothorax
                (e) Pulmonary congestion
            (4) Stimulation of these receptors may result in:
                (a) Bronchoconstriction
                (b) Hyperpnea
                (c) Constriction of larynx (laryngospasm)
                (d) Closure of glottis
                (e) Cough
        c. Type J (juxtapulmonary-capillary) receptors
            (1) Located in the walls of alveoli
            (2) Stimulation is caused by:
                (a) Increased interstitial fluid volume
                (b) Chemical irritants
                (c) Microembolism
            (3) Stimulation of these receptors may result in:
                (a) Rapid, shallow breathing
                (b) Severe expiratory constriction of larynx
                (c) Hypoventilation and bradycardia
                (d) Inhibition of spinal reflexes
VII. Glossopharyngeal Nerve
     A. Innervates the peripheral chemoreceptor cells located in the carotid bodies.
     B. Conducts afferent impulses to the medullary respiratory center.

VIII. Peripheral Chemoreceptors
   A. Chemoreceptor cells can differentiate between concentrations or pressures of various substances.
   B. Two groups of peripheral chemoreceptor cells have been identified.
      1. *Carotid bodies*
         a. Located at the bifurcation of the common carotid artery.
         b. Innervated by the glossopharyngeal (cranial IX) nerve.
         c. Primarily respond to hypoxemia.
      2. *Aortic bodies*
         a. Located in the arch of the aorta.
         b. Innervated by the vagus (cranial X) nerve.
         c. Play a minor role in regulating ventilation.
   B. Peripheral chemoreceptors are stimulated by:
      1. Decreased Pa_{O_2}.
      2. Changes in arterial pH.
      3. A synergistic response occurs if hypoxemia and acidosis are both present.
   C. Effects of Pa_{O_2}:
      1. Initial stimulation occurs at a Pa_{O_2} of 500 mm Hg and gradually increases as Pa_{O_2} decreases.
      2. Maximum stimulation occurs when Pa_{O_2} is between 40 and 60 mm Hg.
      3. A gradual decrease in stimulation is noted when Pa_{O_2} is less than 30 mm Hg.
      4. Additional sources of stimulation:
         a. Decreased blood flow
         b. Increased temperature
      5. These cells are primarily affected by oxygen delivery in the form of dissolved oxygen. Any pathophysiologic situation in which oxygen delivery is inadequate for the metabolic needs of these cells results in stimulation.
      6. Conditions having no stimulating effect:
         a. Carbon monoxide poisoning
         b. Anemia
   D. Effects of Pa_{CO_2} and H^+ concentrations
      1. The cell membrane is permeable to both H^+ and Pa_{CO_2}.
      2. These cells are directly affected only by H^+ concentrations.
      3. Pa_{CO_2} changes cause a change in H^+ concentration, which may stimulate the receptor.
      4. Thus, Pa_{CO_2} has an indirect effect on these cells.
      5. Stimulation is primarily a result of an increase in H^+ concentration.

      6. Decreases in H^+ concentration have only a minimal effect.
      7. Stimulation of these receptors by an increase in $[H^+]$ causes:
         a. Increased respiratory rate
         b. Increased tidal volume
      8. Stimulation of these receptors by a decrease in $[H^+]$ may cause:
         a. Decreased respiratory rate
         b. Decreased tidal volume
      9. The magnitude of the response of the peripheral chemoreceptors to $[H^+]$ changes is grossly less than that of the central chemoreceptors.
    E. These receptors are adaptive over time.
IX. Central Chemoreceptors
    A. A poorly defined group of cells located near the ventrolateral surface of the medulla oblongata.
    B. These cells are in contact with cerebral spinal fluid (CSF) and arterial blood.
    C. Actual stimulation is caused by $[H^+]$ of CSF.
    D. The composition of the CSF differs somewhat from that of blood.
      1. Electrolytes similar in content to those in plasma
      2. Low protein content: 15–45 mg/100 ml
      3. P_{CO_2}: 50.2 ± 2.6 mm Hg
      4. pH: 7.336 ± 0.012
      5. HCO_3^-: 21.5 ± 1.2 mEq/L
    E. Diffusion across blood-brain barrier
      1. The only readily diffusible substance is carbon dioxide.
      2. HCO_3^- and H^+ also move across the membrane, but extremely slowly. Active transport mechanisms and diffusion are believed to be involved in the movement of these two substances.
    F. Mechanism of stimulation
      1. Changes in arterial P_{CO_2} alter diffusion of carbon dioxide across the blood-brain barrier, causing a change in P_{CO_2} of the CSF.
      2. The altered P_{CO_2} level will effect a change in CSF $[H^+]$.
      3. The altered $[H^+]$ either stimulates or inhibits ventilation.
      4. Increased P_{CO_2} (increased H^+) stimulates ventilation, while decreased P_{CO_2} (decreased H^+) inhibits ventilation.
    G. Factors influencing CSF carbon dioxide levels
      1. Cerebral blood flow
      2. CO_2 production
      3. CO_2 content of venous blood

       4. CO_2 content of arterial blood

       5. Alveolar ventilation

  X. Efferent Impulses From the Medulla Oblongata

     A. All efferent impulses are directed via the spinal cord to the various muscles of ventilation.

     B. Skeletal muscle is composed of two types of contractile fibers.

       1. Extrafusal fibers (main muscle): Contraction of these fibers is responsible for actual muscular contraction.

       2. Fusimotor fibers (muscle spindle fibers): These fibers are organs of proprioception that determine the extent of muscle contraction necessary to perform a certain workload.

  XI. Medullary Adjustments in Compensated Respiratory Acidosis

     A. Acute increases in Pa_{CO_2} rapidly cause an increase in CSF P_{CO_2}. This occurs because the blood-CSF barrier is very permeable to CO_2.

     B. The increased P_{CO_2} in the CSF causes the CSF pH to decrease, which stimulates the central chemoreceptors.

     C. If the organism is unable to increase its level of ventilation, the elevated Pa_{CO_2} and CSF P_{CO_2} levels persist.

     D. As a result, the kidney will begin to retain HCO_3^-.

     E. As the serum HCO_3^- level increases, active transport mechanisms and diffusion increase the CSF HCO_3^- level.

     F. The CSF pH eventually returns to normal as the CSF HCO_3^- level increases.

     G. When the CSF pH is returned to normal, the organism responds to changes in Pa_{CO_2} at the new elevated level.

     H. Chronically elevated Pa_{CO_2} and CSF P_{CO_2} levels result in:

       1. Decreased central chemoreceptor drive to ventilate.

       2. Decreased sensitivity to CO_2 changes.

     I. Because of the decreased sensitivity to CO_2, the organism frequently functions on a hypoxic drive (see Chap. 19).

 XII. Medullary Adjustments in Compensated Respiratory Alkalosis

     A. Acute decreases in Pa_{CO_2} rapidly cause a decrease in CSF P_{CO_2}.

     B. This causes the CSF pH to increase, which inhibits the central chemoreceptors.

     C. If the stimulus causing hyperventilation persists, the decreased Pa_{CO_2} and CSF P_{CO_2} levels also persist.

     D. As a result, the kidney will begin to excrete more HCO_3^-.

     E. As the serum HCO_3^- level decreases, active transport mechanisms and diffusion decrease the CSF HCO_3^- level.

     F. The CSF pH eventually returns to normal as the CSF HCO_3^- decreases.

      G. When the CSF pH is returned to normal, the organism responds to changes in Pa_{CO_2} at the new decreased level.

XIII. Medullary Adjustments in Compensated Metabolic Acidosis

      A. Since H^+ does not readily cross the blood-brain barrier, decreases in plasma pH stimulate the peripheral chemoreceptors.

      B. This is interpreted as a rise in Pa_{CO_2}: thus the peripheral chemoreceptors increase the level of ventilation, decreasing Pa_{CO_2}.

      C. The decreased Pa_{CO_2} decreases the CSF P_{CO_2}, which increases the CSF pH, resulting in inhibition to ventilation via the central chemoreceptors.

      D. As a result, the peripheral chemoreceptors stimulate ventilation while the central chemoreceptors inhibit ventilation.

      E. Since the effect on the peripheral chemoreceptors is the predominant stimulus, there is a stepwise readjustment (decrease) in CSF HCO_3^- levels. This allows normalization of CSF pH and a sustained increase in the drive to ventilate.

      F. The maximum response of the respiratory system to a metabolic acidosis does not occur until the CSF pH is normalized.

XIV. Medullary Adjustments in Compensated Metabolic Alkalosis

      A. Since neither H^+ or HCO_3^- readily cross the blood-brain barrier and the peripheral chemoreceptors respond poorly to alkalosis, the respiratory system's response to a metabolic alkalosis is poor unless the alkalosis is significant.

      B. A significant increase in plasma pH causes inhibition of the peripheral chemoreceptors, which inhibits ventilation, resulting in increased Pa_{CO_2}.

      C. The increased Pa_{CO_2} increases the CSF P_{CO_2}, which stimulates ventilation via the central chemoreceptors.

      D. As a result, the peripheral chemoreceptors inhibit ventilation, while the central chemoreceptors stimulate ventilation.

      E. Since inhibition of the peripheral chemoreceptors is the predominant stimulus, there is a stepwise readjustment (increase) in the CSF HCO_3^-. This allows a normalization of the CSF pH and a sustained decrease in the drive to ventilate.

      F. It is rare that the Pa_{CO_2} rises above 50 mm Hg unless the metabolic alkalosis is severe. Remember, if the Pa_{CO_2} increases the alveolar P_{O_2} decreases, possibly resulting in hypoxemia, which stimulates ventilation via the peripheral chemoreceptors.

BIBLIOGRAPHY

Berger A.J., Mitchell R.A., Severinghaus J.W.: Regulation of respiration. *N. Engl. J. Med.* 297:92, 1977.

Cherniack R.M., Cherniack L.: *Respiration in Health and Disease*, ed. 3. Philadelphia, W.B. Saunders Co., 1983.

Comroe J.H.: *Physiology of Respiration,* ed. 2. Chicago, Year Book Medical Publishers, Inc., 1974.

Dejours P.: *Respiration.* New York, Oxford University Press, 1966.

Egan D.F.: *Fundamentals of Respiratory Therapy,* ed. 3. St. Louis, C.V. Mosby Co., 1977.

Guyton A.C.: *Textbook of Medical Physiology,* ed. 7. Philadelphia, W.B. Saunders Co., 1982.

Mitchell R.A., Berger A.J.: Neural regulation of respiration. *Am. Rev. Respir. Dis.* 111:206, 1975.

Murray J.F.: *The Normal Lung.* Philadelphia, W.B. Saunders Co., 1976.

Nunn J.F.: *Applied Respiratory Physiology,* ed. 2. Boston, Butterworth Publishing Co., 1977.

Spearman C.B., Sheldon R.L., Egan D.F.: *Egan's Fundamentals of Respiratory Therapy,* ed. 4. St. Louis, C.V. Mosby Co., 1982.

West J.B.: *Respiratory Physiology: The Essentials,* ed. 2. Baltimore, Williams & Wilkins Co., 1979.

6 / Anatomy of the Cardiovascular System

I. Blood
 A. A heterogeneous substance composed of a fluid (plasma) and a cellular component.
 B. Plasma: Whole blood minus the cellular component.
  1. It is a pale yellow (strawlike) color.
  2. Plasma, the interstitial fluid, and the intracellular fluid are the three major body fluids.
  3. Major constituents are water and chemical compounds (solutes).
   a. Water, the solvent, constitutes approximately 90% of plasma.
   b. The major solutes protein, foodstuffs, and electrolytes constitute about 10% of plasma.
  4. Plasma minus clotting factors is called blood serum.
 C. Cellular components: Red blood cells (RBCs), white blood cells (WBCs), and platelets.
  1. RBCs (erythrocytes): Biconcave disks with a diameter of 7–8 μ and a thickness of about 2 μ.
   a. Mature RBCs have no nucleus.
   b. RBCs are surrounded by a semipermeable membrane.
    (1) Placed in a hypotonic solution (less than 0.9% NaCl), they will swell and can rupture (hemolysis).
    (2) Placed in a hypertonic solution (greater than 0.9% NaCl), they will shrivel (crenation).
   c. RBCs are relatively flexible and are able to accommodate changes in shape without rupturing. This becomes important when they pass through tight spots in the circulation (e.g., capillaries or sinusoids).
   d. RBCs are produced in myeloid tissue (red bone marrow); a process termed erythropoiesis.
   e. The normal number of RBCs is higher in males than in females.
    (1) Female: 4.1–5.1 million RBCs/cu mm.
    (2) Male: 4.8–6.0 million RBCs/cu mm.

f. Reticulocytes are newly released RBCs that retain a small portion of the hemoglobin-forming endoplasmic reticulum.

   (1) In 2–3 days, formation of hemoglobin will be complete. At this point, the endoplasmic reticulum disappears and the cell is a mature erythrocyte.

   (2) The percentage of total RBCs that are reticulocytes indicates the rate of erythropoiesis.

   (3) The normal range (percentage) of reticulocytes is 0.5%–1.5% of the total number of RBCs.

      (a) More than 1.5% usually indicates increased erythropoiesis.

      (b) Less than 0.5% usually indicates decreased erythropoiesis.

g. Hemoglobin is the major solute contained within the RBC.

   (1) The normal amount of hemoglobin contained in the blood is higher in males than females:

      (a) Female: 12–14 gm Hb/100 ml of blood

      (b) Male: 13–16 gm Hb/100 ml of blood

h. The hematocrit is the volume percentage of RBCs in whole blood; i.e., a hematocrit equal to 45 means that 45% of whole blood is RBCs by volume.

   (1) The normal hematocrit is higher in males than females:

      (a) Female: 37–47

      (b) Male: 40–54

i. Normally hemoglobin levels are equal to about one third of the hematocrit.

2. Types of WBCs (leukocytes): Polymorphonuclear neutrophils, eosinophils and basophils, and mononuclear monocytes and lymphocytes.

   a. Polymorphonuclear leukocytes

      (1) Are formed in myeloid tissue.

      (2) Have a multilobed nucleus.

      (3) Are collectively called "polys."

      (4) Appear histologically to possess granulated cytoplasm and are collectively termed granulocytes.

      (5) All can perform phagocytosis.

      (6) Polymorphonuclear neutrophils

         (a) Have a diameter of about 10 μ.

         (b) Have a nucleus that contains one to five lobes.

         (c) Are highly phagocytic.

         (d) Make up 50%–75% of the total number of leukocytes.

    (7) Polymorphonuclear eosinophils
       (a) Readily absorb an acid stain.
       (b) Have a bilobed nucleus.
       (c) Are implicated in parasitic as well as allergic processes.
       (d) Make up 2%–4% of the total number of leukocytes.
       (e) Have a diameter of about 10 μ.
    (8) Polymorphonuclear basophils
       (a) Readily absorb a basic stain.
       (b) Have a three- or four-lobed nucleus.
       (c) Contain heparin, which may serve to prevent coagulation of blood at sites of inflammation.
       (d) Make up less than 0.5% of the total number of leukocytes.
       (e) Have a diameter of about 10 μ.
  b. Mononuclear leukocytes
    (1) Are formed in lymphoid tissue.
    (2) Mononuclear monocytes
       (a) Have a diameter of 10–15 μ.
       (b) Have a crescent-shaped nucleus.
       (c) Have cytoplasm containing very fine granules.
       (d) Are highly phagocytic cells.
       (e) Make up 3%–8% of the total number of leukocytes.
    (3) Mononuclear lymphocytes
       (a) Have a diameter of about 6–9 μ.
       (b) Have a round nucleus.
       (c) Have cytoplasm that appears clear.
       (d) Form antibodies that remain intracellular (cellular antibodies) or form antibodies that are released into the bloodstream (circulating antibodies).
       (e) Make up 20%–40% of the total number of leukocytes.
  c. Total WBC count has the normal range of 5,000–10,000 WBCs/cu mm.
  d. A differential count identifies the percentage of the total WBC count that each WBC type comprises (Table 6–1). (Note normal range [%] in each of the WBC types previously described.)
  e. Megakaryocyte: A special type of blood cell.
    (1) Formed in myeloid tissue.

TABLE 6–1.—NORMAL FUNCTION AND PERCENTAGE
COMPOSITION OF LEUKOCYTES

TYPE	FUNCTION	PERCENTAGE COMPOSITION
Neutrophil	Phagocytosis	50–75
Eosinophil	Hypersensitivity reaction	2–4
Basophil	Anticoagulation	< 0.5
Monocyte	Phagocytosis	3–8
Lymphocyte	Antibody formation	20–40

    (2) Fragments into small irregular pieces of protoplasm called thrombocytes or platelets.
      (a) Are 2–4 μ in diameter.
      (b) Have no nucleus.
      (c) Have a granular cytoplasm.
      (d) Normal platelet count is 200,000–350,000/cu mm.
      (e) Function in clot formation (hemostasis).
D. Total blood volume of an individual.
  1. Equal to about 70–72 ml of blood per kilogram of body weight.
  2. This relationship varies inversely with the amount of excess body fat; i.e., an obese individual has less blood volume per kilogram than a slender individual.
II. The Blood Vessels (Fig 6–1)
A. The blood vessels consist of a closed system of connected arteries, arterioles, capillaries, venules, and veins.
B. *Arteries* contain three characteristic layers: tunica intima, tunica media, and tunica adventitia.
  1. Tunica adventitia (external layer)
    a. Consists of connective tissue surrounding a network of collagenous and elastic fibers.
    b. Supports and protects the blood vessels.
    c. Contains vasa vasorum, very fine vessels that serve the tunica adventitia with its blood supply.
    d. Contains lymphatic vessels and nerve fibers.
  2. Tunica media (middle layer)
    a. Thickest layer of the artery.
    b. Composed of circularly arranged smooth muscle and elastic fibers.
    c. Nerve fibers contained in tunica adventitia terminate in the smooth muscle layer of the tunica media.
  3. Tunica intima (internal layer)

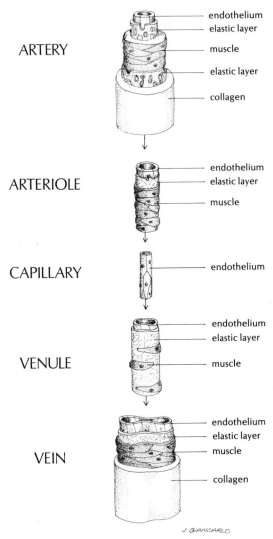

ARTERY

ARTERIOLE

CAPILLARY

VENULE

VEIN

J GIANCARLO

Fig 6–1.—Schematic representation of the anatomic structure of major types of blood vessels (see text). (From Shapiro B.A., Harrison R.A., Kacmarek R.M., et al.: *Clinical Application of Respiratory Care,* ed. 3. Chicago, Year Book Medical Publishers, Inc., 1985. Reproduced by permission.)

    a. Thinnest layer of the artery.
    b. Consists of flat layer of simple squamous cells called the endothelium:
       (1) The endothelium is supported by a fine layer of connective tissue.

(2) The connective tissue is surrounded by a longitudinally placed network of elastic fibers.
c. Common to all blood vessels, the endothelium even being continuous with the endocardium of the heart.
C. Large arteries: Termed "elastic arteries" because the tunica media has less smooth muscle and more elastic fibers.
D. Medium-sized arteries: Sometimes called "nutrient arteries" because they control the flow of blood to various areas of the body. Their ability to regulate blood flow lies in a tunica media, which is almost entirely composed of smooth muscle.
E. *Arterioles* (small arteries)
   1. The arterioles have a thin tunica intima and adventitia but have a thick, smooth muscle layer in the tunica media.
   2. The arterioles range in diameter from 20 μ to 50 μ.
   3. The tunica media is extensively innervated by postsynaptic sympathetic nerve fibers.
   4. Due to the extensive innervation and abundance of smooth muscle, the arterioles control regional blood flow to the capillary beds.
   5. The arterioles are frequently called the "resistance vessels." By vasomotion, they control the rate of arterial runoff (the rate at which blood leaves the arterial tree) and thereby arterial blood volume.
   6. The arterioles terminate in either metarterioles or capillaries.
      a. Metarterioles range in diameter from 10 μ to 20 μ.
      b. Metarterioles can bypass a capillary bed entirely by shunting blood directly to the venules.
      c. Metarterioles can also allow blood to pass from arterioles to capillaries.
F. *Capillaries*
   1. Consist only of tunica intima.
   2. Vary in diameter from 5 μ to 10 μ.
   3. Where capillaries originate from arterioles or metarterioles, there frequently is a small band of smooth muscle called the precapillary sphincter.
      a. This sphincter controls blood flow through the distal capillary.
      b. It is responsive (vasoactive) to local P_{CO_2}, P_{O_2}, pH, and temperature.
   4. Capillaries frequently are called "exchange vessels," because they are the site of gas, fluid, nutrient, and waste exchange.
      a. An intracellular cleft lies between the individual squames comprising the endothelium.

(1) They are about 50–60 Å wide.

(2) They act as pores through which substances can move into and out of the capillaries.

 b. The basement membrane usually is continuous in the capillaries and may limit movement of substances into and out of the capillaries.

G. *Veins* consist of a tunica intima, media, and adventitia, but each layer is thinner than its counterpart in the arteries.

 1. Tunica adventitia

  a. One to five times as thick as the tunica media.

  b. Made up of connective, elastic, and smooth muscle tissue.

 2. Tunica media

  a. Made up of circularly arranged smooth muscle, collagenous, and elastic tissue.

  b. Innervated by postsynaptic fibers of sympathetic nervous system.

   (1) Veins are not as extensively innervated as arteries.

   (2) By venodilation or venoconstriction, veins can alter venous blood volume and "venous return."

 3. Tunica intima

  a. Consists of endothelial cells supported by delicate elastic fibers and connective tissue.

H. In general, all vessels of the venous system have smaller amounts of elastic and smooth muscle tissue than their arterial counterparts.

I. *Venules* (small veins) have the three characteristic layers, but they are very thin and almost indistinguishable.

J. Veins are called "capacitance vessels" or "reservoir vessels" because 70%–75% of the blood volume exists in the venous system.

K. Veins contained in the periphery of the body contain one-way valves.

 1. Valves are formed by duplication of endothelial lining of veins.

 2. Valves are semilunar and prevent retrograde flow of blood.

 3. Valves are found in veins more than 2 mm in diameter and exist in areas subjected to muscular pressure, e.g., arms and legs.

 4. Valves are absent in veins less than 1 mm in diameter and in areas such as the abdominal and thoracic cavities.

III. The Lymphatic Vessels

A. These vessels are a type of circulatory system that collects fluid and other material in the interstitial space and returns them to the venous vasculature.

B. Lymphatic vessels originate as blindly ending vessels called lymphatic capillaries.
  1. They have no basement membrane and consist only of loosely fitting endothelial cells.
  2. They are invested in every tissue of the body except for cartilage, bone, epithelium, and the CNS.
C. Lymphatic capillaries drain into larger lymphatic vessels, which take on three characteristic layers similar to those of the veins.
  1. Larger lymphatic channels contain smooth muscle, elastic, fibrous, and connective tissue.
  2. These vessels resemble the veins except that the three layers composing the lymphatics are much thinner.
  3. One-way semilunar valves are found about every millimeter and are more frequent in the lymphatics than in the veins.
D. The larger lymphatic vessels drain into lymph nodes (Fig 6–2).
  1. Lymph nodes are found in the neck, axilla, groin, thorax, breast, arms, and mouth.
  2. Lymph nodes are bean or oval shaped.
  3. Lymph moves into the lymph nodes via afferent lymphatic channels.
    a. The lymph is exposed to phagocytic reticular endothelial cells lining the sinus of the nodes.
    b. The lymph is filtered and exits from the lymph node via efferent lymphatic channels.
E. The large efferent lymphatic vessels join one of two major lymphatic ducts (Fig 6–3).
  1. Right lymphatic duct
    a. Drains right upper quadrant of the trunk.
    b. Drains right side of the head and neck.
    c. Drains filtered lymph into right subclavian vein.
  2. Thoracic duct
    a. Drains remainder of the body.
    b. Largest lymphatic vessel but smaller than either vena cava.
      (1) The duct is 15–18 in. long.
      (2) It originates in the lumbar region of the abdominal cavity and ascends to the neck.
    c. Drains filtered lymph into left subclavian vein.
IV. The Heart
A. The heart is a muscular pump that maintains circulation of the blood through the vessels to all parts of the body.
B. The heart is located between the lungs in the mediastinum (Fig 6–4).

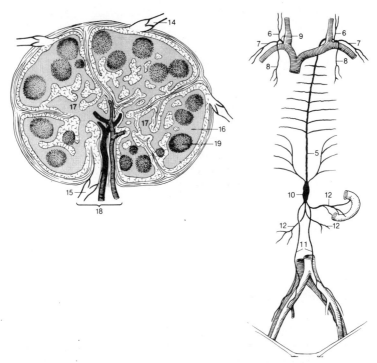

Fig 6–2 (left).—Lymph node (transverse section). 14-afferent lymphatic vessel, 15-efferent lymphatic vessel (From Feneis H.: *Pocket Atlas of Human Anatomy.* New York, Thieme-Stratton, Inc., 1976. Reproduced by permission.)

Fig 6–3 (right).—Thoracic and right lymphatic ducts communicating with the venous system. *5,* Thoracic duct, *9,* right lymphatic duct. (From Feneis H.: *Pocket Atlas of Human Anatomy.* New York, Thieme-Stratton, Inc., 1976. Reproduced by permission.)

    C. The apex is the inferior portion of the heart and is directed inferiorly, anteriorly, and to the left, with most of it left of the midline.

    D. The base is the superior aspect of the heart.

    E. The heart is about the size of the clenched fist.

    F. The heart is encased by a loose nondistensible sac called the pericardium (Fig 6–5).

    G. Layers of pericardium

        1. *Fibrous pericardium*

           a. Outermost layer of pericardium.

           b. Attaches to great vessels (major vessels entering and exiting from the heart) of the heart and loosely encases the heart proper.

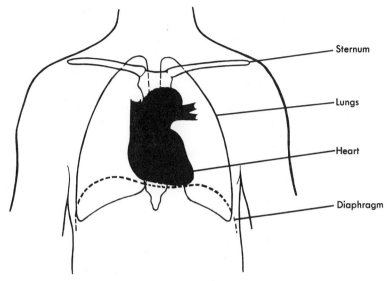

Fig 6–4.—Position of the heart in the thoracic cavity. (From Spearman C.B., Sheldon R.L., Egan D.F.: *Egan's Fundamentals of Respiratory Therapy,* ed. 4. St. Louis, C.V. Mosby Co., 1982. Reproduced by permission.)

    c. Made of white fibrous tissue that protects and anchors the heart to some extent.

    d. Externally attached to sternum, vertebral column, central tendon, and left hemidiaphragm.

  2. *Parietal serous pericardium*

    a. Lines the fibrous pericardium, to which it is closely adherent.

    b. A moist serous membrane that forms a smooth surface to reduce frictional resistances.

    c. Produces a small volume of serous fluid called pericardial fluid.

    d. Becomes continuous with the visceral serous pericardium.

  3. *Visceral serous pericardium*

    a. Directly adherent to the heart.

    b. Commonly called epicardium of the heart.

    c. A serous membrane that produces serous pericardial fluid.

    d. The small space between visceral and parietal serous pericardial layers is called the pericardial space.

  4. The fact that the visceral and parietal serous pericardial layers are smooth membranes with a small volume of lubricating pericardial fluid between them allows the heart to move freely in the pericardial sac opposed by reduced frictional forces.

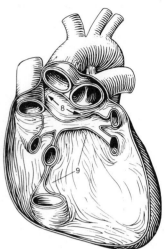

Fig 6–5.—Pericardial sac encases heart and great vessels (posterior view). (From Feneis H.: *Pocket Atlas of Human Anatomy.* New York, Thieme-Stratton, Inc., 1976. Reproduced by permission.)

H. The heart wall has three distinctive layers (Fig 6–6).
   1. *Epicardium* or visceral serous pericardium
      a. Most superficial layer.
      b. A transparent serous sheet lying on a delicate network of connective tissue.
      c. Contains fat, coronary blood vessels, and coronary nerves, which are observable on cardiac surface.
   2. *Myocardium*
      a. Located just deep to the epicardium and is the middle layer of heart wall.
      b. Composed almost exclusively of cardiac muscle with the exception of coronary blood vessels.
      c. Thickest of the three cardiac layers.
   3. *Endocardium*
      a. Deepest cardiac layer, the internal lining of the heart.
      b. Smooth layer of squamous epithelium.
      c. Continuous with endothelial lining of all blood vessels.
      d. Duplication of this layer in the heart forms the cardiac valves.
I. The heart has four chambers (Fig 6–7).
   1. The two superior chambers, or atria.
   2. The two inferior chambers, or ventricles.
   3. Externally the two atria are separated from the two ventricles by a groove that circumscribes the heart, the coronary sulcus.

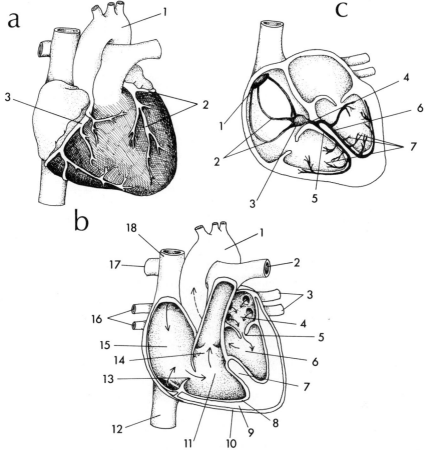

Fig 6–6.—Functional anatomy of the heart: *1,* aorta; *2,* left pulmonary artery; *3,* pulmonary veins from left lung; *4,* left atrium; *5,* mitral valve; *6,* left ventricle; *7,* intraventricular septum; *8,* endocardium; *9,* myocardium; *10,* epicardium; *11,* right ventricle; *12,* inferior vena cava; *13,* tricuspid valve; *14,* pulmonary semilunar valves; *15,* right atrium; *16,* pulmonary veins from right lung; *17,* right pulmonary artery; *18,* superior vena cava. (From Shapiro B.A., Harrison R.A., Kacmarek R.M., et al.: *Clinical Application of Respiratory Care,* ed. 3. Chicago, Year Book Medical Publishers, Inc., 1985. Reproduced by permission.)

4. Externally the two atria are separated from each other by the roots of both the aorta and the pulmonary artery.
5. Externally the two ventricles are separated from each other by a groove, the interventricular sulcus.
6. Internally the two atria are separated from each other by a wall, the interatrial septum.

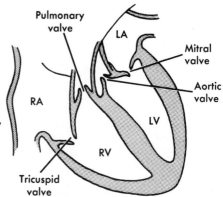

Fig 6–7.—Heart chambers and valves. *RA,* right atrium; *RV,* right ventricle; *LA,* left atrium; *LV,* left ventricle. (From Spearman C.B., Sheldon R.L., Egan D.F.: *Egan's Fundamentals of Respiratory Therapy,* ed. 4. St. Louis, C.V. Mosby Co., 1982. Reproduced by permission.)

    a. The fossa ovalis, a depression in the atrial septal wall, is the remnant of the fetal foramen ovale.

7. Internally the two ventricles are separated from each other by a fibrous and muscular interventricular septum. It is continuous with the interatrial septum through its fibrous portion (see Fig 6–6).

8. Internally the atria are separated from the ventricles by a structure known as the fibroskeleton of the heart (Fig 6–8).

    a. The fibroskeleton consists of fibrous rings [which surround the atrioventricular (AV) cardiac valves, pulmonic semilunar valves, and aortic semilunar valves], fibrous interventricular septum, right and left trigone, and tendon of conus.

        (1) The right fibrous trigone consists of fibrous tissue that connects the two AV rings, fibrous interventricular septum, and ring of the aortic semilunar valve.

        (2) The left fibrous trigone consists of fibrous tissue that connects the fibrous ring of the left AV valve with the aortic semilunar valve.

        (3) The tendon of conus is fibrous tissue that connects the fibrous ring of the pulmonic semilunar valve with the ring surrounding the aortic semilunar valve.

    b. Functions of the fibroskeleton.

        (1) It houses the four cardiac valves.

        (2) It serves as the origin of and point of insertion for atrial and ventricular bands of muscle.

        (3) It electrically isolates atrial muscle bundles from ventricular muscle bundles.

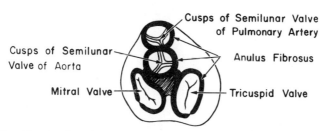

Cusps of Semilunar Valve
of Pulmonary Artery

Cusps of Semilunar—
Valve of Aorta

Anulus Fibrosus

Mitral Valve

Tricuspid Valve

Fig 6–8.—Heart valves formed on the borders of the cardiac fibrous skeleton. View is from the base of the heart. (From Little R.C.: *Physiology of the Heart and Circulation.* ed., 2. Chicago, Year Book Medical Publishers, Inc., 1981. Reproduced by permission.)

     (a) The fibroskeleton is bridged only by the common bundle branch of the electrical conduction system of the heart, called the bundle of His.

     (b) This arrangement allows repolarization and depolarization of the atria separate from the ventricles.

  9. The *right atrium* is positioned atop the right ventricle (Fig 6–9).

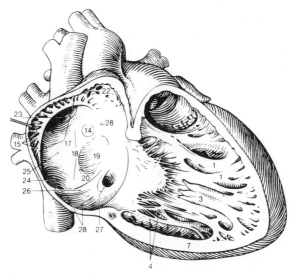

Fig 6–9.—Right atrium and systemic great veins. *1,* trabeculae carneae; *3,* papillary muscles; *4,* chordae tendineae; *14,* right atrium; *23,* opening of superior vena cava; *24,* opening of inferior vena cava; *27,* opening of coronary sinus. (From Feneis H.: *Pocket Atlas of Human Anatomy.* New York, Thieme-Stratton, Inc., 1976. Reproduced by permission.)

a. It is anterior to the left atrium because the heart is rotated to the left.
   (1) Thus, the bulk of the anterior surface of the heart is composed of the right heart (right atrium and ventricle).
   (2) Most of the posterior surface of the heart is composed of the left heart (left atrium and ventricle).
b. The right atrium is larger than the left atrium and has a thinner wall.
   (1) The right atrial wall is about 2 mm thick.
   (2) The atrial musculature is divided into deep atrial muscle, which encircles each atrium individually, and superficial atrial muscle, which encircles both atria.
   (3) The deep and superficial muscle fibers run perpendicularly to one another and originate and insert on the fibroskeleton of the heart.
   (4) Contraction of the two major groups of atrial muscle fibers tends to decrease the size of the respective atria in all dimensions.
c. The cavity of the right atrium consists of two parts:
   (1) The major cavity of the right atrium, or sinus venarum.
   (2) The smaller cavity, which appears externally as a pouch, called the right auricle. (*Note:* Auricle is a term formerly used to denote the entire atrium.)
d. The right atrium accepts venous blood from the following veins:
   (1) The superior vena cava, which opens into the superior and posterior portions of the major cavity of the right atrium.
   (2) The inferior vena cava, which opens into the most inferior portion of the right atrium very near the interatrial septal wall.
   (3) The coronary sinus, which opens into the right atrium between the tricuspid valve and the opening of the inferior vena cava.
10. The *left atrium* is positioned atop the left ventricle (Fig 6–10).
   a. The left atrium is smaller than the right atrium and has a thicker wall.
      (1) The left atrial wall is about 3 mm thick.
      (2) The left atrial muscle fibers are divided into deep and superficial muscle groups and have an arrangement similar to that of the right atrium.

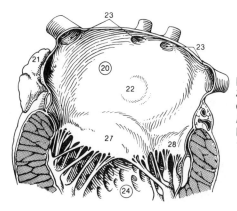

Fig 6–10.—Left atrium and pulmonary veins. *20,* left atrium; *23,* pulmonary veins; *27–28,* cusps of mitral valve. (From Feneis H.: *Pocket Atlas of Human Anatomy.* New York, Thieme-Stratton, Inc., 1976. Reproduced by permission.)

b. The cavity of the left atrium consists of two parts:
   (1) The major cavity of the left atrium.
   (2) The left auricle, which appears externally as a pouch-like structure.
c. The left atrium accepts arterial blood from the four pulmonary veins, which open into its superior and posterior aspects.
11. Right ventricle (Fig 6–11)
   a. It constitutes most of the anterior surface of heart.
   b. The right ventricular wall is one third the thickness of the left ventricular wall.
   c. The ventricular musculature classically is separated into deep and superficial muscle groups.
      (1) Both deep and superficial muscle groups appear to originate on the fibroskeleton of the heart.
      (2) Superficial fibers follow a clockwise spiral course to the apex of the heart. At the apex, these fibers turn inward and follow a spiraled course counterclockwise and upward toward the base of the heart to insert on the fibroskeleton.
      (3) Deep fibers follow a similar course to the superficial ventricular fibers, with three exceptions:
         (a) The spiraled course of the deep fibers is in a direction opposite to that of the superficial fibers.
         (b) Deep fibers may not follow a course all the way to the apex of the heart before starting to ascend.
         (c) Deep fibers may insert into the cardiac fibroskeleton, papillary muscles, or trabeculae carneae.

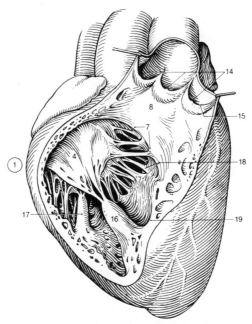

Fig 6–11.—Right ventricle with tricuspid and pulmonic semilunar valves exposed. *1,* right ventricle; *4,* tricuspid valve; *8,* outflow tract of right ventricle; *14,* cusps of pulmonic semilunar valve; *16–18,* papillary muscles. (From Feneis H.: *Pocket Atlas of Human Anatomy.* New York, Thieme-Stratton, Inc., 1976. Reproduced by permission.)

      (i) Papillary muscles are fingerlike projections of cardiac muscle located in the cavity of each ventricle.

      (ii) Trabeculae carneae are irregular bundles of muscle that form ridges along the internal wall of the ventricular cavity.

    (4) Contraction of ventricular muscle fibers tends to decrease the internal anteroposterior and transverse diameter significantly, but leaves the vertical diameter virtually unchanged.

  d. The right ventricle receives venous blood from the right atrium through an opening called the right AV orifice.

    (1) This orifice is surrounded by a fibrous ring that is a part of the cardiac fibroskeleton.

    (2) The right AV orifice is about 4 cm in diameter.

    (3) The right AV orifice contains the tricuspid valve.

(a) The tricuspid valve contains three cusps, each fused at its origin in the AV ring.

(b) The cusps are formed by a duplication of the endocardial layer of the heart and are supported with fibrous tissue.

(c) The three cusps collectively have a funnel shape that projects into the cavity of the right ventricle.

(d) The free borders (inferior border) of each cusp have an attached fibrous cordlike structure, the chordae tendineae.

(e) The chordae tendineae are in turn attached to the intraventricular papillary muscles.

(f) The chordae tendineae commonly cross, passing from one of the cusps to a group of papillary muscles on the opposite side of the ventricle.

e. The cavity of the right ventricle is lined with muscular ridges (trabeculae carneae) and papillary muscle covered by endocardium.

(1) The cavity of the right ventricle has a bellows or U shape.

(2) The muscular arrangement and shape of the right ventricle are well suited to its function of pumping blood under low pressure.

f. Blood exits from the cavity of the right ventricle by passing through the pulmonary artery via an opening called the orifice of the pulmonary trunk.

(1) This orifice is surrounded by a fibrous ring, a component of the cardiac fibroskeleton.

(2) The pulmonary orifice is located in the superior, anterior, and medial section of the right ventricle.

(3) The pulmonary orifice contains the pulmonic semilunar valve.

(a) The pulmonic semilunar valve is composed of three half-moon-shaped cusps.

(b) This valve resembles the type found in the large veins of the periphery.

(c) This valve, like the AV valves, is formed by duplication of the endocardial layer and is supported by fibrous tissue.

12. Left ventricle (Fig 6–12)

a. It constitutes most of the posterior surface of the heart.

b. The left ventricular wall is three times the thickness of the right ventricular wall.

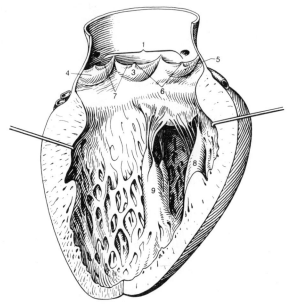

Fig 6–12.—Left ventricle with mitral and aortic semilunar valves exposed. *1,* opening of left ventricle into aorta; *3–5,* cusps of aortic semilunar valve; *8–9,* papillary muscles. (From Feneis H.: *Pocket Atlas of Human Anatomy.* New York, Thieme-Stratton, Inc., 1976. Reproduced by permission.)

    c. Left ventricular muscle fibers are part of the continuum of muscle circumscribing both ventricles and cannot be anatomically separated from right ventricular fibers. (*Note:* The arrangement of the ventricular muscle fibers is described in the foregoing section on the right ventricle.)

    d. The left ventricle receives arterial blood from the left atrium through the left atrioventricular orifice (see Fig 6–6).

      (1) This orifice is surrounded by a fibrous ring, which is one of the components of the cardiac fibroskeleton.

      (2) Contained in the left AV orifice is the bicuspid or mitral valve.

        (a) The mitral valve is composed of two cusps.

        (b) The anatomical structure is very similar to that of the previously discussed tricuspid valve except that the chordae tendineae are thicker and stronger in the left ventricle.

e. The cavity of the left ventricle is lined with muscular ridges (trabeculae carneae), which appear in a more numerous and dense arrangement than in the right ventricle. Papillary muscles with the corresponding thick chordae tendineae, along with the trabeculae carneae, are covered by the endocardial layer.
   (1) The cavity of the left ventricle is conical.
   (2) The arrangement of the left ventricular musculature coupled with its conical shape lends well to its function of pumping blood under high pressure.
f. Blood exits from the cavity of the left ventricle by passing through the aortic opening.
   (1) This opening is surrounded by a fibrous ring, a component of the cardiac fibroskeleton.
   (2) The aortic opening exists in the superior, posterior, and medial section of the left ventricle.
   (3) The aortic opening contains the aortic semilunar valve.
      (a) The aortic semilunar valve is anatomically similar to the pulmonic semilunar valve except that the aortic cusps are stronger, larger, and thicker.

BIBLIOGRAPHY

Ayres S.M., Giannelli S. Jr., Mueller H.S.: *Care of the Critically Ill*, ed. 2. New York, Appleton-Century-Crofts, 1974.

Crowley L.V.: *Introductory Concepts in Anatomy and Physiology*. Chicago, Year Book Medical Publishers, Inc., 1976.

Feneis H.: *Pocket Atlas of Human Anatomy*. Chicago, Year Book Medical Publishers, Inc., 1976.

Gray H., Goss C.M.: *Gray's Anatomy of the Human Body*, ed. 29. Philadelphia, Lea & Febiger, 1973.

Guyton A.C.: *Textbook of Medical Physiology*, ed. 6. Philadelphia, Lea & Febiger, 1981.

Jacob S.W., Francone C.A.: *Structure and Function in Man*, ed. 3. Philadelphia, W.B. Saunders Co., 1974.

Little R.C.: *Physiology of the Heart and Circulation*. Chicago, Year Book Medical Publishers, Inc., 1977.

McLaughlin A.J.: *Essentials of Physiology for Advanced Respiratory Therapy*. St. Louis, C.V. Mosby Co., 1977.

Ruch T.C., Patton H.D.: *Physiology and Biophysics*, ed. 20. Philadelphia, W.B. Saunders Co., 1974.

Rushmer R.F.: *Cardiovascular Dynamics*, ed. 3. Philadelphia, W.B. Saunders Co., 1970.

Shapiro B.A., Harrison R.A., Kacmarek R.M., et al.: *Clinical Application of Respiratory Care*, ed. 3. Chicago, Year Book Medical Publishers, Inc., 1985.

Spearman C.B., Sheldon R.L., Egan D.F.: *Egan's Fundamentals of Respiratory Therapy*, ed. 4. St. Louis, C.V. Mosby Co., 1982.

7 / Physiology of the Cardiovascular System

I. Functions of the Blood
  A. Primary vehicle of transport of substances in the body.
    1. Respiratory gases (e.g., oxygen and carbon dioxide).
    2. Circulating antibodies and leukocytes involved in the body's defense mechanisms.
    3. Platelets and clotting factors involved in hemostasis.
    4. Cellular nutrients to all of the cells.
    5. Cellular waste products away from the cells.
    6. Electrolytes, proteins, water, and hormones, all of which contribute to the numerous complex functions of blood.
II. Anatomical Classification of the Vascular Bed (Fig 7–1)
  A. The typical vascular bed begins with the aorta or pulmonary artery.
  B. Branches from either of these main arteries are called large arteries.
  C. The larger arteries continue to branch to medium arteries.
  D. The medium arteries branch further to the arterioles.
  E. The end of the arteriolar bed is marked by a thick band of smooth muscle called the precapillary sphincter, which marks the initial portion of the microcirculation.
  F. The arterioles branch to metarterioles or directly to capillaries.
  G. Distal to the precapillary sphincter are the capillaries.
  H. Many capillaries join to form venules.
  I. Numerous venules join to form small veins, which in turn join to form large veins.
  J. Large veins join the major veins of the body—either the vena cava or the pulmonary veins.
III. Functional Divisions of the Vascular Bed
  A. Distribution, resistance, exchange, and capacitance vessels.
    1. Distribution vessels begin with the major arteries and include the large and medium arteries.
      a. These vessels distribute the cardiac output to the various organ systems.

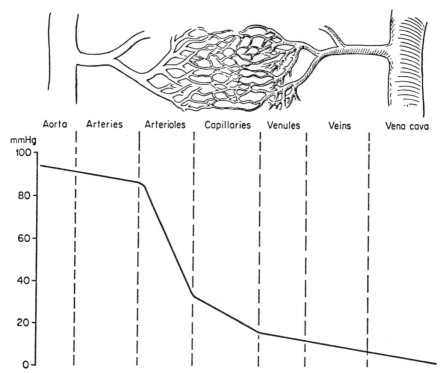

Fig 7–1.—Typical vascular bed with graphic representation of pressure drop across the systemic circulation. (From Ross G.: *Essentials of Human Physiology,* ed. 2. Chicago, Year Book Medical Publishers, Inc., 1982. Reproduced by permission.)

      b. These vessels typically are under an elevated pressure, contain a relatively small percentage of total blood volume, and are very elastic.

    2. Resistance vessels begin with the arterioles and end with the precapillary sphincter.

      a. These vessels have the largest proportion of smooth muscle constituting the vascular wall of any of the blood vessels.

      b. Through contraction and relaxation of the smooth muscle, the resistance vessels can regulate the distribution of blood to the various capillary beds.

      c. The resistance vessels are the major source of peripheral resistance and function in arterial blood pressure regulation.

3. The exchange vessels are the capillaries.
   a. Fluid, gas, nutrient, and waste exchange occurs in these vessels.
   b. Exchange of these substances occurs between capillary blood and interstitial fluid. Exchange then occurs from the interstitial fluid to the cells that make up the tissue.
   c. The major process underlying exchange in the capillaries is diffusion.
   d. Due to the vast distribution of capillary beds, the process of diffusion is fast enough to maintain cellular metabolism.
4. Capacitance vessels include the venules through the large veins and encompass the total venous system.
   a. Capacitance vessels serve as channels for blood return to the heart from the various capillary beds.
   b. These vessels are called "capacitance" or "reservoir vessels" because they contain most (70%–75%) of the total blood volume.
   c. The capacitance vessels are typically under low pressure, contain a large blood volume, and are relatively inelastic compared to their arterial counterparts.

IV. Vascular System: Systemic and Pulmonary Circulations (Fig 7–2)
   A. Systemic circulation

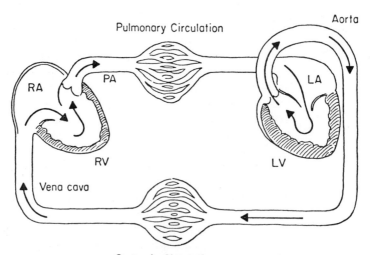

Fig 7–2.—The pulmonary and systemic circulations. (From Ross G.: *Essentials of Human Physiology,* ed. 2. Chicago, Year Book Medical Publishers, Inc., 1982. Reproduced by permission.)

1. Systemic circulation begins with the systemic pump, the left ventricle, and continues to a typical vascular bed, ending with the right atrium.
   a. Functions of systemic circulation:
      (1) To distribute left ventricular cardiac output so that each region of the body receives an adequate volume of blood per unit time.
      (2) To perfuse individual tissues so that cellular metabolism is maintained.
      (3) To return venous blood to the right side of the heart to maintain right ventricular output.
2. Control of systemic circulation is governed by four major mechanisms: autonomic control, hormonal control, local control, and mechanical factors.
   a. The arterial portion of the systemic circulation is basically governed by three mechanisms: The autonomic nervous system, hormonal control, and local control.
      (1) Arteries and arterioles are innervated extensively and virtually exclusively by postganglionic fibers of the sympathetic nervous system.
      (2) The arterial vasculature of different tissues varies in the degree of sympathetic innervation.
         (a) The largest degree of sympathetic innervation is to the arterial vasculature perfusing the skin.
         (b) The degree of sympathetic innervation steadily decreases through the arterial vasculature perfusing spleen, mesenteric vessels, and kidneys.
         (c) A smaller degree of sympathetic innervation exists in the muscles.
         (d) The least degree of sympathetic innervation exists in the vessels perfusing the heart and brain. Furthermore, these vessels have a small degree of parasympathetic innervation.
      (3) Sympathetic stimulation of blood vessels results in smooth muscle contraction and vasoconstriction.
         (a) This principally affects the resistance vessels due to their large component of smooth muscle.
         (b) Tonic sympathetic stimulation of arterial blood vessels results in a given arteriolar caliber.
            (i) Increased sympathetic stimulation above this tonic level results in vasoconstriction and an increase in resistance to flow through these vessels.

(ii) Decreased sympathetic stimulation below
this tonic level results in vasodilation and a
decrease in resistance to flow through these
vessels.
(iii) Because of differing degrees of sympathetic
innervation in the different tissues, general
sympathetic stimulation results in varying
degrees of vasoconstriction and varying resistance to blood flow from tissue to tissue.
(4) Parasympathetic stimulation of the arterial vasculature of the brain and heart results in smooth muscle
relaxation and vasodilation. This phenomenon results
in a decrease in resistance to blood flow.
(5) The adrenomedullary hormones, norepinephrine and
epinephrine, both stimulate the α (alpha) receptors
and produce vasoconstriction.
(6) Acidosis, hypoxemia, hypercarbia, and increased temperature all produce local relaxation of smooth muscle in resistance vessels and resultant vasodilation.
b. The capillary bed of the systemic circulation is governed
almost exclusively by local factors.
(1) In tissues where capillary blood flow is limited by arteriolar constriction, there is local accumulation of
acid and carbon dioxide as well as a deficiency of oxygen.
(2) These local factors result in relaxation of the smooth
muscle and local arteriolar dilation, which reestab-
lishes blood flow.
(3) Blood flow removes the local accumulation of waste
products and replenishes oxygen and nutrient supply,
resulting in arteriolar constriction, which in turn limits blood flow.
(4) Thus the cycle repeats itself, providing blood flow to
tissues intermittently to maintain cellular metabolism.
c. The veins of the systemic circulation are governed by the
autonomic nervous system, hormonal factors, and mechanical factors.
(1) The veins are exclusively innervated by postganglionic fibers of the sympathetic nervous system.
(2) The veins have a less extensive innervation than do
their arterial counterparts. However, unlike that of

the arteries, sympathetic innervation of the venous vasculature does not vary from one tissue to the next.

(a) Thus, sympathetic stimulation causes venoconstriction of all veins of the body.

(b) Generalized venoconstriction decreases the venous vascular space, resulting in increased venous return to the heart.

(c) On the other hand, decreased sympathetic stimulation results in a decrease in venous tone and venodilation.

(d) Generalized venodilation increases the venous vascular space and decreases venous return to the heart.

(3) The adrenomedullary hormones, epinephrine and norepinephrine, both mimic sympathetic stimulation and produce venoconstriction.

(4) Mechanical factors that affect the veins of the systemic venous system are the thoracoabdominal pump, skeletal muscle pump, and semilunar valves.

(a) The thoracoabdominal pump affects the veins by aiding venous return. This is accomplished by exposing the intrathoracic veins to the fluctuating subatmospheric pressure produced by spontaneous ventilation. Coupled with the fact that extrathoracic veins are surrounded by atmospheric or supra-atmospheric pressure, venous return is enhanced.

(b) The veins in the limbs contain semilunar valves that prevent retrograde flow of blood. When skeletal muscle contracts, it compresses the veins, increasing venous pressure. Because these veins have valves, compression of vessels can squeeze blood in only one direction. This mechanism also is responsible for enhancing venous return.

B. Pulmonary circulation (see Fig 7–2)
  1. Pulmonary circulation begins with the pulmonary pump, the right ventricle, and continues to a typical vascular bed, ending with the left atrium.
    a. Functions of pulmonary circulation
      (1) To distribute right ventricular output to pulmonary capillaries, matching the alveolar ventilation with an adequate volume of blood per unit time.

(2) To perfuse the cells on the lung parenchyma with nutrients and rid them of waste products.

(3) To return blood to the left side of the heart to maintain left ventricular output.

2. Control of pulmonary circulation is governed by the same four mechanisms that affect systemic circulation.

   a. In general, the pulmonary vasculature has less smooth muscle and thinner walls than its counterpart in the systemic circulation.

   b. This makes pulmonary circulation susceptible to mechanical factors, e.g., intrathoracic and alveolar pressures, and the effects of gravity on the distribution of blood flow.

   c. Pulmonary vasculature responds to sympathetic stimulation just as does the systemic circulation, but to a much lesser extent.

   d. Three local factors that have profound effects on pulmonary resistance vessels are decreased alveolar PO_2, hypoxemia, and acidemia. All three cause pulmonary vasoconstriction, with increased resistance to blood flow.

   e. Adrenomedullary hormones produce pulmonary vasoconstriction but to a milder degree than in systemic circulation.

   f. Thus, most of the control of pulmonary circulation depends on passive response to mechanical factors as well as on local factors. This is in contrast to the dominance that the sympathetic nervous system displays in controlling systemic circulation.

3. Systemic vascular resistance is normally six to ten times pulmonary vascular resistance.

V. Basic Functions of the Heart (Fig 7–3)

   A. To impart sufficient energy to the blood to provide circulation through the vascular system.

      1. As has been discussed, the vascular resistance of systemic circulation is much greater than that of pulmonary circulation. Therefore the left side of the heart must create greater pressures than the right side to bring about a given flow.

      2. The major principle of circulation (blood flow) is that, for circulation to exist, there must be a pressure gradient. The heart must create that pressure gradient across the respective parts of the vasculature. Therefore, for a given vascular resistance, blood flow is a direct function of the pressure gradient generated by the heart.

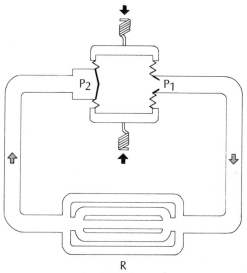

R

Fig 7–3.—Schematic representation of circulation, depicting the heart's function of establishing the pressure gradient. (From Shapiro B.A., Harrison R.A., Kacmarek R.M., et al.: *Clinical Application of Respiratory Care,* ed. 3. Chicago, Year Book Medical Publishers, Inc., 1985. Reproduced by permission.)

VI. Mechanical Events of the Cardiac Cycle
    A. Electric events of the heart are precursors of the mechanical events of the heart.
        1. If the heart is normal, depolarization of the atria causes atrial contraction (systole).
        2. Depolarization of the ventricles causes ventricular contraction (systole).
        3. Repolarization of the atria causes atrial relaxation (diastole).
        4. Repolarization of the ventricles causes ventricular relaxation (diastole).
    B. Atrial systole
        1. Mechanical left and right atrial systole begins at the peak of the P wave of the ECG.
        2. The decrease in size of the respective atria causes left atrial pressure to rise about 7–8 mm Hg and right atrial pressure 5–6 mm Hg. The pressure differential from atria to ventricles causes blood to flow from the atria through the respective AV orifices to the ventricles.
        3. Normal mean right and left atrial pressures are 0–8 mm Hg and 2–12 mm Hg, respectively.
        4. Atrial systole accounts for 20%–40% of the total ventricular

volume. This figure depends on heart rate and atrial contractility. The remaining 60%–80% of ventricular volume is a result of passive filling by venous return.

5. The atria are very weak pumps in comparison to the ventricles and should be thought of as thin-walled blood reservoirs for the respective ventricles. The 20%–40% of ventricular volume added by atrial systole is simply a priming of the ventricles prior to ventricular systole. Atrial systole is not essential for adequate ventricular filling, as can be demonstrated by atrial fibrillation or complete heart block.

6. Atrial systole increases the end-diastolic volume of each ventricle to about 145 ml. It also increases the end-diastolic pressure of the right and left ventricles to 2–8 mm Hg and 4–12 mm Hg, respectively. The ventricles are now prepared for their subsequent contraction.

C. Ventricular systole and atrial diastole

1. Mechanical left and right ventricular systole begins at the peak of the R wave of the ECG and coincides with atrial diastole.

2. Ventricular contraction increases intraventricular pressure. When pressure in the respective ventricles exceeds atrial pressure, the tricuspid and mitral valves close, producing the S_1, or first heart sound.

3. Aortic and pulmonic semilunar valves have been closed during ventricular diastole because pressure in the aorta and pulmonary artery has exceeded left and right ventricular pressure.

4. With both AV and semilunar valves closed, the ventricles are functionally closed chambers. Contraction of the ventricle decreases their size and rapidly increases intraventricular pressure.

5. The first portion of ventricular systole is called isovolumetric contraction. It is characterized by both the AV and semilunar valves being closed and by a rapid increase in intraventricular pressure without a concomitant change in intraventricular blood volume.

6. The second portion of ventricular systole is called the period of ejection. Ejection begins when left and right intraventricular pressure exceeds the pressure in the aorta and pulmonary artery, respectively. It should be noted that this point is the diastolic pulmonary artery and aortic pressure. Previous to ventricular systole, blood has been steadily leaving

both the pulmonary and systemic (aortic) arterial system, and intra-arterial pressure has been steadily dropping. The lowest intra-arterial pressure is attained just prior to actual ventricular ejection and is called diastolic pressure of the respective arteries. Normal diastolic pressure for the aorta and pulmonary artery is 60–90 mm Hg and 5–16 mm Hg, respectively.

7. The period of ejection is characterized by opening of the semilunar valves.

   a. During this time intraventricular pressure steadily increases above intra-arterial pressure, causing blood to leave the ventricles.

   b. Intraventricular pressure attains its maximum value (ventricular systolic pressure), followed by an increase in intra-arterial pressure to its maximum value (arterial systolic pressure).

   c. Normal right and left ventricular systolic pressure is 15–28 mm Hg and 90–140 mm Hg, respectively.

   d. Normal pulmonary artery and aortic systolic pressure is 15–28 mm Hg and 90–140 mm Hg, respectively.

   e. When ejection is complete, intra-arterial pressure and retrograde blood flow cause closing of aortic and pulmonic semilunar valves. This produces the second, or S_2, heart sound.

8. The total period of ejection causes a stroke volume of 70 ml to be added to each arterial system by the respective ventricles.

9. It should be noted that the end-diastolic volume of each ventricle is 145 ml and the stroke volume 70 ml. This results in a residual blood volume of each ventricle equal to 75 ml. The residual volume is called the end-systolic volume. All previous blood volume values are based on the normal resting heart.

10. Closure of aortic and pulmonic semilunar valves marks the beginning of ventricular diastole.

D. Ventricular diastole

   1. Mechanical left and right ventricular diastole begins after completion of the T wave of the ECG.

   2. Ventricular diastole begins with closure of the pulmonic and aortic semilunar valves and ends with onset of atrial systole.

   3. Tricuspid and mitral valves have remained closed all through the preceding ventricular systole and remain closed

in early ventricular diastole. This is because intraventricular pressure exceeds intra-atrial pressure.

4. The ventricles are functionally closed chambers with all cardiac valves remaining closed. Relaxation of the ventricular myocardium precipitates a large decrease in intraventricular pressure without a change in intraventricular blood volume.

5. When right and left intraventricular pressures drop below the respective intra-atrial pressures, the tricuspid and mitral valves open. This results in a rapid filling of each ventricle by intra-atrial blood, followed by passive distention of the ventricles by blood returning from the lung and periphery.

6. It should be noted that blood will continue to passively fill the ventricles through the AV valves, which remain open until the onset of ventricular systole. This slow but steady addition to ventricular volume is evidenced by a small increase in intra-atrial and intraventricular pressures.

7. The ventricular filling occurring during ventricular diastole accounts for 60%–80% of the end-diastolic volume.

8. The entire myocardium remains relaxed until the onset of the P wave and atrial systole initiate another cardiac cycle.

E. Summary of mechanical events of the cardiac cycle

1. After the P wave of the ECG, the atria contract, propelling blood through the open AV valves to the ventricles.

2. During the height of the following QRS complex, the ventricles contract in unison. It is during this same time that atrial relaxation occurs.

3. Intraventricular pressure soon rises above atrial pressure and causes the AV valves to close. This prevents retrograde flow of the blood from the ventricles to atria. Closure of the AV valves produces the S_1 heart sound.

4. Intraventricular pressure continues to rise rapidly and soon exceeds intra-arterial pressure. This causes the semilunar valves to open and provides blood flow from the ventricles to the arteries.

5. Relaxation of the ventricles occurs after completion of the T wave of the ECG.

6. As the ventricles relax, intraventricular pressure drops below the respective intra-arterial pressures. This causes the semilunar valves to close, preventing retrograde flow of blood from arteries to respective ventricles. Closure of the semilunar valves produces the S_2 heart sound.

7. Intraventricular pressure continues to drop until intraven-

tricular pressure falls below intra-atrial pressure. This causes the respective AV valves to open and provides blood flow from atria to ventricles.

8. Blood returning from pulmonary and systemic circulations continues to flow through the atria and open AV valves passively, filling the relaxed ventricles. This passive filling continues until the onset of the subsequent atrial contraction, which begins the next cardiac cycle.

VII. Cardiac Output
   A. The amount of blood pumped out of each ventricle is termed the cardiac output.
   B. The cardiac output of the right and left ventricles is equal and identical over a period of time.
   C. The cardiac output (CO) is equal to the stroke volume (SV) times the heart rate (HR):

$$CO = SV \times HR \qquad (1)$$

   1. The cardiac output is conventionally expressed in liters per minute.
      a. The normal range of cardiac output in a resting individual is 4–8 L/minute.
      b. *With stress or exercise, the cardiac output can increase five to six times its normal resting value.*
   2. The stroke volume is the amount of blood ejected from the ventricle with each ventricular systole.
      a. The stroke volume is expressed in milliliters per contraction.
      b. The normal range for the stroke volume of a resting individual is 60–130 ml per contraction.
   3. The heart rate is the number of times the heart contracts per minute. The normal range for the heart rate of a resting individual is 60–100 contractions per minute.
   4. *Example:*
      An individual with a stroke volume equal to 70 ml per contraction and a heart rate of 80 contractions per minute would have a cardiac output of 5,600 ml/minute or 5.6 L/minute by the following calculation:

$$\frac{70 \text{ ml}}{\text{contraction}} \times \frac{80 \text{ contractions}}{\text{minute}} = \frac{5,600 \text{ ml}}{\text{minute}} \text{ or } \frac{5.6 \text{ L}}{\text{minute}} \qquad (2)$$

   5. It should be evident that increases in cardiac output are brought about by increases in the heart rate and/or stroke

volume, and that decreases in cardiac output are brought
about by decreases in heart rate and/or stroke volume.

D. Control of heart rate

1. It should be recalled that heart rate is set by the pacemaker
of the heart (SA node). The number of times per minute that
the SA node depolarizes is largely governed by neural and
chemical factors.

2. The neural factors that affect heart rate are mediated
through the two divisions of the autonomic nervous system,
i.e., the parasympathetic and sympathetic nervous systems.

  a. Parasympathetic impulses are conducted to the SA node
through cranial nerve X (vagus nerve).

    (1) Parasympathetic effects on the SA node are inhibitory
and decrease the heart rate.

    (2) The result of decreasing the heart rate is called neg-
ative chronotropism. Thus the parasympathetic nervous system exhibits negative chronotropic effects.

  b. Sympathetic impulses are conducted to the SA node
through sympathetic nerve fibers originating from the
upper thoracic (T1–T5) segment of the spinal cord.

    (1) Sympathetic effects on the SA node are excitatory
and increase the heart rate.

    (2) The result of increasing the heart rate is called posi-
tive chronotropism. Thus the sympathetic nervous
system exhibits positive chronotropic effects.

  c. The sympathetic and parasympathetic nervous systems
are generally considered antagonists. However, in bringing about changes in heart rate, the two divisions of the
autonomic nervous system complement each other.

    (1) However, each nervous system can perform both
positive and negative chronotropism. Under certain
clinical conditions, heart rate is altered by selective
activities of one division of the autonomic nervous
system.

    (2) In general, the parasympathetic nervous system is
the dominant division of the neural input into the SA
node. This is evidenced by total autonomic blockade,
resulting in mild tachycardia.

  d. Neural control of heart rate also is mediated through
higher brain centers, e.g., the cerebral cortex and hypothalamus.

    (1) The cerebral cortex is responsible for changes in

heart rate in response to emotional factors, e.g., anxiety, fear, anger, and grief.

    (2) The hypothalamus appears responsible for changes in heart rate in response to alterations in both local and environmental temperature.

  3. Major chemical factors that affect heart rate: electrolytes, exogenously administered drugs, and hormones.

    a. The three major electrolytes having effects on the heart rate are potassium, sodium, and calcium.

      (1) Excess potassium and sodium have the effect of decreasing the heart rate.

      (2) Excess calcium causes an increase in the heart rate.

      (3) Potassium and sodium imbalance can alter cardiac membrane permeability and thus slow or speed the rate of electric conduction through the myocardium.

      (4) However, only electrolyte *imbalance* brings about such changes in heart rate.

    b. Classes of drugs that exert an effect on heart rate by either mimicking or inhibiting the activity of the sympathetic or parasympathetic nervous system:

      (1) Sympathomimetics such as isoproterenol or epinephrine mimic the activity of the sympathetic nervous system and cause positive chronotropism.

      (2) Sympatholytics such as dichloroisoproterenol or propranolol inhibit the activity of the sympathetic nervous system and cause negative chronotropism.

      (3) Parasympathomimetics such as metacholine, pilocarpine, or neostigmine mimic the activity of the parasympathetic nervous system and cause negative chronotropism.

      (4) Parasympatholytics such as atropine inhibit the activity of the parasympathetic nervous system and cause positive chronotropism.

    c. The major hormones that affect the heart rate are the adrenomedullary hormones.

      (1) The adrenal medulla secretes epinephrine and norepinephrine into the circulating blood.

      (2) These two naturally occurring catecholamines have direct positive chronotropic effects on the heart.

  4. *Heart rate is under many influences,* ranging from conscious control by the cerebral cortex to exogenously administered pharmacologic agents. The most important regulatory con-

trol of heart rate is mediated through the autonomic nervous system.

E. Control of stroke volume

    1. Size of stroke volume: Governed by preload, afterload, and state of contractility of ventricles.

        a. *Preload:* Degree of ventricular diastolic filling before ejection begins, or the presystolic ventricular loading force.

            (1) The Frank-Starling law states that the more the heart is filled during diastole, the greater the subsequent force of contraction. This results in increased stroke volume (Fig 7–4, curve A).

            (2) This relationship is primarily related to presystolic myocardial fiber length.

            (3) Presystolic fiber length is directly related to end-diastolic volume, for it is the actual intraventricular blood volume coupled with the compliance characteristics of the ventricle that results in myocardial fiber stretch.

            (4) Since myocardial fiber length is virtually impossible to measure in the intact heart, it would seem that end-diastolic volume is an appropriate parameter for assessing preload.

                (a) The first factor affecting end-diastolic volume is the presence of a total blood volume sufficient for

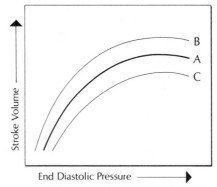

Fig 7–4.—The Frank-Starling relationship. *A,* control; *B,* positive inotropism; *C,* negative inotropism (see text). (From Shapiro B.A., Harrison R.A., Kacmarek R.M., et al.: *Clinical Application of Respiratory Care,* ed. 3. Chicago, Year Book Medical Publishers, Inc., 1985. Reproduced by permission.)

an effective vascular volume to vascular space relationship. There must be an adequate blood volume within the vascular space for the heart to cir-
culate blood effectively. It is the *relationship*
between vascular volume to vascular space that is
crucial, not the absolute values of either vascular
volume or vascular space.

(b) The state of the venous tone is the second factor
affecting end-diastolic volume. The relationship
between vascular volume and vascular space is
essential to ensure adequate venous return and
ventricular filling. It should be noted that 60%–
80% of ventricular filling is accomplished by passive return of blood from the veins. The state of
venous tone regulates venous vascular space, and
it is therefore as crucial as blood volume in determining adequacy of venous return.

(c) The third major factor that affects end-diastolic
volume is force of atrial systole. As mentioned,
20%–40% of ventricular filling is accomplished
by atrial systole. This is not of critical importance
in the normal heart but becomes paramount in
any cardiac dysfunction where ventricular compliance is decreased (i.e., ventricular hypertrophy
or myocardial infarction).

(d) The fourth major factor that affects end-diastolic
volume is compliance of the ventricle. As mentioned, this factor is not of importance in the normal heart, but decreases in ventricular compliance require a greater filling pressure per unit
volume change. Thus, increased filling pressure
is necessary or the end-diastolic volume will have
a reduced value.

(e) End-diastolic volume is an acceptable parameter
for assessing preload; however, this too is difficult
to measure with any accuracy in the intact heart.
The most easily measured parameter that reflects
preload is ventricular end-diastolic pressure.

(5) Given a constant ventricular compliance, it may be
inferred that ventricular end-diastolic pressure should
correlate well with ventricular end-diastolic volume.
Accepting the latter as true, myocardial fiber length

can be expressed as a function of end-diastolic pressure.

   (a) In clinical practice, preload is assessed by measuring ventricular end-diastolic pressure.

   (b) Right ventricular preload is assessed by end-diastolic pressure measurements taken from a central venous pressure (CVP) catheter as central venous pressure (see Chap. 14).

   (c) Left ventricular preload is assessed by end-diastolic pressure measurements taken from a pulmonary artery catheter as pulmonary wedge pressure (see Chap. 14).

   (d) In general, the higher the end-diastolic pressure (preload), the greater the subsequent ventricular contraction and resulting stroke volume.

(6) The Frank-Starling relationship is the basis for (1) matching cardiac output to venous return and (2) balancing the output of right and left ventricles. For example, if venous return to the right atrium has suddenly increased because increased venous tone has altered the vascular volume/vascular space relationship:

   (a) Increased venous return to the right ventricle would increase the right ventricular end-diastolic volume.

   (b) Increased end-diastolic volume would result in an increased myocardial fiber length.

   (c) Increased myocardial fiber length would in turn result in an increased force of contraction of the right ventricle.

   (d) Increased force of contraction of the right ventricle would result in an increased right ventricular stroke volume, all other factors remaining equal.

   (e) It should be noted that two phenomena have occurred. (1) Venous blood has been mobilized back to the heart, and the increased venous return has been matched by an increase in right ventricular stroke volume. This is one of the major ways that cardiac output is increased. (2) Right ventricular output now exceeds left ventricular output.

   (f) Increased right ventricular output will result in

increased venous return to the left atrium and left ventricle.

(g) In similar fashion, increased venous return to the left ventricle increases left ventricular end-diastolic volume.

(h) The increased end-diastolic volume would result in increasing the left ventricular myocardial fiber length. This in turn would result in an increase in the force of contraction of the left ventricle.

(i) The increased force of contraction of the left ventricle would result in an increased left ventricular stroke volume.

(j) At this point venous blood has been mobilized from the venous reservoirs and has resulted in increased output from both the right and left sides of the heart. Furthermore, left ventricular output is in equilibrium with right ventricular output—all in accordance with the Frank-Starling relationship.

(k) The regulatory function of the Frank-Starling mechanism is frequently referred to as "autoregulation" in that it is an intrinsic factor based on the architecture of the myocardial fibers, which automatically regulate cardiac output to equal venous return. Thus it has led physiologists over the years to make the statement that "within the physiologic limits of the heart, it will pump out all the blood it receives without allowing a backup of blood into the venous system."

b. *Afterload:* Resistance to flow from the ventricles.

(1) The work the heart must perform in order to pump blood out of the ventricles and into the circulation depends on three major factors: resistance of the semilunar valves, blood viscosity, and arterial blood pressure.

(a) As resistance of the semilunar valves (i.e., pulmonic or aortic stenosis) increases, afterload will be increased.

(b) As blood viscosity increases (i.e., hyperproteinemia or polycythemia), afterload will be increased.

(c) As arterial blood pressure increases (pulmonary

or systemic hypertension), afterload will be increased.

  (d) Decreases in any of these three parameters result in decreasing the afterload.

(2) Increases in afterload result in increases of ventricular work:

  (a) The greater the resistance against which the ventricle must contract to eject blood, the more slowly it contracts.

  (b) Increased afterload results in a decreased stroke volume, which initially increases end-systolic volume. The normal venous return will then be added to the already increased end-systolic volume and increase the end-diastolic volume above normal. This allows a more forceful contraction against an increased afterload as a result of the Frank-Starling mechanism. This enables the ventricle to pump a given stroke volume against an increased afterload. *This compensation is at the expense of an increase in ventricular size.* The larger the heart the greater the work necessary to develop the myocardial tension required to produce a given intraventricular pressure (Laplace's law).

  (c) Both the slower rate of contraction and the increased ventricular size result in greater oxygen requirements to perform a given amount of work than that of the normal heart.

(3) Thus, increases in afterload may or may not cause a decrease in stroke volume, but will cause increases in myocardial work.

(4) Decreases in afterload, commonly called "after-load reduction," may or may not cause an increase in stroke volume, but will cause decreases in myocardial work.

(5) In general, the poorer the cardiac function, the more dependent is the stroke volume on afterload.

  (a) Increases in afterload tend to decrease stroke volume in the patient with poor cardiac function.

  (b) Increases in afterload do not cause decreases in stroke volume in the patient with normal cardiac function.

(c) Decreases in afterload tend to increase stroke volume in the patient with poor cardiac function.

(d) Decreases in afterload generally do not cause increases in stroke volume in the patient with normal cardiac function.

(6) In the absence of valvular disease, afterload is clinically assessed by measuring mean arterial blood pressure.

(a) Right ventricular afterload is assessed by mean pulmonary artery measurements taken via a pulmonary artery catheter.

(b) Left ventricular afterload is assessed by mean systemic arterial pressure measurements taken via an intra-arterial (systemic) catheter.

c. *State of ventricular contractility:* Force with which the ventricles contract.

(1) The force of contraction of the ventricles at any given preload and afterload depends on the state of contractility (see Fig 7–4).

(a) An increase in the state of ventricular contractility for a given preload and afterload is termed positive inotropism.

(b) A decrease in the state of ventricular contractility for a given preload and afterload is termed negative inotropism.

(c) The net effect of positive inotropism is generally a greater volume output per unit time.

(d) The net effect of negative inotropism is generally a smaller volume output per unit time.

(2) Ventricular contractility is altered by the sympathetic and parasympathetic nervous systems, blood gases (PO_2, PCO_2), pH, hormones, and exogenously administered drugs.

(3) The sympathetic nervous system extensively innervates the atrial and ventricular myocardium.

(a) Postganglionic nerve fibers of the sympathetic nervous system release norepinephrine to β (Beta) receptor sites in the atrial and ventricular myocardium.

(b) This increases contractility of the myocardium; positive inotropism. Thus the sympathetic nervous system displays positive inotropic effects.

(c) Alterations in sympathetic discharge to the myocardium are believed to constitute the most important regulatory control of ventricular contractility.

(4) The parasympathetic nervous system only minutely innervates the atrial myocardium, and the ventricular myocardium is innervated even more sparsely.

(a) Postganglionic nerve fibers of the parasympathetic nervous system release acetylcholine to the muscarinic receptor sites of the atrial and ventricular myocardium.

(b) As previously mentioned, due to the scantiness of parasympathetic innervation, the result is only a mild decrease in myocardial contractility, or a slight negative inotropism. Thus the parasympathetic nervous system displays minor negative inotropic effects.

(5) Effects of blood gases on myocardial contractility:

(a) Mild decreases in PO_2 result in increased contractility, whereas severe drops in PO_2 result in decreased myocardial contractility.

(b) Increases in PCO_2 result in decreased contractility, whereas decreases in PCO_2 result in increased myocardial contractility.

(c) Metabolic or respiratory acidosis results directly in decreased contractility, whereas metabolic and respiratory alkalosis may alter contractility through electric conduction dysfunction and arrhythmia.

(6) The most important hormones affecting myocardial contractility are the adrenomedullary hormones.

(a) As previously stated, the adrenal medulla secretes epinephrine and norepinephrine into the circulating blood.

(b) These two naturally occurring catecholamines have direct positive inotropic effects on the myocardium.

(c) The major differences between the effects of the catecholamines and direct sympathetic stimulation are that the effects of catecholamines take longer to establish but last longer.

(d) This is true of the effect of catecholamines on both contractility and heart rate.

(7) The following exogenously administered drugs can alter myocardial contractility:

    (a) The sympatholytics (e.g., propranolol) produce negative inotropic effects through β-receptor blockade.

    (b) The sympathomimetics (e.g., isoproterenol or epinephrine) produce positive inotropic effects through β-receptor stimulation.

    (c) Some antiarrhythmics (e.g., quinidine or procainamide) produce negative inotropic effects.

    (d) Derivatives of digitalis produce positive inotropic effects.

(8) Myocardial contractility is an elusive parameter to assess clinically. However, controversial attempts have been made to quantitate it.

(9) It should be remembered that the stroke volume is under a gamut of influences. However, any stroke volume is determined by the interrelation of preload, afterload, and the state of ventricular contractility.

VIII. Control of Arterial Blood Pressure

  A. Under normal circumstances, arterial blood volume exceeds arterial vascular space. This relationship results in an intravascular pressure dictated by the absolute arterial blood volume and the elastic properties of the arterial vasculature.

  B. The arterial system is continually receiving blood (inflow) from the left ventricle as cardiac output and continually allowing blood to leave the arterial system (outflow) as arterial runoff.

  C. It is the balance or imbalance between cardiac output (inflow) and arterial runoff (outflow) that results in any given arterial blood volume.

  D. The relationship between arterial blood volume and arterial vascular space is the primary determinant of arterial blood pressure.

  E. Thus, by the equation $P = \dot{Q} \times R$, it can be demonstrated that cardiac output ($\dot{Q}$) and peripheral resistance (R) are directly related to arterial blood pressure (P). Arterial blood pressure is dependent on alteration of the blood volume to vascular space relationship by cardiac output and/or peripheral resistance, as follows:

    1. Increases in peripheral resistance (i.e., vasoconstriction) re-

sult in decreasing the arterial runoff. If cardiac output remains the same, then inflow exceeds outflow from the arterial vasculature. This results in an increase in the arterial blood volume to vascular space relationship and a concomitant increase in arterial blood pressure.

2. Decreases in peripheral resistance (i.e., vasodilation) result in decreasing the arterial blood pressure by the exact opposite mechanism.

3. Increases in cardiac output result in increasing the rate of inflow to the arterial system. If peripheral resistance remains the same, then inflow exceeds outflow from the arterial vasculature. This results in an increase in the arterial blood volume to vascular space relationship and an increase in arterial blood pressure.

4. Decreases in cardiac output result in decreasing arterial blood pressure by the exactly opposite mechanism.

5. It should be noted that in the four examples above the imbalance between inflow and outflow is only temporary. It is by these mechanisms that arterial blood pressure can be increased or decreased. Once the desired arterial pressure is attained, the balance between inflow and outflow will maintain the pressure at that level.

F. As has been described, cardiac output and peripheral resistance are for a large part under neural control. Therefore it becomes apparent that regulation of arterial blood pressure is mediated through neural alterations in cardiac output and peripheral resistance.

G. Neural regulation of arterial blood pressure is mediated through autonomic fibers that originate from an area of the medulla oblongata. This area of the medulla is sometimes called the "cardiovascular center."

H. The cardiovascular center may be functionally divided into four subcenters: The vasomotor excitatory (vasoconstrictor) center, vasomotor inhibitory (vasodilator) center, cardiac excitatory center, and cardiac inhibitory center.

1. The vasomotor excitatory center influences the arterioles through the sympathetic nervous system. The degree of vasoconstriction or vasodilation is directly related to the amount of sympathetic stimulation.

2. The vasomotor inhibitory center does not influence the arterioles directly but acts by inhibiting the activity of the vasomotor excitatory center.

3. The cardiac excitatory center influences the heart through the sympathetic nervous system. Sympathetic stimulation originating from this center results in positive inotropic and chronotropic effects.

4. The cardiac inhibitory center influences the heart through the parasympathetic nervous system. Parasympathetic stimulation originating from this center results in a negative chronotropic effect and a mild negative inotropic effect.

I. The cardiovascular center in the medulla receives sensory input from the entire body. The most important sources of sensory input are the exteroceptors, higher brain centers, local factors, peripheral chemoreceptors, and baroreceptors.

1. Exteroceptors (e.g., proprioceptors, thermal receptors, and pain receptors) are sources of sensory input. Stimulation of the proprioceptors, pain receptors, and thermal receptors through muscular activation, pain, and heat, respectively, results in an increase in heart rate. This potentially will increase arterial blood pressure. Cold and muscular inactivity slow the heart rate and potentially decrease arterial blood pressure.

2. Higher brain centers (e.g., the cerebral cortex and hypothalamus) have medullary input.

   a. Emotional factors alter blood pressure by mediation through the cerebral cortex. Fear or anger usually increases the blood pressure by stimulating the vasomotor and cardiac excitatory centers. This stimulation results in vasoconstriction and an increase in heart rate. However, decreases in blood pressure can be mediated through the cerebrum by stimulation of the vasomotor inhibitory center, as in fainting or blushing.

   b. The hypothalamus mediates its control on the vasomotor inhibitory center in response to increases in body temperature. This causes vasodilation of the vessels of the skin and loss of body heat. A decrease in body temperature will result in vasoconstriction of the vessels of the skin with heat conservation as mediated through the hypothalamus.

   c. Direct stimulation of the anterior portion of the hypothalamus produces bradycardia and a decrease in arterial blood pressure, whereas stimulation of the posterior portion of the hypothalamus produces tachycardia and an increase in arterial blood pressure.

3. The vasomotor inhibitory and excitatory centers are sensitive to local and direct effects of pH and P_{CO_2} of arterial blood perfusing these centers.
   a. Local increases in arterial pH and decreases in P_{CO_2} cause depression of the vasomotor excitatory center by the vasomotor inhibitory center. This results in vasodilation, a decrease in peripheral resistance, and a decrease in arterial blood pressure.
   b. Local decreases in arterial pH and increases in P_{CO_2} cause direct excitation of the vasomotor excitatory center. This results in vasoconstriction, an increase in peripheral resistance, and an increase in arterial blood pressure.
   c. A local drop in P_{O_2} of arterial blood potentiates the vasoconstrictor effect but alone has no local effect.
4. Peripheral chemoreceptors (aortic and carotid bodies) are responsible for initiating the vasomotor chemoreflex.
   a. Hypoxemia, hypercapnia, and acidemia all stimulate the peripheral chemoreceptors.
   b. The stimulated chemoreceptors in turn send an increased number of afferent impulses to the vasomotor excitatory center, with resultant vasoconstriction. This increases peripheral resistance and arterial blood pressure.
   c. When hypoxemia and hypercapnia or hypoxemia and acidemia exist, the chemoreceptors display a synergistic effect. That is, the stimulation arising from the chemoreceptors secondary to two simultaneous stimuli is greater than the mathematical sum of the two stimuli when they act alone. This results in a more profound vasoconstriction and an increase in blood pressure.
5. Baroreceptors are by far the most important short-acting regulator of arterial blood pressure.
   a. Baroreceptors (pressoreceptors) are stretch receptors located in the arch of the aorta and carotid sinus.
   b. They respond to changes in pressure, which stretch them to different degrees. The greater the pressure, the greater the number of impulses the baroreceptors will send.
   c. With a drop in arterial blood pressure, the number of impulses sent by the baroreceptors decreases. This decreased number of inhibitory impulses causes the vasomotor excitatory and cardiac excitatory centers to become more active. This results in increased cardiac output and

increased peripheral resistance, thus restoring arterial blood pressure to normal.

d. With an increase in arterial blood pressure, the number of impulses sent out by the baroreceptors increases. This increased number of inhibitory impulses causes the vasomotor excitatory center to become depressed directly and indirectly through increased activity of the vasomotor inhibitory center. In addition, the increased number of inhibitory impulses depresses the cardiac excitatory center and stimulates the cardiac inhibitory center, resulting in a decreased heart rate. Thus, peripheral resistance and cardiac output decrease, restoring normal blood pressure.

BIBLIOGRAPHY

Anthony C.P., Kolthoff N.J.: *Textbook of Anatomy and Physiology*, ed. 8. St. Louis, C.V. Mosby Co., 1971.

Ayres S.M., Giannelli S.J., Mueller H.S.: *Care of the Critically Ill*, ed. 2. New York, Appleton-Century-Crofts, 1974.

Crowley L.V.: *Introductory Concepts in Anatomy and Physiology*. Chicago, Year Book Medical Publishers, Inc., 1976.

Gray H., Goss C.M.: *Gray's Anatomy of the Human Body*, ed. 29. Philadelphia, Lea & Febiger, 1973.

Guyton A.C.: *Textbook of Medical Physiology*, ed. 5. Philadelphia, W.B. Saunders Co., 1976.

Jacob S.W., Francone C.A.: *Structure and Function in Man*, ed. 3. Philadelphia, W.B. Saunders Co., 1974.

Little R.C.: *Physiology of the Heart and Circulation*. Chicago, Year Book Medical Publishers, Inc., 1977.

McLaughlin A.J.: *Essentials of Physiology for Advanced Respiratory Therapy*. St. Louis, C.V. Mosby Co., 1977.

Mountcastle V.B.: *Medical Physiology*, ed. 14. St. Louis, C.V. Mosby Co., 1980.

Ross G.: *Essentials of Human Physiology*. Chicago, Year Book Medical Publishers, Inc., 1978.

Ruch T.C., Patton H.D.: *Physiology and Biophysics*, ed. 20. Philadelphia, W.B. Saunders Co., 1974.

Rushmer R.F.: *Cardiovascular Dynamics*, ed. 3. Philadelphia, W.B. Saunders Co., 1970.

Schroeder J.S., Daily E.K.: *Techniques in Bedside Hemodynamic Monitoring*. St. Louis, C.V. Mosby Co., 1976.

Shapiro B.A., Harrison R.A., Kacmarek R.M., et al.: *Clinical Application of Respiratory Care*, ed. 3. Chicago, Year Book Medical Publishers, Inc., 1985.

8 / Anatomy and Physiology of the Nervous System

I. Structure of the Nerve Fiber
   A. Each nerve fiber has three components.
      1. Cell body or soma: Primary metabolic area, site of initial synthesis of transmitter substance.
      2. Dendrite: Normally the structures that carry impulses *to* the cell body. A single neuron may contain 10,000 dendrites.
      3. Axon: Normally the structure that conducts impulses *away* from the cell body. Usually only one axon leaves a cell body; however, it may branch extensively.
II. Classification of Neurons
   A. Each neuron is classified by the direction of impulse transmission.
      1. Sensory (afferent) neurons: Transmit nerve impulses to the spinal cord or brain.
      2. Motor (efferent) neurons: Transmit nerve impulses from the brain or spinal cord to muscles or glands (effector organ).
      3. Interneurons (internuncial): Conduct impulses from sensory to motor neurons entirely within central nervous system (CNS).
III. Nerve Cell Membrane Potential
   A. In the resting state, the inner surface of the cell membrane is negative as compared to the positive outer surface. This sets up an electric potential across the cell membrane (normal polarity).
      1. Intracellular: The primary cation, potassium (K^+), is readily diffusible across the cell membrane.
      2. Extracellular: The primary cation, sodium (Na^+), is poorly diffusible across the cell membrane.
      3. High extracellular Na^+ and low extracellular K^+ levels, along with high intracellular K^+ and low intracellular Na^+ levels, are maintained in the resting state by the *Na pump* (active transport).
      4. The continual diffusion of K^+ to the outside of the membrane sets up a negative intracellular membrane charge and a positive extracellular membrane charge.

142

IV. Action Potential
   A. In order for a nerve impulse to be transmitted, an alteration in the cell's resting membrane potential must be achieved.
   B. An action potential is a stimulus that is capable of significantly increasing the cell membrane's permeability to sodium.
   C. The action potential is an all-or-nothing phenomenon. That is, the stimulus must be strong enough to allow for a reversal in membrane potential; if it is not, an action potential does not occur.
   D. An action potential may be caused by:
      1. Electric stimulation
      2. Chemicals
      3. Mechanical damage to membrane
      4. Heat or cold
      5. Decreased serum calcium (Ca^{+2}), which increases the tendency for development of an action potential (low calcium tetany).

V. Nerve Impulse Propagation
   A. The nerve impulse is a self-propagating wave of electric charge that travels along the surface of the neuron's membrane. The nerve impulse travels in one direction only, from dendrite to cell body to axon.
   B. Depolarization: Stage 1 of the action potential, in which an impulse travels along the nerve fiber.
      1. Sodium ions rush to the inside of the cell membrane.
      2. A positive intracellular membrane charge is set up with a negative extracellular membrane charge.
      3. There is a complete reversal of the membrane potential.
   C. Repolarization: Stage 2 of the action potential, in which the membrane returns to the normal resting membrane potential.
      1. Immediately after the impulse passes a point on the membrane, the membrane's permeability to Na^+ is again decreased.
      2. Na^+ ions are actively removed from the cell by the Na pump.
      3. The resting membrane potential is reestablished.

VI. Nerve Synapse
   A. The nerve synapse (synaptic cleft) is the junction between one neuron and another neuron, muscle, or gland. It is an actual space between nerve fibers.
   B. Transmission of an impulse from the axon of one nerve to a dendrite, soma, or effector organ is a chemical process occurring

across the synapse. The distance across the synapse is about 200 Å.

C. Presynaptic terminals are located on the axon and contain vesicles that synthesize, store, and secrete a transmitter substance into the synapse. The transmitter substance stimulates the dendrite or soma of the next nerve, causing an action potential.
1. Primary transmitter substances of the peripheral nervous system are:
   a. Acetylcholine
   b. Norepinephrine

D. Postsynaptic terminals are located on dendrites, somas, or effector organs. After being stimulated, these terminals secrete a substance into the synapse to metabolize the transmitter substance.

E. Acetylcholine as the transmitter substance (Fig 8–1)
1. Acetylcholine is synthesized, stored, and released from the presynaptic vesicles. It is formed from the reaction of acetyl coenzyme A with choline.

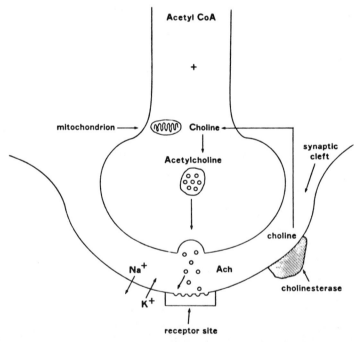

Fig 8–1.—Synthesis, storage, release, and inactivation of acetylcholine (see text). (From Rau J.L.: *Respiratory Therapy Pharmacology,* ed. 2. Chicago, Year Book Medical Publishers, Inc., 1984. Reproduced by permission.)

2. These vesicles are formed in the cell body and migrate to the surface of the presynaptic terminal.

3. When an action potential reaches the presynaptic terminal, acetylcholine is released into the synapse.

4. The acetylcholine moves across the synapse and stimulates a receptor on the postsynaptic terminal.

5. After stimulation the acetylcholine is released back into the synapse and the postsynaptic terminal releases cholinesterase (acetylcholinesterase, or acetylcholine esterase are terms synonymous with cholinesterase) which metabolizes acetylcholine, forming choline and acetic acid.

6. The choline is reabsorbed into the presynaptic terminal and is available to form more acetylcholine.

F. Norepinephrine as the transmitter substance (Fig 8–2)

1. Norepinephrine is synthesized, stored, and released from the presynaptic vesicles.

2. The synthesis of norepinephrine proceeds via three reactions:

$$\text{Tyrosine} \rightarrow \text{Dopa}$$
$$\text{Dopa} \rightarrow \text{Dopamine}$$
$$\text{Dopamine} \rightarrow \text{Norepinephrine}$$

3. Norepinephrine is released via a mechanism identical to acetylcholine (see section VI-E).

4. After stimulation, norepinephrine has two possible immediate fates:

a. Metabolism in the synapse by catechol-o-methyl-transferase (COMT).

b. Reabsorption into the presynaptic terminal.

5. Within the presynaptic terminal, norepinephrine has one of two fates:

a. Reabsorption by the presynaptic vesicles.

b. Metabolism in the cytoplasm by monoamine oxidase (MAO).

6. Complete metabolism of products formed in the synapse occurs in the liver via both MAO and COMT.

VII. Alteration of Nerve Impulse Transmission

A. Acidosis decreases transmission across the synapse.

B. Alkalosis increases transmission across the synapse.

VIII. Neuromuscular Junction

A. This junction is the site of transmission of impulses from nerves to skeletal muscle fibers.

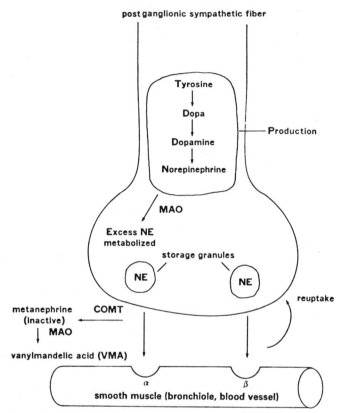

Fig 8–2.—Synthesis, storage, release, and inactivation of norepinephrine (see text). (From Rau J.L.: *Respiratory Therapy Pharmacology,* ed. 2, Chicago, Year Book Medical Publishers, Inc., 1984. Reproduced by permission.)

    B. The axon of the nerve branches at its end to form a structure called the motor end-plate, which invaginates into muscle fiber but does not penetrate the muscle membrane.

    C. The motor end-plate's terminal aspects are referred to as sole feet.

    D. Sole feet provide a large area of "contact" on the muscle surface. It is from the sole feet that the transmitter substance acetylcholine is secreted.

    E. After stimulation, cholinesterase is secreted to metabolize acetylcholine.

IX. Reflex Arc or Reflex Action

    A. The reflex arc is a functional process of the nervous system. Most neuromuscular and neuroglandular mechanisms are controlled by it.

B. The reflex arc consists of a series of neurons in which impulses are transmitted from a receptor to the CNS, and then to a motor neuron to elicit a response.

C. Most simple reflexes consist of an impulse from a sensory neuron being transmitted (normally in the spinal cord) to a motor neuron.

D. Complex reflexes may involve many internuncial neurons.

E. Reflex actions are involuntary, specific, predictable, and adaptive.

X. Organization of the Nervous System

    A. The nervous system is composed of the brain, spinal cord, ganglia (aggregations of nerve cell bodies), and nerves, which regulate and coordinate bodily activities.

    B. Divisions of the nervous system

        1. The CNS is composed of the brain and spinal cord, which acts as a switchboard, receiving and sending impulses to all areas of the body.

        2. The peripheral nervous system is composed of neurons that enter and leave the CNS. The peripheral nervous system has two main divisions:

            a. Somatic nervous system, which is responsible for voluntary bodily functions.

            b. Autonomic nervous system (ANS), which is responsible for involuntary bodily functions.

    C. Central nervous system

        1. The CNS is subdivided into the following structures:

            a. Cerebral cortex

            b. Diencephalon

                (1) Thalamus

                (2) Subthalamus

                (3) Hypothalamus

            c. Brain stem

                (1) Medulla

                (2) Pons

                (3) Midbrain

                (4) Cerebellum

            d. Spinal cord

        2. The cerebral cortex is primarily responsible for:

            a. All higher brain functions (i.e., memory, reasoning, sight, hearing, etc.)

b. Integration of all sensory stimuli

c. Voluntary control of bodily activities

3. The diencephalon is located between the cerebral cortex and the brain stem between the hemispheres of the cerebral cortex. It contains the following structures:

   a. Thalamus

      (1) Primary relay station of the brain for:

         (a) Hearing

         (b) Touch

         (c) Pressure

         (d) Position

         (e) Pain

      (2) Site of action of many psychoactive drugs.

   b. The subthalamus is responsible for the coordination of fine motor activity (extrapyramidal) with the cerebellum.

   c. Hypothalamus

      (1) It is responsible for many of the organism's vegetative functions via the ANS and hormonal control.

         (a) Eating

         (b) Drinking

         (c) Sleeping

         (d) Temperature

         (e) Sexual behavior

         (f) Fluid and electrolyte balance

      (2) The hypothalamus assists in the modulation of emotion and behavior.

      (3) Many psychoactive drugs are active at the hypothalamus.

4. The brain stem lies within the cranium and connects the diencephalon with the spinal cord. It contains the following structures:

   a. Medulla

      (1) The medulla contains control centers for the following:

         (a) Respiration

         (b) Peripheral vasoconstriction

         (c) Gastrointestinal function

         (d) Sleeping

         (e) Walking

      (2) The ascending reticular activating system (ARAS) travels through the medulla. The ARAS helps to modulate behavior.

      b. The pons contains two centers that effect respiration (see Chap. 5).

        (1) Apneustic center

        (2) Pneumotaxic center

      c. The midbrain acts as a relay station, controlling vision and hearing.

      d. The cerebellum coordinates fine motor activity with the subthalamus.

    5. Spinal cord

      a. Channels information from the brain to the periphery.

      b. Most reflexes are coordinated via the spinal cord.

D. Somatic nervous system (Fig 8–3).

    1. Responsible for all voluntary muscular activities.

    2. Contains both sensory and motor neurons.

    3. Ganglia are located within the spinal cord.

E. Autonomic nervous system

    1. Contains only motor neurons (see Fig 8–3).

    2. Uses input via the somatic nervous system that is coordinated by the CNS.

    3. Each nerve of the ANS has a ganglion outside of the spinal cord.

    4. The ANS is responsible for all involuntary bodily activities.

    5. It is subdivided into:

      a. Parasympathetic (craniosacral) nervous system.

      b. Sympathetic (thoracolumbar) nervous system.

    6. The two divisions are basically antagonistic.

    7. The ANS is activated and controlled primarily by:

      a. Spinal cord

      b. Brain stem

      c. Hypothalamus

    8. It is activated secondarily by:

      a. Cerebral cortex

      b. Visceral reflexes

    9. Sympathetic nervous system: Nerves of the SNS originate from the spinal cord at levels T–1 (thoracic) through L–2 (lumbar).

      a. Nerve fibers that transmit SNS impulses are either:

        (1) Preganglionic fibers

        (2) Postganglionic fibers

      b. The SNS fibers synapse primarily at ganglia located along the spinal cord. Here they form a chain of interconnecting ganglia referred to as the sympathetic chain.

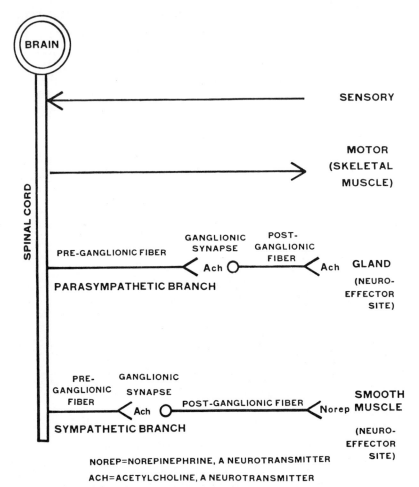

Fig 8–3.—Functional comparison of the central nervous system and the peripheral nervous system. (From Rau J.L.: *Respiratory Therapy Pharmacology*, ed. 2. Chicago, Year Book Medical Publishers, Inc., 1984. Reproduced by permission.)

    c. Some SNS fibers synapse at peripheral ganglia (celiac ganglion and hypogastric plexus), bypassing the sympathetic chain.

    d. Transmitter substances of the SNS:

        (1) Preganglionic fiber: Acetylcholine.

        (2) Postganglionic fiber: Norepinephrine.

    e. Transmitter substance metabolism:

(1) Acetylcholine: Metabolized by cholinesterase.
(2) Norepinephrine: Metabolized by MAO or COMT.
10. Parasympathetic nervous system (PNS): Nerves of the PNS originate from sacral nerves 1 through 4 and cranial nerves III, VII, IX, and X. Eighty percent (80%) of all PNS impulses originate from *cranial nerve X (vagus nerve)*.
   a. Nerve fibers that transmit PNS impulses are either:
      (1) Preganglionic fiber
      (2) Postganglionic fiber
   b. These fibers synapse at the ganglia of the PNS, which are located very close to the organs they innervate.
   c. The transmitter substance for both preganglionic and postganglionic fibers is acetylcholine (metabolized by cholinesterase) (Table 8–1).
F. Adrenal medulla: Secretes epinephrine (75% by volume) and norepinephrine (25% by volume) into the bloodstream, resulting in stimulation of the SNS.
   1. Innervation is via specific preganglionic fibers of the SNS.
   2. Adrenal secretions assist in maintaining normal tone of the SNS.
G. Effects of activation of the SNS and PNS:
   1. Adrenergic effect: An effect activated or transmitted by norephinephrine or epinephrine
   2. Adrenergic receptor: A receptor stimulated by norepinephrine or epinephrine
   3. Cholinergic effect: An effect activated or transmitted by acetylcholine

TABLE 8–1.—COMPARISON OF THE SYMPATHETIC NERVOUS SYSTEM AND THE PARASYMPATHETIC NERVOUS SYSTEM

FEATURE	SNS	PNS
Origin of nerve fibers from the CNS	T-1 to L-2	S-1 to S-4; cranial nerves III, VII, IX, X
Relative length:		
Preganglionic fiber	Short	Long
Postganglionic fiber	Long	Short
Transmitter substance:		
Preganglionic fiber	Acetylcholine	Acetylcholine
Postganglionic fiber	Norepinephrine	Acetylcholine
Transmitter substance metabolized by:		
Preganglionic fiber	Cholinesterase	Cholinesterase
Postganglionic fiber	Monamine oxidase & catechol-o-methyl-transferase	Cholinesterase

4. Cholinergic receptor: A receptor stimulated by acetylcholine
5. Effects of PNS and SNS on various organs:
   a. Lung
      (1) Bronchi
          SNS: Relaxes smooth muscles (bronchodilation)
          PNS: Contracts smooth muscles (bronchoconstriction)
      (2) Mucosal arterioles
          SNS: Vasoconstriction
          PNS: No effect
      (3) Pulmonary arterioles
          SNS: Vasoconstriction or dilation
          PNS: No effect
   b. Heart
      SNS: Increased rate (+ chronotropic effect) and force of
          contraction (+ inotropic effect)
      PNS: Decreased rate (− chronotropic effect) and force
          of contraction (− inotropic effect)
   c. Systemic blood vessels
      SNS: Vasoconstriction or dilation
      PNS: No effect
   d. Gastrointestinal tract
      SNS: Decreased general motility
          Decreased glanular secretion
          Increased sphincter tone
      PNS: Increased general motility
          Increased glanular secretion
          Decreased sphincter tone
   e. Salivary gland
      SNS: Produces viscid secretions
      PNS: Produces profuse watery secretions
   f. Eye
      SNS: Relaxes ciliary muscle and dilates pupil
      PNS: Contracts ciliary muscle and constricts pupil

BIBLIOGRAPHY

Carrier O.: *Pharmacology of the Peripheral Autonomic Nervous System.* Chicago, Year Book Medical Publishers, Inc., 1972.
Ganong W.F.: *Review of Medical Physiology*, ed. 7. Los Altos, Calif., Lange Medical Publications, 1979.
Goodman L.S., Gilman A. (eds.): *The Pharmacological Basis of Therapeutics*, ed. 5. New York, Macmillan Publishing Co., Inc., 1975.
Guyton A.C.: *Textbook of Medical Pharmacology*, ed. 6. Philadelphia, W.B. Saunders Co., 1981.

Julian R.M.: *A Primer of Drug Action,* ed. 3. San Francisco, W.H. Freeman and Co., 1981.

Lehnert B.E.: *The Pharmacology of Respiratory Care.* St. Louis, C.V. Mosby Co., 1980.

Rau J.L.: *Respiratory Therapy Pharmacology,* ed. 2. Chicago, Year Book Medical Publishers, Inc., 1984.

Spearman C.B., Sheldon R.L., Egan D.F.: *Egan's Fundamentals of Respiratory Therapy,* ed. 4. St. Louis, C.V. Mosby Co., 1982.

9 / Renal Anatomy and Physiology

I. Gross Anatomy (Fig 9–1)
   A. The kidneys are located outside the peritoneal cavity, on each side of the spinal column within the posterior abdominal wall.
   B. Renal vessels and nerves enter on the medial border.
   C. The renal pelvis is a continuation of the ureter.
      1. The outer border of the renal pelvis is divided into major calices.
      2. Each major calyx is subdivided into minor calices.
      3. Each minor calyx is cupped about a renal pyramid.
      4. Nephrons, the functional aspect of the kidney, are located within each renal pyramid (Fig 9–2).
   D. A dissection of the kidney from top to bottom demonstrates two major regions:
      1. The outer region, called the renal cortex
      2. The inner region, called the renal medulla
   E. A single ureter leaves the medial border of each kidney and enters the bladder.
   F. A single urethra leaves the bladder.
II. The Nephron (Fig 9–3; see also Fig 9–2)
   A. The nephron is the functional unit of the kidney.
   B. Each kidney is composed of about 1 million nephrons.
   C. Each nephron is composed of a kidney tubule and its corresponding blood supply.
   D. The site of initial formation of urine is the glomerulus. The glomerulus filters blood into Bowman's capsule, forming the glomerular filtrate.
   E. The kidney tubule itself begins with Bowman's capsule and continues sequentially with the following structures:
      1. Proximal convoluted tubule
      2. Loop of Henle
         a. Descending limb
         b. Ascending limb
      3. Distal convoluted tubule
      4. Collecting duct
   F. The circulatory supply of the nephron is provided by the arcuate artery.

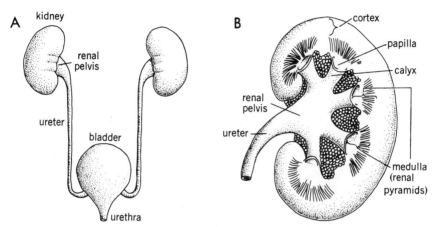

Fig 9–1.—Gross anatomy of the kidney. (From Vander A.J., et al.: *Human Physiology.* New York, McGraw-Hill Book Co., Inc., 1970. Reproduced by permission.)

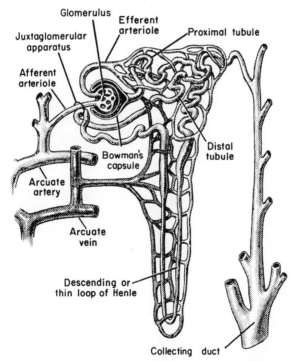

Fig 9–2.—Gross anatomy of the nephron. (From Smith: *The Kidney: Structure and Functions in Health and Disease.* New York, Oxford University Press, 1951. Reproduced by permission.)

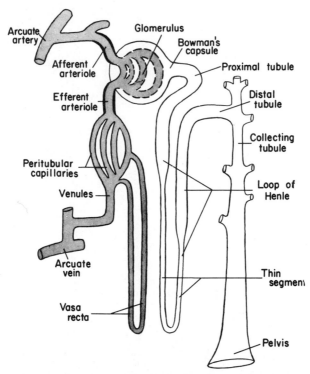

Fig 9–3.—Gross anatomy of the kidney tubular system and corresponding circulatory system. (From Guyton A.C.: *Textbook of Medical Physiology,* ed. 6. Philadelphia, Lea & Febiger, 1981. Reproduced by permission.)

    1. From this artery an afferent arteriole leads to the glomerulus.
    2. Blood exits the glomerulus via an efferent arteriole.
    3. The efferent arteriole forms the peritubular capillaries which intertwine about the distal and proximal convoluted tubules.
    4. The efferent arterioles also form the vasa recta, a long looping capillary that forms about the loop of Henle.
    5. Blood leaves the peritubular capillaries and the vasa recta via the arcuate veins.

  III. Major Functions of the Kidney
    A. Formation of the glomerular filtrate (see section IV)
    B. Tubular reabsorption (see section V)
    C. Tubular secretion (see section VI)
    D. Renin secretion (see section XI)
    E. Erythropoietic factor secretion: In the presence of hypoxemia,

the kidney secretes erythropoietic factor, which stimulates red blood cell production.

F. Activation of vitamin D: Vitamin D is necessary for appropriate absorption of calcium via the gastrointestional tract.

G. Gluconeogenesis: The formation of glucose from fats and protein during periods of significant physiologic stress.

IV. Glomerular Filtration

A. Filtration of fluid and electrolytes at the glomerulus follows Starling's law of fluid exchange (see Chap. 15).

B. However, since protein is poorly filterable across the glomerulus, except under pathologic conditions, only three forces normally control fluid exchange.

   1. Forces moving fluid out of the glomerulus
      a. Glomerular hydrostatic pressure   60 mm Hg
      b. Total outward force   60 mm Hg

   2. Forces maintaining fluid in the glomerulus
      a. Glomerular colloid osmotic pressure   28 mm Hg
      b. Bowman's capsule hydrostatic pressure   + 18 mm Hg
      c. Total inward force   46 mm Hg

   3. Net filtration pressure
      a. Total outward force   60 mm Hg
      b. Total inward force   − 46 mm Hg
      c. Filtration pressure   14 mm Hg

C. In the average adult about 125 ml/min of fluid is filtered across the glomerulus.

D. This filtrate is essentially protein free and has concentrations of dissolved crystalloids similar to that of plasma.

E. The kidney receives about 20% of the cardiac output, of which about 55% is fluid.

   1. If cardiac output is 5.5 L, 1.1 L perfuses the kidney each minute.
   2. 55% of 1.1 L = 605 ml/min of fluid.
   3. From this fluid volume, 125 ml/min of glomerular filtrate is formed.
   4. The glomerular filtration fraction is the percent of the plasma volume filtered:

$$\frac{125 \text{ ml/min}}{605 \text{ ml/min}} \approx .20, \text{ or } 20\%$$

   5. Normally, 20% of the fluid presented to the kidney is filtered.

    F. Alterations in the tone of the afferent arteriole and the efferent arteriole affect the volume of glomerular filtrate formed.
      1. Increased tone of the afferent arteriole decreases glomerular hydrostatic pressure and thus filtration volume.
      2. Increased tone of the efferent arteriole increases glomerular hydrostatic pressure and thus filtration volume.

  V. Tubular Reabsorption: The movement of filtered substances back into the bloodstream.
    A. Of the 125 ml/min of glomerular filtrate formed, only 1 ml/min of urine is formed; the remainder is reabsorbed. Normally, urinary output is about 40–60 ml/hour.
    B. Reabsorption occurs via simple diffusion, facilitated diffusion, and active transport mechanisms (see Chap. 15).
    C. The vast majority of the electrolytes in the glomerular filtrate are reabsorbed. Less than 1.0% of the following filtered substances are excreted:
      1. Sodium
      2. Chloride
      3. Potassium
      4. Bicarbonate
      5. Phosphate
      6. Sulfate
      7. Calcium
      8. Magnesium
      9. Albumin
    D. All filtered glucose is reabsorbed, unless the blood glucose level is above 375 mg/dl (mg%). The threshold for the spillage of glucose in the urine is 375 mg/dl (mg%).
    E. About 50% of the urea filtered is reabsorbed.
    F. Little of the creatinine and creatine filtered is reabsorbed.

 VI. Tubular Secretion
    A. The movement of substances from the blood into the kidney tubule.
    B. The following substances are secreted into the kidney tubule:
      1. Potassium
      2. Hydrogen
      3. Urea
      4. Creatinine

VII. Renal Clearance
    A. Clearance of a substance refers to the volume of plasma cleared of the substance per unit time.
    B. Every substance in the blood has its own clearance rate.

C. Renal clearance of a substance is equal to the glomerular filtration rate (GFR) if the substance is:
1. Freely diffusible at the glomerulus.
2. Not chemically altered in the kidney.
3. Not secreted.
4. Not reabsorbed.
5. Thus, all of the substance that is filtered is excreted.
D. Renal clearance is equal to:

$$C = \frac{(U)(V)}{P} \tag{1}$$

where C = clearance of substance X, U = urine concentration of X, V = urine volume per unit time, and P = arterial plasma concentration of X.
E. Normally, renal clearance is determined from a 24-hour urine sample.
F. Inulin, an inert polysaccharide, is the standard for determining the GFR because its renal clearance is equal to the GFR.
D. Clinically, plasma creatinine and urea levels are used as indicators of GFR changes.
1. Creatinine results from the breakdown of voluntary muscle. As muscle breaks down, creatine is produced, which is converted to creatinine in the blood.
2. Urea is produced from the metabolism of amino acids.
3. Plasma creatinine levels are indirectly affected by the GFR.
4. All creatinine filtered is excreted.
5. In addition, a small quantity of creatinine is secreted.
6. Thus, as the GFR decreases, the plasma creatinine level increases.
7. Urea plasma levels are also indirectly affected by the GFR.
8. Plasma concentrations of creatinine are affected by the following:
   a. GFR
   b. Breakdown of voluntary muscle
   c. Hypermetabolic states
9. Plasma concentrations of urea are affected by the following:
   a. GFR
   b. Breakdown of voluntary muscle
   c. Hypermetabolic state
   d. Metabolism of sequestered (third space) blood

VIII. Counter Current Multiplier
A. The configuration of the nephron allows for the concentrating of urine.
B. In the descending limb of the loop of Henle, water is reabsorbed. However, Na^+ and Cl^- are not reabsorbed. Thus, the concentration of the filtrate increases toward the tip of the nephron.
C. In the ascending limb of the loop of Henle, Na^+ and Cl^- are reabsorbed. However, water is not reabsorbed. Thus, the concentration of the filtrate decreases toward the top of the loop of Henle.
D. This arrangement causes a variation in the osmolarity of the interstitium from the top to the bottom of the loop of Henle. This variation is maintained by the arrangement of the circulatory system.
E. The collecting duct passes through the interstitium parallel to the loop of Henle. As a result, fluid moving through the collecting duct can be concentrated if the permeability of the collecting duct to water and Na^+ reabsorption are increased.

IX. Antidiuretic Hormone (ADH)
A. ADH affects the reabsorption of water in the distal convoluted tubule and the collecting duct.
B. Increased ADH increases the reabsorption of water.
C. Decreased ADH decreases the reabsorption of water.
D. ADH levels are controlled by the hypothalamus.
E. ADH is actually released by the posterior pituitary via stimulation from the hypothalamus.
F. ADH levels are controlled by:
1. Pressure in the atria
a. Increased atrial pressure is viewed by the body as an increased extracellular fluid volume: therefore ADH levels are decreased.
b. Decreased atrial pressure is viewed by the body as a decreased extracellular fluid volume; therefore ADH levels are increased. (Positive pressure ventilation normally decreases atrial pressure.)
2. Osmolarity of the extracellular fluid
a. Decreased osmolarity is viewed by the body as an increase in extracellular fluid volume; therefore ADH levels are decreased.
b. Increased osmolarity is viewed by the body as a decrease

in extracellular fluid volume; therefore ADH levels are increased.

X. Aldosterone
  A. Controls the reabsorption of Na^+ and the secretion of K^+.
  B. Increased aldosterone increases the reabsorption of Na^+ and the secretion of K^+.
  C. Decreased aldosterone decreases the reabsorption of Na^+ and the secretion of K^+.
  D. Aldosterone affects Na^+ and K^+ movement at the distal convoluted tubule and the collecting duct.
  E. Aldosterone is secreted by the adrenal cortex. Its levels are increased by:
    1. Decreased serum Na^+
    2. Increased serum K^+
    3. Increased ACTH (see Chap. 34)
    4. Increased angiotensin II (see section XI)

XI. Renin-Angiotensin
  A. Renin is secreted by the kidney in response to a decrease in the delivery of sodium chloride to a group of cells located between the afferent and efferent arterioles, the macula densa cells.
  B. Essentially, a decrease in perfusion of the kidney increases the release of renin.
  C. Renin converts angiotensinogen formed by the liver to angiotensin I.
  D. Angiotensin I is converted to angiotensin II by the pulmonary endothelium.
  E. Figure 9–4 summarizes the effects of angiotensin II.
  F. Angiotensin II is converted to angiotensin III. Most of the effects in Figure 9–4 can also be attributed to angiotensin III.
  G. Angiotensin levels facilitate Na^+ and H_2O retention and elevate arterial blood pressure. Angiotensin is the strongest vasopressor produced by the body.
  H. Angiotensin levels increase in response to physiologic stress.

XII. Secretion of H^+ and Reabsorption of HCO_3^-
  A. Figure 9–5 illustrates the sequence of reactions maintaining normal H^+ secretion and HCO_3^- reabsorption.
  B. Carbonic anhydrase is present in kidney tubule cells, increasing the hydration of CO_2, which dissociates into H^+ and HCO_3^-.
  C. As CO_2 enters the kidney cell, H^+ and HCO_3^- are formed. The HCO_3^- formed moves into the blood and the H^+ moves into the glomerular filtrate. As each H^+ moves into the glomerular

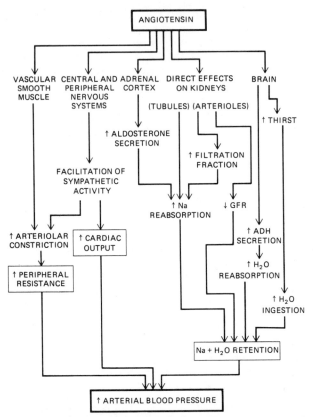

Fig 9–4.—The direct and indirect effects of an increase in angiotensin. Note that all responses are directed toward an increase in Na⁺ and H₂O retention and an increase in arterial blood pressure. (From Vander A.J.: *Renal Physiology,* ed. 2. New York, McGraw-Hill Book Co., Inc., 1980. Reproduced by permission.)

filtrate, a Na^+ is reabsorbed into the bloodstream.
D. In the glomerular filtrate, the H^+ is buffered by:
 1. HCO_3^-
 2. HPO_4^{-2} (dibasic phosphate)
 3. NH_3 (ammonia)
E. Note that for every HCO_3^- reabsorbed, one H^+ is secreted.
F. This series of reactions (see Fig 9–5) continues in the presence of normal acid-base balance.
G. If a decrease in plasma Pa_{CO_2} occurs, there is a decrease in the amount of HCO_3^- reabsorbed and H^+ excreted.

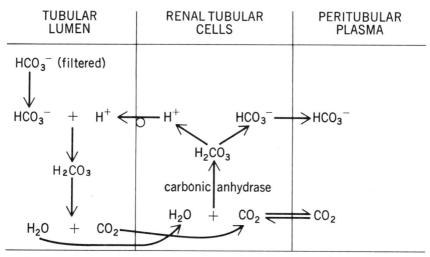

Fig 9–5.—The normal mechanism for the reabsorption of filtered HCO_3^-. For every HCO_3^- reabsorbed, one H^+ ion is secreted. O indicates that movement of H^+ is via an active transport mechanism. (From Vander A.J.: *Renal Physiology*, ed. 2. New York, McGraw-Hill Book Co., Inc., 1980. Reproduced by permission.)

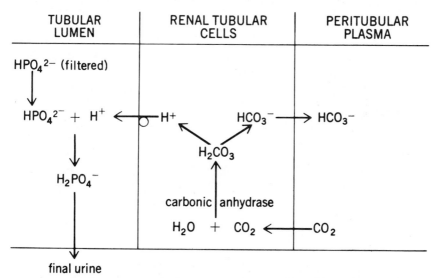

Fig 9–6.—The use of HPO_4^{-2} as a buffer of secreted H^+. This system is primarily active in the presence of excess Pa_{CO_2} creating a larger quantity of H^+ to be secreted than normal. With each H^+ ion secreted a HCO_3^- is reabsorbed, thus increasing total extracellular $[HCO_3^-]$. (From Vander A.J.: *Renal Physiology*, ed. 2. New York, McGraw-Hill Book Co., Inc., 1980. Reproduced by permission.)

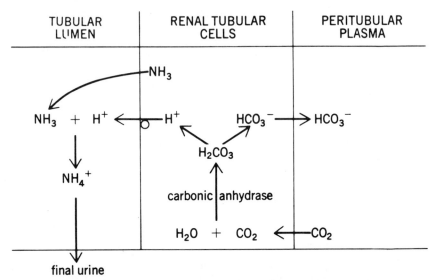

Fig 9–7.—The reaction of secreted H^+ with NH_3. This system is primarily active in the presence of excess Pa_{CO_2}. The additional H^+ formed is buffered and HCO_3^- is reabsorbed, increasing the total extracellular $[HCO_3^-]$. (From Vander A.J.: *Renal Physiology*, ed. 2. New York, McGraw-Hill Book Co., Inc., 1980. Reproduced by permission.)

  H. If Pa_{CO_2} levels are increased, there is an increase in the amount of HCO_3^- reabsorbed and H^+ excreted.
  I. When this occurs, the HCO_3^- in the tubular lumen is rapidly depleted. HPO_4^{-2} and NH_3 are used to buffer the excess H^+ excreted (Figs 9–6 and 9–7).
  J. The kidney can continue to buffer acid until the pH of the urine decreases to about 4.0.
  K. The quantity of HCO_3^- reabsorbed over normal is equal to the amount of acid excreted in the form of $H_2PO_4^{-1}$ and NH_4^+.
  L. Compensation for respiratory acid-base imbalances.
   1. If P_{CO_2} level increases, more HCO_3^- is formed and moved into the blood. This normalizes the acidic pH caused by the increased P_{CO_2} level.
   2. If P_{CO_2} level decreases, less HCO_3^- is formed and moved into the blood. This normalizes the alkalotic pH caused by the decreased P_{CO_2} level.
   3. Compensation by the kidney is relatively complete, but the mechanism may take hours to normalize the pH (24–48 hours).

BIBLIOGRAPHY

Ellerbe S.: *Fluid and Blood Component Therapy in the Critically Ill and Injured.* New York, Churchill Livingstone, Inc., 1981.

Gabow P.A.: *Fluids and Electrolytes: Clinical Problems and Their Solution.* Boston, Little, Brown & Co., 1983.

Guyton A.C.: *Textbook of Medical Physiology,* ed. 6. Philadelphia, Lea & Febiger, 1981.

Rose B.D.: *Clinical Physiology of Acid-Base and Electrolyte Disorders.* New York, McGraw-Hill Book Co., 1977.

Schrier R.W. (ed.): *Renal and Electrolyte Disorders,* ed. 2. Boston, Little, Brown & Co., 1980.

Smith K.: *Fluids and Electrolytes: A Conceptual Approach.* New York, Churchill Livingstone, Inc., 1980.

Sullivan L.P.: *Physiology of the Kidney.* Philadelphia, Lea & Febiger, 1975.

Tepperman J.: *Metabolic and Endocrine Physiology: An Introductory Text,* ed. 3. Chicago, Year Book Medical Publishers, Inc., 1973.

Vanatta J.C., Fogelman M.J.: *Moyers Fluid Balance: A Clinical Manual,* ed. 2. Chicago, Year Book Medical Publishers, Inc., 1976.

Vander A.J.: *Renal Physiology,* ed. 2. New York, McGraw-Hill Book Co., 1980.

Weldy N.J.: *Body Fluids and Electrolytes: A Programmed Presentation,* ed. 3. St. Louis, C.V. Mosby Co., 1980.

10 / Neonatal and Pediatric Anatomy and Physiology

I. Embryologic Development of the Lung
  A. Normal gestation: About 38–42 weeks
    1. Premature births: Gestational periods of less than 38 weeks.
    2. Postmature births: Gestational periods of more than 42 weeks.
  B. Gestational development of the lung
    1. Week 4: Lungs start to form as an outpouching of the esophagus.
    2. Week 7: Diaphragm starts to form.
    3. Week 10: Cartilaginous rings of trachea and the lymphatics of the respiratory system start to form.
    4. Week 12: Mucosal glands appear.
    5. Week 14: Mucosal glands begin to secrete mucus.
    6. Week 24: Significant development of cartilaginous support of the conducting airways.
    7. Weeks 24–26: Lung parenchyma starts to develop. The pulmonary capillary network also develops. In some cases, development is sufficient to support extrauterine life.
    8. Week 28: Alveolar ducts and sacs have developed and alveolar type II cells begin to appear. The number of alveoli necessary to support extrauterine life is now present.
    9. At normal birth: The number of alveoli is about 24 million and the surface area of the lung is about 2.8 sq m.
    10. During the first 3 years of life there is a tremendous increase in the number and size of alveoli.
    11. By adulthood, there are about 300 million alveoli with a total surface area of about 80 sq m.
  C. Surfactant development
    1. Surfactant first appears between gestational weeks 22 and 24. At this time lecithin and sphingomyelin appear in the pulmonary and amniotic fluid.
    2. As gestation proceeds, the volume of lecithin in the pulmonary fluid increases, whereas sphingomyelin levels remain relatively constant.

    3. At about 35 weeks of gestation, lecithin levels increase significantly.

    4. Normally, after 35 weeks of gestation, the ratio of lecithin to sphingomyelin (L/S ratio) is above 2:1. An L/S ratio of 2:1 is indicative of pulmonary maturity; i.e., the fetus should be able to support extrauterine life.

    5. L/S ratios can be determined intrauterinely by analysis of amniotic fluid (amniocentesis).

    6. If L/S amniotic fluid ratios are less than 2:1, the incidence of respiratory distress syndrome increases.

    7. L/S ratios of less than 1:1 normally are incompatible with extrauterine existence.

II. Fetal Circulation (Fig 10–1)

    A. During intrauterine life, gas exchange, nutrient exchange, and waste elimination are accomplished by the placenta.

    B. The placenta also serves as a rich vascular bed that can accommodate large volumes of blood. The placenta is in part responsible for the low systemic vascular resistance in the fetus.

    C. The lung is fluid filled to about the FRC level and does not participate in external gas exchange.

    D. Lung fluid tends to compress the pulmonary capillary beds. This, coupled with low intrauterine PO_2 causing vasoconstriction, tends to make the pulmonary capillary beds high in vascular resistance.

    E. Thus, pressures within the heart are completely opposite in utero to those after birth; i.e., pressures within the right side of the heart are greater during fetal life than the pressures within the left side of the heart.

    F. In utero, pulmonary blood flow need not be as high as is necessary during extrauterine life.

    G. For this reason, blood flow is diverted from the lung by two different routes: the foramen ovale and the ductus arteriosus.

    H. The foramen ovale is a flaplike valve between the right and left atria.

    I. The foramen ovale allows blood to flow directly between the right and left atria, bypassing the lung; a right-to-left shunt.

    J. Blood flows from right to left atria through the foramen ovale because of the existence of (1) a rudimentary valve called the crista intervenans, which actually directs and routes blood to the foramen ovale, and (2) a pressure gradient between the right and left sides of the heart.

    K. The ductus arteriosus is a fetal communicating vessel between the pulmonary artery and aorta.

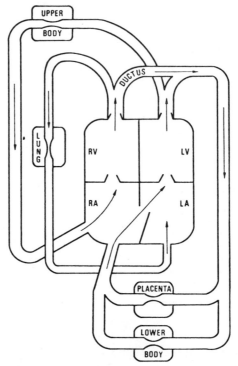

Fig 10–1.—Fetal circulation. Right ventricle *(RV);* left ventricle *(LV);* left atrium *(LA);* right atrium *(RA);* the foramen ovale between RA and LA; ductus arteriosus shunts blood from high-resistance lung vessels. (From Lough M.D., Doershuk C.F., Stern R.C. (eds.): *Pediatric Respiratory Therapy.* Chicago, Year Book Medical Publishers, Inc., 1974. Reproduced by permission.)

L. Blood is pumped from the right ventricle into the pulmonary artery. Since pulmonary artery pressure in utero exceeds systemic (aortic) vascular pressure, much of the blood is directed through the ductus arteriosus, (the path of least resistance), enters the aorta, and again bypasses the lung (a right-to-left shunt).

M. The remainder of the blood passes through the pulmonary capillary bed, through the left side of the heart, and out into the aorta.

N. In utero, about 10% of cardiac output passes through the lung.

O. The remaining 90% bypasses the lung by either the foramen ovale or the ductus arteriosus.

P. Blood in the aorta eventually reaches the umbilical arteries and enters the placenta where it undergoes exchange of gases, nutrients, and wastes.

Q. Blood leaves the placenta by the umbilical vein, carrying oxygenated blood.

R. The umbilical vein travels to the liver where most of the blood bypasses the liver via the ductus venosus.

S. The ductus venosus drains into the inferior vena cava.

T. The inferior vena cava drains into the right atrium and the blood is again circulated as described, beginning with section II, I.

III. Circulatory Changes at Normal Birth (Fig 10–2)

A. Following clamping of the cord at birth, the supply of oxygenated blood from the placenta is stopped.

B. In order for the neonate to sustain life, fetal circulation must be altered and blood must perfuse the lung to become oxygenated.

C. There is a significant decrease in pulmonary vascular resistance after birth. This occurs as a result of elimination of fetal lung fluid and the presence of oxygen in the lung.

D. With lung fluid eliminated, the pulmonary capillary bed is no longer compressed by hydrostatic forces.

E. When ventilation begins, oxygen diffuses into the pulmonary

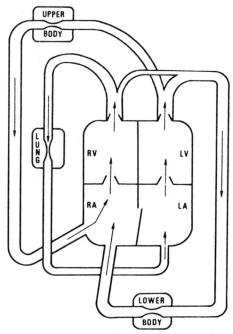

Fig 10–2.—Transitional circulation at birth. The ductus arteriosus begins to close. The foramen ovale closes from rising left atrial pressure. (From Lough M.D., Doershuk C.F., Stern R.C. (eds.): *Pediatric Respiratory Therapy*. Chicago, Year Book Medical Publishers, Inc., 1974. Reproduced by permission.)

capillary blood. As pulmonary capillary blood oxygen tensions begin to rise, the vasoconstriction present in the fetal pulmonary vascular bed is gradually reversed.

F. With pulmonary vascular resistance reduced, larger portions of the cardiac output begin to perfuse the lung.

G. At the same time, there is a significant increase in systemic vascular resistance. This occurs in part from loss of the placenta as a blood reservoir, which also results in a decrease in venous return to the right side of the heart.

H. The increase in peripheral vascular resistance results in an increase in pressure in the left side of the heart.

I. The reduction in venous return and the decrease in pulmonary vascular resistance result in a decrease in pressure in the right side of the heart.

J. Now pressure in the left side of the heart exceeds pressure in the right side. This pressure change causes a functional closure of the foramen ovale.

K. In addition, the rise in oxygen tension in the ductus arteriosus causes it to begin to constrict.

L. Blood flow through the ductus arteriosus is also reversed, due to the change in pressures.

M. The ductus arteriosus usually closes functionally within the first 24 hours of life.

N. The ductus arteriosus anatomically closes within the first 3 weeks of life and becomes the ligamentum arteriosus.

IV. Pulmonary Changes at Birth

A. In order for the neonate to sustain extrauterine life, fetal lung fluid must be eliminated from the lung. This occurs through several mechanisms.

   1. The compliant chest wall of the neonate is compressed in the birth canal during the birth process, forcing much of the fluid out of the lung.

   2. Fetal lung fluid is low in protein content. When pulmonary blood flow increases at birth, some of the fluid is moved into the blood by osmosis.

   3. The lymphatic system also absorbs a portion of lung fluid.

B. The first breath of the neonate is stimulated by several factors.

   1. The change in temperature between intrauterine and extrauterine conditions

   2. The bright light and sounds in the delivery room

   3. The hypoxemia, acidemia, and hypercapnia that develop during the birth process

C. Intrathoracic pressures of -40 to -90 cm H_2O must be generated to initiate the first breath.
D. During the first several breaths, the inspiratory tidal volume exceeds the expiratory tidal volume. The difference in volumes occurs because the functional residual capacity is being established.
V. Clinical Evaluation of the Neonate
  A. Apgar score: This scoring system is used to evaluate the neonatal
  cardiopulmonary status after birth.
    1. Apgar scores are normally determined 1 and 5 minutes after
    birth.
    2. Scores are based on a scale of 0 to 10.
      a. Scores 7–10: Few, if any, supportive measures are
      needed.
      b. Scores 4–6: Mild to moderate asphyxia; the infant should
      be suctioned, oxygenated, and possibly ventilated.
      c. Scores 0–3: Full cardiopulmonary resuscitation should
      be initiated.
    3. Scoring is performed in five areas, each area scored from 0
    to 2.
      a. Heart rate
        (1) Absent: 0
        (2) Less than 100 per minute: 1
        (3) Greater than 100 per minute: 2
      b. Respiratory rate
        (1) Absent: 0
        (2) Slow, irregular: 1
        (3) Good cry: 2
      c. Muscle tone
        (1) Limp: 0
        (2) Some flexion of the extremities: 1
        (3) Active movement: 2
      d. Reflex irritability to stimulation
        (1) No response: 0
        (2) Grimace: 1
        (3) Cough or sneeze: 2
      e. Color
        (1) Blue or pale: 0
        (2) Pink body, blue extremities: 1
        (3) Completely pink: 2
  B. Silverman score: This system is used to evaluate the level of respiratory distress of a neonate.

    1. Scores are based on a scale of 0 to 10.
        a. Scores of 0 to 3: No respiratory distress to mild respiratory distress
        b. Scores of 4 to 6: moderate respiratory distress
        c. Scores of 7 to 10: severe respiratory distress
    2. Scoring is performed in five areas, scored from 0 to 2.
        a. Upper chest movement
            (1) Synchronized movement: 0
            (2) Lag of upper chest on inspiration: 1
            (3) Seesaw movement of upper chest: 2
        b. Lower chest movement
            (1) No retractions: 0
            (2) Retractions just visible: 1
            (3) Marked retractions: 2
        c. Xiphoid retractions
            (1) No retractions: 0
            (2) Retractions just visible: 1
            (3) Marked retractions: 2
        d. Dilation of nares
            (1) None: 0
            (2) Minimal dilation: 1
            (3) Marked dilation: 2
        e. Expiratory grunt
            (1) None: 0
            (2) Heard only with stethoscope: 1
            (3) Heard with naked ear: 2
VI. Prenatal Conditions That Increase Neonatal Mortality and Morbidity
    A. Prematurity
    B. Maternal factors
        1. Drug and alcohol abuse
        2. Extreme emotional stress
        3. Obstetric complications
        4. Cigarette smoking
        5. Placental insufficiency
        6. Multiple pregnancy
        7. Third trimester viral infection
        8. First pregnancy late in life
        9. Diabetes
      10. Maternal age over 35 or under 16
      11. Anemia
      12. Hypertension
      13. Thyroid disease

14. Isoimmunization—red blood cell antigens or platelet antigens
15. Fever
16. Infection
17. Past history of infant with jaundice, respiratory distress, or anomalies
18. Medications: Steroids, antimetabolites, salicylates, warfarin, reserpine, thyroid medication

VII. Blood Gases of the Neonate
   A. Blood gases at birth usually show metabolic and respiratory acidosis along with severe hypoxemia.

   | pH | 7.20–7.25 | HCO_3^- | 18–19 mEq/L |
   | P_{CO_2} | 53–58 mm Hg | P_{O_2} | 20–25 mm Hg |

   B. Within the first hour after birth, P_{O_2} in the term infant is about 60 mm Hg, and in the premature infant, 40–60 mm Hg.
   C. Twenty-four hours after birth, P_{CO_2} values range from 35 to 40 mm Hg, but P_{O_2} values may take weeks to normalize to the 80–100 mm Hg range.

VIII. Respiratory Patterns of the Neonate
   A. Respiratory rate is usually two to three times that of the average adult, 30–50/minute
      1. In general the more premature the neonate the greater its respiratory rate.
      2. As the child's age increases the respiratory rate decreases:
         a. 6 months: 28/min
         b. 1 year: 24/min
         c. 3 years: 22/min
         d. 5 years: 20/min
         e. 8 years: 18/min
         f. 12 years: 16/min
         g. 15 years: 14/min
   B. The neonate shows little movement of the thoracic cage, with ventilation being primarily diaphragmatic in nature. The diaphragm's motion is limited in the neonate due to the large size of the abdominal viscera.
   C. Tidal volumes of the neonate average 6–8 ml/kg.
   D. Periodic breathing patterns in the premature infant.
      1. Periods of apnea lasting 5–10 seconds, followed by a period of tachypnea lasting 10–15 seconds, are frequently seen.
      2. The neonate's overall ventilatory rate remains at 30–50 per minute, but during the actual ventilatory periods the rate accelerates to 50–60 per minute.

    3. Periodic breathing patterns occur more often during wakeful states.

    4. The pattern does not develop until after the first 24 hours of life; the more premature the infant, the more common the pattern.

    5. This pattern usually is not considered serious if periods of apnea do not exceed 10 seconds.

  E. True apneic spells in premature neonates.

    1. Apneic spells are defined as true periods of apnea if longer than 15–20 seconds.

    2. A high mortality is associated with apneic spells of this length.

    3. The etiology is unclear, but the spells seem to be a result of CNS problems.

IX. Hemodynamic Values

  A. Heart rate is usually twice that of the average adult, 140 ± 50/minute.

    1. Generally, the more premature the neonate, the faster the heart rate.

    2. As the child's age increases, the heart rate decreases:

      a. 6 months: 120 ± 40/min

      b. 1 year: 110 ± 40/min

      c. 3 years: 105 ± 35/min

      d. 5 years: 100 ± 35/min

      e. 8 years: 95 ± 30/min

      f. 12 years: 90 ± 30/min

      g. 15 years: 80 ± 25/min

  B. Blood pressure is normally much lower in the neonates than in adults, averaging 70/50 mm Hg.

    1. Generally, the more premature the neonate, the lower the blood pressure.

    2. As the child's age increases, the blood pressure also increases:

      a. 3 months: 90/60 mm Hg

      b. 1 year: 100/60 mm Hg

      c. 5 years: 105/60 mm Hg

      d. 8 years: 110/60 mm Hg

      e. 12 years: 118/60 mm Hg

      f. 15 years: 120/65 mm Hg

X. Fetal Monitoring

  A. Ultrasound: The use of mechanical radiant energy with a frequency greater than 20,000 cycles per second to visually display images (echoes) of the fetus.

      1. Generally used to determine gestational age

      2. Also used to:

         a. Estimate growth of fetus

         b. Identify multiple pregnancies

         c. Identify fetal abnormalities

         d. Determine amount of amniotic fluid

         e. Determine location of placenta

B. Amniocentesis: The withdrawal of amniotic fluid by insertion of a needle through the mother's abdominal and uterine walls into the amniotic cavity. Used to:

      1. Evaluate chromosomal makeup

      2. Perform protein and enzyme analysis

      3. Evaluate creatinine levels

      4. Determine L/S ratios

      5. Identify presence of meconium

C. Continuous external fetal heart rate monitors

      1. Used primarily during labor and delivery

      2. Provides beat-by-beat monitoring during maternal contractions

      3. Used to evaluate cardiovascular status of fetus

D. Blood gas monitoring

      1. Scalp vein or buttocks vein pH

         a. During delivery of infants at risk, a venous sample from the scalp or buttocks (whichever presents) is taken to assess pH.

         b. pH ranges

            (1) Greater than 7.25 is considered normal

            (2) 7.20–7.25 is considered abnormal, monitor carefully

            (3) Less than 7.20, significant reduction, deliver immediately

      2. Umbilical cord gases

         a. Sample is taken immediately after birth from the clamped umbilical artery.

         b. Normal values:

            (1) pH, greater than 7.20

            (2) P_{CO_2}, 45–50 mm Hg

            (3) P_{O_2}, less than 40 mm Hg

      3. Arterial blood gases

         a. In neonates at risk an umbilical artery catheter is frequently placed.

         b. In addition to monitoring blood gases, fluid and nutritional levels can be managed via this catheter.

c. Normal arterial blood gas levels:
  (1) 500 gm to 1,500 gm neonate
    pH,   7.35–7.45
    PCO_2, 35–45 mm Hg
    PO_2, 50–60 mm Hg
  (2) 1,500 gm to 2,500 gm neonate
    pH,   7.35–7.45
    PCO_2, 35–45 mm Hg
    PO_2, 60–70 mm Hg
  (3) Greater than 2,500 gm neonate
    pH,   7.35–7.45
    PCO_2, 35–45 mm Hg
    PO_2, 70–90 mm Hg
4. Capillary blood gases
  a. Capillary blood samples are normally taken from the neonate's heal.
  b. Values may differ from arterial blood gases.
    (1) PO_2 values are about 10–15 mm Hg less than actual arterial.
    (2) PCO_2 values may be consistent with actual arterial or up to 3 mm Hg higher.
    (3) pH values tend to be consistent with actual arterial but may be 0.01–0.02 pH units lower.
  c. Arterial and capillary samples may differ considerably:
    (1) If poor technique is employed.
    (2) If the neonate becomes agitated during the procedure.
    (3) During the first 24 hours after birth perfusion to the heal is poor and results are unreliable.
    (4) In neonates with shock or poor peripheral perfusion.
  d. Blood gas samples from any artery will have values consistent with umbilical artery samples unless a right-to-left shunt of significant magnitude exists. Specifically, persistent fetal circulation results in marked differences in PO_2 values.
  e. If persistent fetal circulation is present, gases from the right upper quadrant of the body will have PO_2 values much higher than the rest of the organism because the right common carotid artery leaves the aorta before the ductus arteriosus enters the aorta.
    (1) To determine if persistent fetal circulation exists, PO_2 values from the right upper quadrant are compared to PO_2 values from outside this quadrant.

(2) Sites of right upper quadrant arterial blood gas sampling:
   (a) Right radial artery
   (b) Right brachial artery
   (c) Right temporal artery
(3) Sites outside right upper quadrant for arterial blood gas sampling:
   (a) Umbilical artery
   (b) Left radial artery
   (c) Left brachial artery
(4) If PO_2 determinations differ by more than 10%, persistent fetal circulation or other right-to-left shunt-producing anomalies may exist.

XI. Transcutaneous PO_2 and PCO_2 Monitoring
  A. A Clark electrode (PO_2) or a Severinghaus electrode (PCO_2) is used which provides a continuous readout.
  B. Electrodes are maintained at 44° C and are placed on any flat surface, normally the chest or abdomen.
  C. Electrode position must be changed every 3–4 hours, or skin burns or blisters may develop.
  D. Even when the site is changed every 4 hours, erythema is common; however, it usually disappears within 6–12 hours.
  E. Readings of either monitor are affected by:
    1. Changes in arterial PO_2 or PCO_2
    2. Peripheral perfusion
    3. Skin conditions, anatomical anomalies

XII. Transillumination
  A. The passage of light through body tissues for the purpose of examination.
  B. Used in neonates to identify pneumothoraces or identify an artery for arterial puncture.
  C. When the appearance of one side of the infant's chest is compared to the appearance of the other side of the chest, a marked difference in the halo developed by the light may indicate a pneumothorax. The larger the halo, the greater the likelihood of a pneumothorax.
  D. To identify an artery for puncture, the light source is placed on the side of the limb opposite that to be punctured. The artery will be visualized as a line lighter than surrounding structures.

XIII. Comparative Neonatal Respiratory Anatomy (Table 10–1)
  A. Neonatal head: Very large, about one fourth of total body length, in contrast to the adult head, which is about one eighth of body height.

TABLE 10–1.—COMPARISON OF NEONATAL AND ADULT
RESPIRATORY ANATOMY

STRUCTURE	NEONATE	ADULT
Head to body size ratio	1:4	1:8
Tongue size	Large	Proportional
Laryngeal shape	Funnel-shaped	Rectangular
Narrowest portion of upper airway	Cricoid cartilage	Rima glottidis
Shape and location of epiglottis	Long, C1	Flat, C4
Level of tracheal bifurcation	T3-4	T5
Compliance of trachea	Compliant, flexible	Noncompliant
Angle of mainstem bronchi	10 degrees right, 30 degrees left	30 degrees right, 50 degrees left
Anteroposterior transverse diameter ratio	1:1	1:2
Thoracic shape	Bullet-shaped	Conical
Resting position of diaphragm	Higher than adult	Normal
Location of heart	Center of chest, midline	Lower portion of chest, left of midline
Ratio of body surface area to body size	9 times adult	Normal

B. Neonatal tongue
   1. Very large in relation to size of oral cavity.
   2. Size is primary factor forcing neonates to be obligate nose breathers. Normally only during crying will an infant actively ventilate through the mouth.
   3. Because of tongue size, nasal continuous positive airway pressure (CPAP) without use of endotracheal intubation can be accomplished.
   4. Positive end expiratory pressure (PEEP) levels up to about 8–10 cm H_2O can be used. PEEP levels above this usually cause an oral leak and are difficult to maintain nasally.
C. Neonatal neck: Very short and normally is creased.
D. Neonatal larynx
   1. The length is about 2 cm, compared to 5–6 cm in the adult.
   2. The neonatal larynx is funnel shaped, whereas the diameter of the adult larynx is more or less constant.
   3. The narrowest portion of the neonate's upper airway is the cricoid cartilage; in the adult, the rima glottidis is the narrowest point. The normal anteroposterior diameter of the neonatal glottis is about 7–9 mm, the anteroposterior diameter of the cricoid cartilage about 4–6 mm.

       a. Endotracheal tube size must be based on the diameter of cricoid cartilage.

       b. The larynx is much higher in relation to the oral pharynx and the opening of the larynx is more in a straight line that in the adult.

       c. Therefore, an infant frequently extends the neck when in respiratory distress, whereas the adult will thrust the head forward.

E. Neonatal epiglottis

   1. Stiffer, relatively longer, and U or V shaped, compared to a flatter and much more flexible epiglottis in the adult.

   2. Located at the level of 1st cervical vertebra; in the adult, at 4th cervical vertebra.

F. Neonatal trachea

   1. About 4 cm long, compared to 10–13 cm in the adult.

   2. Anteroposterior diameter about 3.5 mm, lateral diameter about 5 mm.

   3. Normally located to right of midline.

   4. Bifurcation of neonatal trachea at 3rd or 4th thoracic vertebra; in the adult, at 5th thoracic vertebra.

   5. The angle of right and left mainstem bronchi widens with age. At birth the angles from the midline are 10 degrees for the right and 30 degrees for the left; in adulthood the angles are about 30 and 50 degrees, respectively.

   6. Cartilage of the trachea may not be fully formed and often is more flexible than in the adult.

       a. As a result, hyperextension of the head may cause compression of the trachea and result in airway obstruction.

       b. Thus, during artificial ventilation without an endotracheal tube, the neonate's head should be maintained in a neutral position.

G. Neonatal mainstem bronchi

   1. Short and relatively wide compared to those of the adult.

H. Neonatal thoracic cage.

   1. This has nearly equal anteroposterior and transverse diameters, and in general appearance is bullet shaped.

   2. Range of movement is limited, and the ribs are basically fixed in a horizontal position.

   3. The diaphragm is much higher than in the adult because of the relative size of the abdominal viscera. Diaphragm shows minimal movement during ventilation.

4. The heart is located in the center of the chest and slightly higher than in the adult. When external cardiac massage is performed, compression should be applied over the middle of the body of the sternum.

XIV. Body Surface Area

A. The neonate's body surface area in relation to its size is about nine times that of the adult.

B. Maintenance of body heat is thus a significant problem in the neonate, and even more so in the premature infant.

C. The skin of the neonate plays a much greater role in water and heat balance than does that of the adult. This is a result of the large body surface area, which allows significant evaporation of water. In the neonate, 80% of body weight is water; in the adult, only 55%–60%.

BIBLIOGRAPHY

Abramson H.: *Resuscitation of the Newborn Infant.* St. Louis, C.V. Mosby Co., 1973.

Avery G.B.: *Neonatology, Pathophysiology and Management of the Newborn.* Philadelphia, J.B. Lippincott Co., 1975.

Avery M.E.: *The Lung and Its Disorders in the Newborn Infant.* Philadelphia, W.B. Saunders Co., 1974.

Biller J.A., Yeager A.M.: *The Harriet Lane Handbook,* ed. 6. Chicago, Year Book Medical Publishers, 1981.

Bruyn H.B., Kempe C.H., Silver H.K.: *Handbook of Pediatrics,* ed. 11. Los Altos, Calif., Lange Medical Publications, 1975.

Cabal L., Hodgman J., Siassi B., et al.: Factors affecting heated transcutaneous Po_2 and unheated transcutaneous Po_2 in preterm infants. *Crit. Care Med.* 9:298–304, 1981.

Cassady G.: Transcutaneous monitoring in the newborn infant. *J. Pediatr.* 10:837–848, 1983.

Cherniack R.M., Cherniack K.: *Respiration in Health and Disease,* ed. 3. Philadelphia, W.B. Saunders Co., 1983.

Cloherty J.R., Start A.C.: *Manual of Neonatal Care.* Boston, Little, Brown & Co., 1981.

Crouch J.E.: *Functional Human Anatomy,* ed. 2. Philadelphia, Lea & Febiger, 1972.

Daily E.K., Schroeder J.S.: *Techniques in Bedside Hemodynamic Monitoring,* ed. 2. St. Louis, C.V. Mosby Co., 1981.

Eigen H.: Croup or epiglottitis: Differential diagnosis and treatment. *Respir. Care* 20:1158, 1975.

Goodwin J.W., et al.: *Perinatal Medicine—The Basic Science Underlying Clinical Practice.* Baltimore, Williams & Wilkins Co., 1976.

Gregory G.A.: *Respiratory Failure in the Child.* New York, Churchill Livingstone, Inc., 1981.

Guertin S.R., Gordon G.L., Levinsohn M.W., et al.: Intracranial volume pressure response in infants and children: Preliminary report of a predictive marker in metabolic coma. *Crit. Care Med.* 10:1–4, 1982.

Keuskamp D.H.G.: *Neonatal and Pediatric Ventilation*. Boston, Little, Brown & Co., 1974.

Korones S.B.: *High-Risk Newborn Infants*. St. Louis, C.V. Mosby Co., 1976.

Lauersen H.H., Hochberg H.M., George M.E.: Continuous intrapartum monitoring of fetal scalp pH: An adjunct to fetal heart rate monitoring. A Scientific Exhibit—Roche Medical Electronics. Cranbury, New Jersey, 1977.

Lough M.D., Williams T.J., Rawson J.E. (eds.): *Newborn Respiratory Care*. Chicago, Year Book Medical Publishers, Inc., 1979.

Lough M.D., Doershuk C.F., Stern R.C. (eds.): *Pediatric Respiratory Therapy*, ed. 2. Chicago, Year Book Medical Publishers, Inc., 1979.

Meyer C.L., Gresham E.L., Moye L., et al.: Evaluation of a system for continuous neonatal blood pressure monitoring. *Crit. Care Med.* 10:689–691, 1982.

Mindt W., Eberhard P., Hoffman F.: Skin sensors for monitoring oxygen tension of newborns. A Scientific Exhibit—Roche Medical Electronics. Cranbury, New Jersey, 1977.

Nowakowski L.: *Pediatrics: Specific Anatomic Variables, Newborn Respiratory Tract*. Washington, D.C., Robert J. Brady Co., 1974.

Scarpelli E.E.: *Pulmonary Physiology of the Fetus, Newborn and Child*. Philadelphia, Lea & Febiger, 1975.

Slonim N.B., et al.: *Pediatric Respiratory Therapy: An Introductory Text*. Sarasota, Glenn Educational Medical Services, Inc., 1974.

Storer J.S.: Respiratory problems unique to the newborn. *Respir. Care* 20:1146, 1975.

Strang L.B.: *Neonatal Respiration: Physiologic and Clinical Studies*. Philadelphia, J.B. Lippincott Co., 1974.

William J.W.: *Handbook of Neonatal Respiratory Care*. Riverside, Calif., Bourns, Inc., 1977.

11 / Oxygen and Carbon Dioxide Transport

I. Oxygen Cascade

The partial pressure of oxygen (PO_2) decreases significantly from the 159.6 mm Hg in dry air at sea level to less than 3–23 mm Hg in the mitochondria of the cell (Table 11–1).

II. Role of Oxygen in the Cell

   A. About 90% of the oxygen consumed is a result of oxygen being the final electron acceptor of the electron transport chain in the mitochondria of the cell.

   B. The actual reaction produces H_2O:

$$\tfrac{1}{2}\,O_2 + 2\,H^+ \rightarrow H_2O \qquad\qquad (1)$$

   C. Without the presence of O_2, aerobic metabolism is stopped while anaerobic metabolism continues, resulting in the production of lactic acid.

   D. The reaction of O_2 with H^+ to form H_2O allows the formation of the high-energy phosphate group, adenosine triphosphate (ATP).

   E. The yield of ATP molecules from aerobic metabolism significantly exceeds that from anaerobic metabolism.

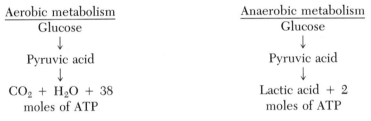

Aerobic metabolism	Anaerobic metabolism
Glucose	Glucose
↓	↓
Pyruvic acid	Pyruvic acid
↓	↓
CO_2 + H_2O + 38 moles of ATP	Lactic acid + 2 moles of ATP

   F. Mitochondrial PO_2 values of less than 2 mm Hg inhibit aerobic metabolism.

III. Carriage of Oxygen in the Blood

   A. Oxygen is carried in two distinct compartments in the blood:
      1. Physically dissolved in plasma
      2. Chemically attached to hemoglobin molecules

   B. Volume physically dissolved in plasma

TABLE 11–1.—THE OXYGEN CASCADE

LOCATION	PARTIAL PRESSURE (mm Hg)	REASON FOR CHANGE
Dry atmospheric air	159.6	
Conducting airways	149.6	Addition of H_2O vapor
End-expiratory gas	114	Mixing of deadspace gas with alveolar gas
Ideal alveolar gas	101	Addition of CO_2
Arterial blood	97	Intrapulmonary shunting
Mean systemic capillary	40	O_2 diffusion into cell
Cellular cytoplasm	<40	O_2 diffusion into mitochondria
Mitochondria	3–23	Metabolic rate

1. According to the Bunsen solubility coefficient for oxygen, 0.023 ml of oxygen can be dissolved in 1 ml of plasma for every 760 mm Hg Po_2.

2. Simplifying this factor to the number of milliliters of oxygen per milliliter of plasma per mm Hg Po_2:

$$0.023 \text{ ml } O_2/760 \text{ mm Hg } =$$
$$0.00003 \text{ ml } O_2/1 \text{ ml plasma/mm Hg } Po_2 \qquad (2)$$

3. Since the oxygen content normally is expressed in volumes percent, multiplying 0.00003 ml of oxygen per milliliter of plasma by 100 gives the factor:

$$(0.00003 \text{ ml } O_2/\text{ml plasma})(100)/1 \text{ mm Hg } Po_2 =$$
$$0.003 \text{ ml } O_2/100 \text{ ml plasma/1 mm Hg } Po_2 \qquad (3)$$

4. Thus, multiplying the Po_2 of blood by 0.003 will yield the number of milliliters of oxygen physically dissolved in every 100 ml of blood (vol%):

$$(Po_2)(0.003) = \text{ml of oxygen physically dissolved} \qquad (4)$$

C. Hemoglobin (Hb): Structure and carrying capacity
   1. Composition of the normal hemoglobin molecule:
      a. Four porphyrin rings, called hemes, each with a central iron atom.
      b. Four polypeptide chains: two α (alpha) chains and two β (beta) chains, called the globin portion of the molecule.
      c. Each chain is twisted and folded into a basket in which a heme is located.
      d. Each iron atom of the heme is bonded via four covalent bonds to the porphyrin ring and via one covalent bond to

the globin portion. One bond is available to combine with oxygen.

e. The four chains are held together by chemical bonds between unlike chains (α to β, β to α).

f. The hemoglobin molecule undergoes structural changes when it reacts with O_2.

g. The total molecule contracts when it combines with O_2 and expands when O_2 is released.

h. The site of CO_2 attachment is the amino groups (R-NH$_2$) on the porphyrin rings.

i. Also, the terminal imidazole (R-NH) groups are available to buffer H$^+$ (see Chap. 13).

    (1) The importance of hemoglobin as a buffer is second only to that of the HCO_3^-/H_2CO_3 buffer system.

    (2) The buffering capacity of the hemoglobin molecule depends on attachment of oxygen to the iron portion of the molecule.

    (3) Oxygenated hemoglobin (oxyhemoglobin) is a stronger acid but weaker buffer than unoxygenated hemoglobin (deoxyhemoglobin).

    (4) Thus the buffering capacity of venous blood is greater than that of arterial blood.

2. The molecular weight of hemoglobin is about 64,500 gm.

3. Since oxygen attaches to each of the four iron atoms in the hemoglobin molecule, four gram molecular weights of oxygen combine with 64,500 gm of hemoglobin.

4. Simplifying and restating No. 3, one gram molecular weight of oxygen combines with 16,125 gm of hemoglobin.

5. Since one gram molecular weight of oxygen at STP will occupy 22.4 L:

$$\frac{22{,}400 \text{ ml of } O_2}{16{,}125 \text{ gm of Hb}} = 1.34 \text{ ml of } O_2/\text{gm of Hb} \qquad (5)$$

6. Thus, at 100% saturation, 1.34 ml of oxygen can combine with each gram of hemoglobin.

7. The actual volume of oxygen carried attached to hemoglobin is equal to:

$$\text{(Hb content)}(1.34)(HbO_2\% \text{ sat.}) =$$
$$\text{vol\% of } O_2 \text{ carried attached to Hb} \qquad (6)$$

8. As Hb combines with O_2 to form HbO_2, the complex takes on a negative charge and as a result it forms a salt with K$^+$, KHbO$_2$.

9. When O_2 is released at the tissue level, the K^+ is also released and the Hb buffers H^+, forming HHb (reduced hemoglobin).

D. Oxygen content
  1. The total oxygen content of blood is equal to the volume of oxygen physically dissolved in plasma plus the amount chemically combined with hemoglobin (Fig 11–1).
  2. Mathematically the above statement is equal to

$$O_2 \text{ content in vol\%} =$$
$$(P_{O_2})(0.003) + (Hb \text{ content})(1.34)(HbO_2\% \text{ sat.}) \qquad (7)$$

E. Oxyhemoglobin dissociation curve (Fig 11–2)
  1. The overall sigmoidal shape of the curve is a result of the varied affinities of the four oxygen-bonding sites on the hemoglobin molecule.
    a. In general, the affinity of the last site bound is considerably less than the other three sites.

THE PHYSIOLOGY OF RESPIRATION

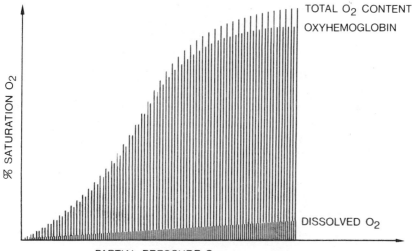

Fig 11–1.—Volume of oxygen dissolved, as oxyhemoglobin, and total oxygen content are indicated. The overall sigmoidal shape of the curve demonstrates varying bonding affinities for oxygen molecules as oxyhemoglobin saturation is increased. (From Shapiro B.A., Harrison R.A., Walton J.R.: *Clinical Application of Blood Gases,* ed. 3. Chicago, Year Book Medical Publishers, Inc., 1982. Reproduced by permission.)

Oxygenation

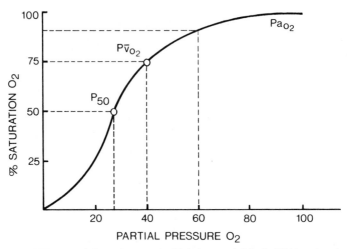

Fig 11–2.—The partial pressure at which hemoglobin is 50% saturated is 27 mm Hg. This is referred to as P_{50}. Normal venous Po_2 of 40 mm Hg and 75% oxyhemoglobin saturation are also indicated. A Po_2 of 60 mm Hg results in 90% saturation of the hemoglobin, whereas the normal arterial Po_2 of 97 mm Hg results in 97% saturation of the hemoglobin. (From Shapiro B.A., Harrison R.A., Walton J.R.: *Clinical Application of Blood Gases*, ed. 3. Chicago, Year Book Medical Publishers, Inc., 1982. Reproduced by permission.)

    b. In addition, the affinity of the first site is less than that of the second or third sites.

2. The steep aspect of the curve is that portion where minimal changes in Po_2 normally will cause significant increases in $HbO_2\%$ saturation and therefore O_2 content.

    a. Increasing the saturation from 50% to 75% normally necessitates only a 13 mm Hg Po_2 increase, whereas increasing the saturation from 75% to 100% normally necessitates well over a 100 mg Hg Po_2 increase.

3. P_{50} is defined as that Po_2 at which the hemoglobin is 50% saturated with oxygen. Normally the P_{50} is equal to 27 mm Hg (see Fig 11–2).

    a. An increased P_{50} indicates a shift of the oxyhemoglobin dissociation curve to the right, resulting in a decreased hemoglobin affinity for oxygen (greater unloading of oxygen at the tissue and decreased loading at the alveoli).

    b. A decreased P_{50} indicates a shift of the oxyhemoglobin dissociation curve to the left, resulting in an increased hemoglobin affinity for oxygen (decreased unloading of oxygen at the tissue and decreased loading at the alveoli).

    c. Hemoglobin is considered an allosteric enzyme because of the two conformational structures it assumes (deoxyhemoglobin and oxyhemoglobin). Allosteric enzymes are substances with two binding sites, one active site and one secondary site. The binding of substances at the secondary site can affect the affinity of binding at the active site.

    d. The following alter the affinity of hemoglobin for oxygen by affecting the secondary site.

        (1) P_{CO_2}

        (2) H^+ or pH

        (3) Temperature

        (4) 2,3-Diphosphoglycerate (2,3-DPG)

        (5) Carbon monoxide

        (6) Abnormal forms of hemoglobin

4. The oxyhemoglobin curve is shifted to the right by:

    a. Increased P_{CO_2}

    b. Increased $[H^+]$ or decreased pH

    c. Increased temperature

    d. Increased 2,3-DPG

5. The oxyhemoglobin curve is shifted to the left by:

    a. Decreased P_{CO_2}

    b. Decreased $[H^+]$ or increased pH

    c. Decreased temperature

    d. Decreased 2,3-DPG

    e. Increased CO

    f. Fetal hemoglobin

    g. Methemoglobin

F. *The Bohr effect:* The effect of carbon dioxide or $[H^+]$ on uptake and release of oxygen from the hemoglobin molecule. The effect is relatively mild.

1. As seen above, carbon dioxide and $[H^+]$ will cause a shift in the oxyhemoglobin dissociation curve.

2. At the systemic capillary bed, increased carbon dioxide and $[H^+]$ moving into the blood decreases hemoglobin affinity for oxygen and increases the volume of oxygen released at the tissue level.

3. At the pulmonary capillary bed, decreased carbon dioxide and $[H^+]$ levels increase hemoglobin affinity for oxygen, thus increasing the volume of oxygen picked up at the pulmonary level.

G. Carbon monoxide (CO)
   1. CO attaches to hemoglobin at the same site as O_2.
   2. The affinity of hemoglobin for CO is 200 times greater than its affinity for O_2.
   3. In addition, carboxyhemoglobin (HbCO) shifts the oxyhemoglobin dissociation curve to the left, decreasing the ability of hemoglobin to unload oxygen.
H. Abnormal hemoglobins
   1. There are over 100 abnormal forms of hemoglobins.
   2. Twelve of these have an effect on the affinity of hemoglobin for oxygen.
   3. Fetal hemoglobin has two γ (gamma) chains instead of β chains, which results in a decreased P_{50} (shift to the left).
   4. Methemoglobin is formed by Fe atoms being oxidized from the ferrous to the ferric state; this also results in a decreased P_{50} (shift to the left).
IV. O_2 Availability
   A. The quantity of O_2 available to the tissue is dependent on O_2 content and cardiac output.
   B. The amount of O_2 transported to tissue is equal to:

$$(O_2 \text{ content in vol\%}) \ (10) \ (\text{cardiac output in L/min}) \qquad (8)$$

   C. In the normal healthy adult, O_2 content equals about 20 vol% and cardiac output is about 5 L/min. Thus:

$$O_2 \text{ transport} = (20 \text{ vol\%}) \ (10) \ (5 \text{ L/min}) = 1,000 \text{ ml/min}$$

   D. O_2 availability is most significantly affected by the hemoglobin level and cardiac output.
   E. Normal O_2 transport ranges from about 900 to 1,200 ml/min at rest.
V. Oxygen Consumption
   A. The normal arterial O_2 content is 20 vol%.
   B. The normal mixed venous O_2 content is about 15 vol%.
   C. Thus, $Ca_{O_2} - C\bar{v}_{O_2}$ is 5 vol%.
   D. If the cardiac output is 5 L/min, the organism consumes 250 ml/min of oxygen.
   E. O_2 consumption in the adult varies from about 200 to 350 ml/min (basal metabolic level).
   F. O_2 consumption is altered by:
      1. Physical activity (metabolic rate)
      2. Physiologic stress
      3. Temperature

    4. Alterations in microcirculation

  G. In the adequately perfused normothermic patient who is not shivering or seizing, O_2 consumption is equal to about 3.5 ml/kg of body weight.

VI. Production of Carbon Dioxide

  A. CO_2 is produced by the metabolism of all food.

  B. In addition, CO_2 is produced in the conversion of glucose to fatty acids.

  C. Normal CO_2 production is about 160–280 ml/min.

VII. Carriage of Carbon Dioxide in the Blood

  A. Carriage in plasma occurs in three distinct ways (Fig 11–3):

    1. Carbon dioxide is dissolved in plasma as P_{CO_2}, which is in equilibrium with the P_{CO_2} in RBCs.

    2. Carbon dioxide is carried predominantly as bicarbonate (HCO_3^-) formed in the RBCs and by the kidney. The HCO_3^- levels in plasma are in equilibrium with the HCO_3^- in RBCs.

      a. Plasma carbon dioxide reacts minimally with water, forming carbonic acid, which dissociates into H^+ and HCO_3^-:

$$CO_2 + H_2O \leftrightharpoons H_2CO_3 \rightleftarrows H^+ + HCO_3^- \qquad (9)$$

      b. The H^+ formed is buffered in the plasma and therefore causes a mild decrease in pH (venous blood).

      c. The above reaction's point of equilibrium is shifted to the left in the plasma, therefore favoring formation of reactants.

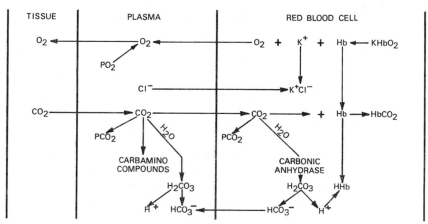

Fig 11–3.—Overall scheme of O_2 and CO_2 transport in blood (see text).

    d. The mathematical relationship between dissolved CO_2 and H_2CO_3 is:

$$(\text{Pco}_2 \text{ mm Hg})(0.0301) = H_2CO_3 \text{ mEq/L or mmoles/L} \tag{10}$$

  3. Carbon dioxide is attached to plasma proteins, forming carbamino compounds.

    a. Carbon dioxide reacts with the terminal amino groups on the plasma proteins ($R-NH_2$):

$$
\begin{array}{c}
H \\
\diagup \\
R-N \\
\diagdown \\
H
\end{array}
+ CO_2 \rightleftarrows
\begin{array}{c}
H \\
\diagup \\
R-N \\
\diagdown \\
COO^-
\end{array}
+ H^+ \tag{11}
$$

      (R—indicates the remainder of the plasma protein)

    b. Most of the H^+ liberated is buffered and therefore causes a mild decrease in the pH (venous blood).

    c. The ionization state of the amino groups affects their ability to bond with carbon dioxide. If the NH_2 groups are oxidized to $NH_3{}^+$, their ability to combine with carbon dioxide is significantly decreased.

B. Carriage of carbon dioxide in RBCs occurs in three distinct ways (see Fig 11–3):

  1. As dissolved Pco_2 in equilibrium with plasma Pco_2

  2. As $HCO_3{}^-$ formed in the RBC

    a. The reaction shown in equation 9 is significantly increased as a result of the presence of the enzyme carbonic anhydrase (CA). The point of equilibrium is shifted to the right, favoring formation of the products:

$$CO_2 + H_2O \overset{CA}{\rightleftarrows} H_2CO_3 \rightleftarrows H^+ + HCO_3{}^- \tag{12}$$

    b. As increasing levels of $HCO_3{}^-$ are formed in the RBC, $HCO_3{}^-$ diffuses into the plasma. As $HCO_3{}^-$ diffuses, there is an imbalance of electric charges inside the RBC, causing Cl^- to move into the RBC. This process is referred to as the *chloride shift* or *Hamburger phenomenon*. The Cl^- diffusing into the RBC associates with the K^+ released as the Hb molecule gives up O_2 and buffers H^+.

  3. As carbon dioxide attached to the terminal amino ($R\text{-}NH_2$) groups of the hemoglobin molecule. This reaction is the same as that shown in equation 11. Again, the H^+ released from the formation of $HCO_3{}^-$ must be buffered.

    a. In RBCs the primary buffer is the imidazole groups on the hemoglobin molecule.

    b. The ability of the imidazole groups to buffer is affected by oxyhemoglobin saturation. With oxygen bound to the heme, the imidazole groups are poor buffers. Without oxygen attached to the heme, the imidazole groups are good buffers.

    c. As oxygen attaches to the heme, more $R\text{-}NH_2$ groups will exist in the $R\text{-}NH_3^+$ form. The tendency for carbon dioxide to attach to the $R\text{-}NH_3^+$ form is less than to the $R\text{-}NH_2$ form.

VIII. The Haldane Effect

    A. Figure 11–4 illustrates the Haldane effect, which is defined as the effect of oxygen on carbon dioxide uptake and release.

    B. As P_{O_2} increases at the pulmonary capillary bed, the ability of hemoglobin to carry carbon dioxide is decreased because more amino groups exist in the oxidized $R\text{-}NH_3^+$ state. This allows large volumes of carbon dioxide to be released at the pulmonary capillary bed.

    C. As the P_{O_2} decreases at the tissue level, the ability of hemoglobin to carry carbon dioxide is increased because more amino groups exist in the reduced $R\text{-}NH_2$ form. This allows large volumes of carbon dioxide to be picked up at the systemic capillary bed (see Fig 11–4).

    D. The Haldane effect facilitates carriage of the normal 4 vol% (200 ml/min) of carbon dioxide picked up from the tissue and released at the lung.

IX. Quantitative Distribution of Carbon Dioxide

    A. Percentage of carbon dioxide carried in each compartment:

       1. 90% of carbon dioxide in blood exists as HCO_3^-.

       2. 5% of carbon dioxide in blood exists as carbamino compounds.

       3. 5% of carbon dioxide in blood exists as dissolved P_{CO_2}.

    B. Percentage of carbon dioxide exhaled from various compartments:

       1. 60% of the carbon dioxide exhaled is carried as HCO_3^-.

       2. 30% of the carbon dioxide exhaled is carried as carbamino compounds.

       3. 10% of the carbon dioxide exhaled is carried as dissolved P_{CO_2}.

X. Total CO_2

    A. Total CO_2 is an expression of the sum of HCO_3^- plus dissolved CO_2.

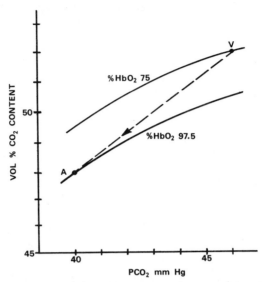

Fig 11–4.—Effect of oxyhemoglobin saturation on volume of CO_2 carried in blood. The carrying capacity of blood for CO_2 is decreased as oxyhemoglobin saturation is increased (Haldane effect). The arrow from *V* to *A* depicts change of CO_2 content from venous to arterial blood.

    B. Total CO_2 may be expressed in millimoles per liter (mmoles/L), milliequivalents per liter (mEq/L), or vol%.

    C. $(P_{CO_2})(0.0301)$ equals mmoles/L or mEq/L of H_2CO_3

    D. Vol% of CO_2 equals (mEq/L)(2.23) or (mmoles/L)(2.23)

    E. mmoles/L or mEq/L of CO_2 equals vol%/2.23

    F. In arterial blood

        1. Total CO_2 = $[HCO_3^-]$ + [dissolved P_{CO_2}]

        2. 25.2 mmoles/L = 24 mmoles/L + 1.2 mmoles/L

        3. 56.2 vol% = 53.52 vol% + 2.68 vol%

 XI. Respiratory Quotient, Respiratory Exchange Ratio, and Ventilation/ Perfusion Ratio

    A. The respiratory quotient (RQ) is defined as the volume of carbon dioxide produced divided by the volume of oxygen consumed per minute:

$$RQ = \frac{4 \text{ vol\% } CO_2}{5 \text{ vol\% } O_2} \text{ or } \frac{200 \text{ ml } CO_2}{250 \text{ ml } O_2} = 0.8 \qquad (12)$$

    B. The RQ is an expression of *internal* respiration.

    C. The respiratory exchange ratio (R) is defined as the volume of carbon dioxide moving from the pulmonary capillaries to the lung divided by the volume of oxygen moving from the lung into the pulmonary capillaries:

$$R = \frac{4 \text{ vol\% } CO_2}{5 \text{ vol\% } O_2} = \frac{200 \text{ ml } CO_2}{250 \text{ ml } O_2} = 0.8 \qquad (13)$$

D. The R is an expression of *external* respiration.
E. Under normal circumstances RQ and R are equal, with a mean value of about 0.8.
F. The ventilation/perfusion ($\dot{V}/\dot{Q}$) ratio is equal to the minute alveolar ventilation divided by the minute cardiac output:

$$\dot{V}/\dot{Q} = \frac{4 \text{ L alveolar minute volume}}{5 \text{ L minute cardiac output}} = 0.8 \qquad (14)$$

G. $\dot{V}/\dot{Q}$ is equal to RQ and R under normal circumstances.
H. It is the alveolar ventilation and the cardiac output that maintain the RQ and R equal.

BIBLIOGRAPHY

Bendixen H.H., et al.: *Respiratory Care.* St. Louis, C.V. Mosby Co., 1965.
Cherniack R.M., Cherniack L.: *Respiration in Health and Disease,* ed. 3. Philadelphia, W.B. Saunders Co., 1983.
Comroe J.H.: *Physiology of Respiration,* ed. 2. Chicago, Year Book Medical Publishers, Inc., 1974.
Des Jardins T.R.: *Clinical Manifestations of Respiratory Disease.* Chicago, Year Book Medical Publishers, Inc., 1984.
Guyton A.C.: *Textbook of Medical Physiology,* ed. 6. Philadelphia, W.B. Saunders Co., 1981.
Murray J.F.: *The Normal Lung.* Philadelphia, W.B. Saunders Co., 1976.
Nunn J.F.: *Applied Respiratory Physiology,* ed. 2. London, Butterworth & Co., Ltd., 1977.
Shapiro B.A., Harrison R.A., Kacmarek R.M., et al.: *Clinical Application of Respiratory Care,* ed. 3. Chicago, Year Book Medical Publishers, Inc., 1985.
Shapiro B.A., Harrison R.A., Walton J.R.: *Clinical Application of Blood Gases,* ed. 3. Chicago, Year Book Medical Publishers, Inc., 1982.
Spearman C.B., Sheldon R.L., Egan D.F.: *Egan's Fundamentals of Respiratory Therapy,* ed. 4. St. Louis, C.V. Mosby Co., 1982.
West J.B.: *Respiratory Physiology: The Essentials.* Baltimore, Williams & Wilkins Co., 1981.
Young J.A., Crocker D.: *Principles and Practice of Respiratory Therapy,* ed. 2. Chicago, Year Book Medical Publishers, Inc., 1976.

12 / Acid-Base Balance and Blood Gas Interpretation

I. Electrolytes
   A. An electrolyte is a substance that is capable of conducting an electrical current when placed into solution.
   B. When an electrolyte dissolves in solution, it dissociates, producing ions. For example, sodium chloride (NaCl) dissociates into sodium (Na^+) and chloride (Cl^-) ions.

$$NaCl \rightarrow Na^+ + Cl^- \tag{1}$$

   C. Strong electrolytes dissociate completely when dissolved in solution.
   D. Weak electrolytes only partially dissociate, with the majority of electrolyte remaining dissolved but undissociated.
   E. A weak acid electrolyte produces H^+ when dissolved.
   F. A weak basic electrolyte produces OH^- when dissolved.
II. Law of Mass Action
   A. The basic chemical and mathematical relationships involved in blood gas interpretation are based on the law of mass action (also referred to as the law of electrolyte dissociation and law of chemical equilibrium).
   B. *The law of mass action* states that when a weak electrolyte is placed into solution, only a small percentage of it dissociates, the vast majority remaining undissociated. Determining the product of the molar concentrations of the dissociated species and dividing that by the molar concentration of the undissociated weak electrolyte yields a dissociation constant for that weak electrolyte. This constant is true for the particular electrolyte at the temperature it was originally determined.
   C. If the weak acid HA is placed into solution, it will reversibly dissociate to H^+ and A^- (the negative ion formed whenever H^+ dissociates from an acid).

$$HA \rightleftharpoons H^+ + A^- \tag{2}$$

D. If 0.01 moles/L of HA were added to solution and 5% of HA dissociated, the following quantities of all three species would exist in solution:

$$HA \quad 95\% \text{ of } 0.01 \text{ or } .0095 \text{ moles/L}$$
$$H^+ \quad 5\% \text{ of } 0.01 \text{ or } .0005 \text{ moles/L}$$
$$A^- \quad 5\% \text{ of } 0.01 \text{ or } .0005 \text{ moles/L}$$

Note: One H^+ and one A^- are formed as every HA molecule dissociates.

E. According to the law of mass action:

$$K = \frac{[H^+][A^-]}{[HA]} \tag{3}$$

where K = the dissociation constant.

F. Inserting the molar concentrations of the individual species and calculating the dissociation constant yields the following:

$$.0000263 = \frac{[0.0005][0.0005]}{[0.0095]}$$

Thus, $K = 2.63 \times 10^{-5}$

G. As explained in sections II above and IV below, the dissociation constant indicates the pH at which a buffer functions most efficiently.

H. The law of mass action applied to water is the basis for the pH scale.

   1. H_2O (water) dissociates into H^+ plus OH^-

$$H_2O \rightleftharpoons H^+ + OH^- \tag{4}$$

   2. The molar concentration of both H^+ and OH^- is 10^{-7} moles/L.

   3. Since the concentration of the undissociated water is so large in comparison to the $[H^+]$ and $[OH^-]$, it is considered a constant.

$$\frac{[H^+][OH^-]}{K_{H2O}} = K \tag{5}$$

   4. This relationship is frequently written as

$$[H^+][OH^-] = K_w \tag{6}$$

where K_w is the dissociation constant for H_2O.

5. The value of K_w is

$$[10^{-7}][10^{-7}] = 10^{-14}$$

6. Thus, a neutral solution is one with 10^{-7} moles of H^+ per liter.
7. Since the H^+ concentration can vary from 10^{-1} to 10^{-14} in this relationship, the limits of the pH scale are defined.
8. pH is equal to $-\log[H^+]$.
9. The pH scale therefore goes from a pH of 1.0 ($[H^+] = 10^{-1}$ moles/L) to a pH of 14.0 ($[H^+] = 10^{-14}$ moles/L).
10. Remember the product of $[H^+]$ and $[OH^-]$ must equal 10^{-14}. As a result, as the $[H^+]$ increases, the $[OH^-]$ decreases, and vice versa.

I. The law of mass action when applied to carbonic acid (H_2CO_3) dissolved in plasma at 37° C yields the following:
1. H_2CO_3 dissociates into $H^+ + HCO_3^-$ (bicarbonate ion)

$$H_2CO_3 \rightleftarrows H^+ + HCO_3^- \tag{7}$$

2. Taking the molar concentration of H^+ and multiplying it by the molar concentration of HCO_3^- and dividing this by the molar concentration of H_2CO_3, the dissociation constant for H_2CO_3 in plasma is calculated:

$$\frac{[H^+][HCO_3^-]}{[H_2CO_3]} = K \tag{8}$$

3. K for the above reaction in blood is equal to 7.85×10^{-7}.
J. The mathematical manipulation of the law of mass action results in the development of the Henderson-Hasselbalch equation.

III. Henderson-Hasselbalch Equation (Standard Buffer Equation)
A. Derivation of the Henderson-Hasselbalch equation from equation 8.
1. Rearranging equation 8 and solving for $[H^+]$ results in the following:

$$[H^+] = \frac{K[H_2CO_3]}{[HCO_3^-]} \tag{9}$$

2. Taking the log to the base 10 of each side of equation 9 yields the following:

$$\log[H^+] = \log K + \log\frac{[H_2CO_3]}{[HCO_3^-]} \tag{10}$$

3. Multiplying each side of equation 10 by -1 yields the following:

$$-\log [H^+] = -\log K - \log \frac{[H_2CO_3]}{[HCO_3^-]} \qquad (11)$$

4. Rearranging $-\log \frac{[H_2CO_3]}{[HCO_3^-]}$ in equation 11 yields the following:

$$-\log [H_2CO_3] (-) -\log [HCO_3^-]$$
$$= -\log [H_2CO_3] + \log [HCO_3^-]$$
$$= +\log [HCO_3^-] - \log [H_2CO_3]$$
$$= +\log \frac{[HCO_3^-]}{[H_2CO_3]} \qquad (12)$$

5. Inserting equation 12 in equation 11 yields the following:

$$-\log H^+ = -\log K + \log \frac{[HCO_3^-]}{[H_2CO_3]} \qquad (13)$$

6. $-\log H^+ = pH$ and $-\log K$ is termed the pK (refer to section IV below). Equation 13 is rewritten as:

$$pH = pK + \log \frac{[HCO_3^-]}{[H_2CO_3]} \qquad (14)$$

7. Equation 14 is the classic buffer equation (see section V) as applied to the HCO_3^-/H_2CO_3 buffer system.
8. A universal representation of the classic buffer equation as applied to a weak acid electrolyte is

$$pH = pKa + \log \frac{[conjugate\ base]}{[undissociated\ acid]} \qquad (15)$$

where pKa is the pK of a weak acid electrolyte
9. If the derivation were carried out for a weak basic electrolyte, the standard equation would be:

$$pOH = pKb + \log \frac{[conjugate\ acid]}{[undissociated\ base]} \qquad (16)$$

10. However, the type of buffer systems used in describing pulmonary physiology are all weak acid electrolytes.

IV. pK (− Log of the Dissociation Constant)
   A. This value represents the pH at which a buffer functions most efficiently.
   B. When the pH of a solution equals the pK, 50% of the buffer exists in the form of the conjugate base and 50% as the undissociated acid.
   C. All buffers have a narrow pH range, identifying where they function appropriately.
   D. In general, if the pH of a solution is above its pK, the solution will buffer acid more effectively than base.
   E. If the pH of a solution is below its pK, the solution will buffer base more effectively than acid.
   F. The further away a solution's pH moves from its pK, the poorer its buffering capabilities.
   G. If the pH of a buffered solution is outside the 1–1.5 pH range about the buffer's pK, the system's buffering capabilities are lost.

V. Buffers
   A. A buffer is a weak acidic or basic electrolyte that has the capability of determining the pH of a solution.
   B. Buffers are used to prevent significant changes in a solution pH.
   C. One should always choose a buffer whose pK is numerically near the pH of the solution to be buffered.
   D. Chemical functioning of buffers:
      1. If the buffer HA from section II is titrated into solution until the pH of the solution is equal to the pK of the buffer, an ideally buffered solution is established. The pK of this system is 4.58 (−log of 2.63×10^{-5}, see section II–F).
      2. After titration the final concentrations of HA and A⁻ are equal to 0.01. Thus the classic buffer equation would be:

$$pH = pK + \log \frac{[A^-]}{[HA]} \qquad (17)$$

or

$$4.58 = 4.58 + \log \frac{0.01}{0.01}$$

Note: The log of $\frac{0.01}{0.01}$ is 0.

3. If acid is added to this buffer, it reacts with the conjugate base (A^-) and forms more undissociated acid (HA).

$$A^- + H^+ \rightarrow HA \qquad (18)$$

This should result in only a minimal change in the pH.
   a. If 0.001 mole/L of H^+ is added to the buffer, the H^+ would react with 0.001 mole/L of A^-.

$$A^- + H^+ \rightarrow HA$$
$$0.001 + 0.001 \rightarrow 0.001$$

Note: 100% efficiency assumed.
   b. As a result, the concentration of A^- would decrease by 0.001 and the concentration of HA would increase by 0.001.

$$pH = 4.58 + \log \frac{0.01 - 0.001}{0.01 + 0.001} \text{ or } \frac{0.009}{0.011}$$

   c. The resulting pH of this solution would be 4.49, or a 0.09 pH unit change.
   d. By comparison, if 0.001 mole/L of H^+ were added to water with a pH of 7.0, the resulting pH would be about 2.99, over a 4.0 pH unit change.
4. If base is added to a buffer, it reacts with free H^+, allowing more HA to dissociate,

$$H^+ + OH^- \rightarrow H_2O \qquad (19)$$

causing the following:

$$HA \rightarrow H^+ + A^-$$

resulting in a minimal change in the pH.
   a. If 0.001 mole/L of OH^- is added to the buffer in equation 17, the OH^- would react with 0.001 mole/L of H^+, causing 0.001 mole/L of HA to dissociate.

$$H^+ + OH^- \rightarrow H_2O$$
$$0.001 + 0.001 \rightarrow 0.001$$

causing the following:

$$HA \rightarrow H^+ + A^-$$
$$0.001 \rightarrow 0.001 + 0.001$$

   b. As a result, the concentration of HA is decreased by 0.001 and the concentration of A^- is increased by 0.001.

$$pH = 4.58 + \log \frac{0.01 + 0.001}{0.01 - 0.001} \text{ or } \frac{0.011}{0.009}$$

    c. The resulting pH of the solution would be 4.67, a 0.09 pH unit change.

    d. By comparison, if 0.001 mole/L of OH^- were added to water with a pH of 7.0, the resulting pH would be about 10.99, almost a 4.0 pH unit change.

VI. The HCO_3^-/H_2CO_3 Buffer System

    A. The most important buffer system in the body is the HCO_3^-/H_2CO_3 system.

$$pH = pK + \log \frac{HCO_3^-}{H_2CO_3} \tag{20}$$

    B. The pK of this system is 6.1 ($K = 7.85 \times 10^{-7}$).

    C. Arterial HCO_3^- levels are about 24 mEq/L.

    D. Arterial H_2CO_3 levels are about 1.2 mEq/L.

    E. Thus, arterial pH is about 7.4:

$$7.4 = 6.1 + \log \frac{24 \text{ mEq/L}}{1.2 \text{ mEq/L}}$$

    F. The ratio of HCO_3^- to H_2CO_3 is 20:1:

$$\frac{HCO_3^-}{H_2CO_3} = \frac{24}{1.2} = \frac{20}{1}$$

    G. If this ratio increases (30:1), the arterial pH increases.

    H. If this ratio decreases (10:1), the arterial pH decreases.

    I. Clinically, HCO_3^- and H_2CO_3 concentrations are extremely time-consuming and costly to determine.

      1. Since the (P_{CO_2}) × (0.0301) is equivalent to the H_2CO_3 concentration, this value can be substituted into equation 20 for H_2CO_3:

$$pH = 6.10 + \log \frac{[HCO_3^-]}{(P_{CO_2})(0.0301)} \tag{21}$$

      2. Clinically the pH of the blood is easily measured, as is the P_{CO_2} (see Chap. 29).

      3. $[HCO_3^-]$ is always the calculated value when blood gas results are reported.

    J. In this buffer system $[HCO_3^-]$ is regulated and controlled by the kidney and P_{CO_2} is regulated and controlled by the lung with the pH a result of the $[HCO_3^-]$ and P_{CO_2}.

K. The HCO_3^-/H_2CO_3 buffer system in blood is a poor chemical buffer.

   1. This is true because of the pK (6.1) of the buffer in relation to the pH (7.4) of the blood.

   2. The pH of blood is outside the chemical buffering range of the HCO_3^-/H_2CO_3 system.

   3. However, this system is considered an essential *physiologic* buffer. That is, the lungs can control the excretion or retention of large quantities of acid in the form of CO_2.

   4. The following reversible reaction illustrates the relationship:

$$CO_2 + H_2O \rightleftharpoons H_2CO_3 \rightleftharpoons H^+ + HCO_3^- \qquad (22)$$

   5. If there is an increase in H^+ the reaction is shifted to the left, increasing plasma CO_2 levels, which are exhaled.

   6. If there is a decrease in H^+ the reaction is shifted to the right, decreasing plasma CO_2 levels.

   7. The effectiveness of HCO_3^- administration in the face of a metabolic acidosis is based on equation 22 shifting to the left, allowing acid to be exhaled as CO_2. If ventilation cannot eliminate the increased CO_2 produced, the acidosis changes from metabolic to respiratory.

VII. Actual versus Standard HCO_3^-

  A. Actual HCO_3^-: Value calculated from actual, measured P_{CO_2} and pH of arterial blood.

   1. Value normally given with arterial blood gas results.

   2. Indicative of nonrespiratory acid-base imbalances.

  B. Standard HCO_3^-: Value calculated from measured pH and P_{CO_2} of venous blood after P_{CO_2} of blood has been equilibrated to 40 mm Hg.

   1. Value usually reported with electrolyte studies by clinical laboratory.

   2. Indicative of a change in acid-base balance, but not precise as to magnitude when compared with arterial pH and P_{CO_2}.

   3. Arterial pH and P_{CO_2} most closely correlate with actual HCO_3^-.

VIII. Base Excess/Base Deficit

  A. The total buffering capacity of the body can be broken down approximately as follows:

   1. 60% by the HCO_3^-/H_2CO_3 system

   2. 30% by hemoglobin buffering system

      3. 10% by all other blood buffers (e.g., phosphates, plasma proteins, ammonia)

B. Of the total body buffers, HCO_3^- and all proteins (including Hb) are the most important.

C. These two systems may be chemically depicted as follows:

$$CO_2 + H_2O \rightleftharpoons H_2CO_3 \rightleftharpoons HCO_3^- + H^+ \qquad (23)$$

$$H \; Prot \rightleftharpoons H^+ + Prot^- \qquad (24)$$

D. If a respiratory acidosis were to develop, the reaction shown in equation 23 would be driven to the right, causing an equal shift of the reaction shown in equation 24 to the left. As a result, the total amount of base in the body would remain unchanged.

E. If a respiratory alkalosis were to develop, the reaction shown in equation 23 would be driven to the left, causing an equal shift of the reaction shown in equation 24 to the right. As a result, the total amount of base in the body would remain unchanged.

F. The sum of $[HCO_3^-] + [Prot^-]$ is the buffer base, which (as demonstrated in VIII–D and VIII–E) remains unchanged in all pure acute respiratory acid-base disturbances.

G. However, if metabolic acid is added to the body, the reactions shown in equations 23 and 24 would both be driven to the left, and the quantity of buffer base would decrease and if metabolic base were added to the body, both reactions (23 and 24) would be driven to the right and the quantity of buffer base would increase.

H. Base excess/base deficit (BE/BD) is defined as the actual buffer base (BB) minus the normal BB.

$$BE/BD = actual \; BB - normal \; BB \qquad (25)$$

  I. In all pure acute respiratory acid-base disturbances, the BE/BD is normal. However, once compensation occurs, the BE/BD becomes positive or negative.

J. All metabolic acid-base disturbances are accompanied by a change in the BE/BD.

K. The BE/BD is the most reliable index of metabolic acid base disorders.

L. The normal BE/BD is zero, with a range of ± 2 mEq/L. The normal total buffer base is 54 mEq/L.

IX. Normal Ranges for Blood Gases

  A. *Absolute* normals: Arterial blood (mean population values)

      1. pH   7.40

      2. P_{CO_2} 40 mm Hg

3. Po_2 100 mm Hg
4. HCO_3^- 24 mEq/L
5. Base excess   0
6. Hemoglobin content   14 gm%
7. Oxyhemoglobin saturation   97.5%
8. Oxygen content   19.8 vol%
9. Carboxyhemoglobin saturation   0%

B. *Normal* ranges: Arterial blood (± 2 standard deviations from the population mean)
1. pH   7.35–7.45
2. Pco_2 35–45 mm Hg
3. Po_2 80–100 mm Hg
4. HCO_3^- 22–27 mEq/L
5. Base excess ± 2
6. Hemoglobin content   12–15 gm%
7. Oxyhemoglobin saturation $\geqq 95\%$
8. Oxygen content >16 vol%
9. Carboxyhemoglobin saturation $<2\%$

C. *Absolute normals:* Venous blood (mean population values)
1. pH   7.35
2. Pco_2 46 mm Hg
3. Po_2 40 mm Hg
4. HCO_3^- 27 mEq/L
5. Oxyhemoglobin saturation   75%

D. *Clinical ranges:* Arterial blood (± 3 standard deviations from the population mean)
1. pH   7.30–7.50
2. Pco_2 30–50 mm Hg
3. The ranges for arterial blood values given in section IX-B indicate the "normal" variation in arterial pH and Pco_2. Slight variations outside these normal ranges may not indicate a clinically significant change.
4. The clinical ranges above indicate an acceptable pH and Pco_2 from a *patient management* point of view. Results outside these ranges normally indicate situations requiring clinical intervention.

X. Mathematical Interrelationships Between pH, Pco_2 and HCO_3^-
A. If the constants and log relationship are eliminated in the HCO_3^-/H_2CO_3 buffer equation, the equation may be simplified to:

$$pH \approx \frac{HCO_3^-}{Pco_2} \qquad (26)$$

This relationship demonstrates the mathematical interrelationship between these variables.

B. In general, under all clinical circumstances the pH will be a result of the HCO_3^- and PCO_2 levels.

C. In a pure respiratory abnormality where the HCO_3^- remains essentially constant, the PCO_2 and pH are indirectly related:

$$HCO_3^- \approx (pH)(PCO_2) \qquad (27)$$

D. In a pure metabolic abnormality where the PCO_2 remains essentially constant, the HCO_3^- and pH are directly related:

$$PCO_2 \approx \frac{HCO_3^-}{pH} \qquad (28)$$

E. These interrelationships provide the basis for blood gas interpretation.

XI. Compensation for Primary Acid-Base Abnormalities

A. Compensation involves the various mechanisms used by the body to normalize the pH after a primary acid-base abnormality. Compensation does not imply correction of the primary abnormalities.

B. Compensation for primary respiratory acid-base imbalances is via the kidney (see Chap. 9).

C. Compensation for primary metabolic acid-base abnormalities is via the respiratory system (see Chap. 5).

XII. Estimation of pH Changes Based Purely on PCO_2 Changes

A. Since the pK of the HCO_3^-/H_2CO_3 system is 6.10 and the quantity of HCO_3^- is 20 times greater than the quantity of H_2CO_3, the body buffers acid more efficiently than base.

B. If, starting at a baseline pH of 7.40 and a PCO_2 of 40 mm Hg, for every 10 mm Hg PCO_2 increase there is an approximate 0.05 pH unit decrease,

1. PCO_2 50: pH 7.35: HCO_3^- 25
2. PCO_2 60: pH 7.30: HCO_3^- 26
3. PCO_2 70: pH 7.25: HCO_3^- 27
4. PCO_2 80: pH 7.20: HCO_3^- 28

This relationship holds if *no* compensation by the kidney has occurred. The HCO_3^- increases as a result of a shifting of the components of the buffer base (see section VIII).

C. If, starting at a baseline pH of 7.40 and a PCO_2 of 40, for every 10 mm Hg PCO_2 decrease there is an approximate 0.10 pH unit increase,

1. PCO_2 35: pH 7.45: HCO_3^- 23

2. P_{CO_2} 30: pH 7.50: HCO_3^- 22
3. P_{CO_2} 25: pH 7.55: HCO_3^- 21
4. P_{CO_2} 20: pH 7.60: HCO_3^- 20

This relationship holds if no compensation by the kidney has occurred. The HCO_3^- decreases as a result of a shifting of the components of the buffer base (see section VIII).

XIII. Interpretation of Arterial Blood Gases

Blood gas interpretation is performed in three steps:

  A. Interpretation of acid-base status

  B. Assessment of level of hypoxemia

  C. Assessment of tissue hypoxia

XIV. Interpretation of Acid-Base Status

  A. Tables 12–1 and 12–2 list ranges for interpretation of blood gases using the classic and clinical methods.

  B. The classic method uses the terminology uncompensated, partially compensated, and compensated, along with the normal ranges for P_{CO_2} and pH.

  C. The clinical method, developed by Shapiro, uses the classic terminology only for metabolic disturbances and acute or chronic alveolar hyperventilation and ventilatory failure for respiratory acid-base imbalances. In addition, the clinical ranges for pH and P_{CO_2} are used.

TABLE 12–1.—Classic Textbook Method of Blood Gas Interpretation

STATUS	pH	P_{CO_2}	HCO_3^-	BE
RESPIRATORY ACIDOSIS				
Uncompensated	↓ 7.35	↑ 45	Normal	Normal
Partially compensated	↓ 7.35	↑ 45	↑ 27	↑ +2
Compensated	7.35–7.45	↑ 45	↑ 27	↑ +2
RESPIRATORY ALKALOSIS				
Uncompensated	↑ 7.45	↓ 35	Normal	Normal
Partially compensated	↑ 7.45	↓ 35	↓ 22	↓ −2
Compensated	7.40–7.45	↓ 35	↓ 22	↓ −2
METABOLIC ACIDOSIS				
Uncompensated	↓ 7.35	Normal	↓ 22	↓ −2
Partially compensated	↓ 7.35	↓ 35	↓ 22	↓ −2
Compensated	7.35–7.40	↓ 35	↓ 22	↓ −2
METABOLIC ALKALOSIS				
Uncompensated	↑ 7.45	Normal	↑ 27	↑ +2
Partially compensated*	↑ 7.45	↑ 45	↑ 27	↑ +2
Compensated*	7.40–7.45	↑ 45	↑ 27	↑ +2
COMBINED RESPIRATORY AND METABOLIC ACIDOSIS	↓ 7.35	↑ 45	↓ 22	↓ −2
COMBINED RESPIRATORY AND METABOLIC ALKALOSIS	↑ 7.45	↓ 35	↑ 27	↑ +2

*In general, partially compensated or compensated metabolic alkalosis is rarely seen clinically because of the body's mechanism to prevent hypoventilation, as outlined in Chapter 5.

TABLE 12–2.—Clinical Method of Blood Gas Interpretation

STATUS	pH	Pco₂	HCO₃⁻	BE
VENTILATORY FAILURE				
(Respiratory acidosis)				
Acute	↓ 7.30	↑ 50	Normal	Normal
Chronic	7.30–7.50	↑ 50	↑ 27	↑ +2
ALVEOLAR HYPERVENTILATION				
(Respiratory alkalosis)				
Acute	↑ 7.50	↓ 30	Normal	Normal
Chronic	7.40–7.50	↓ 30	↓ 22	↓ −2
METABOLIC ACIDOSIS				
Uncompensated	↓ 7.30	Normal	↓ 22	↓ −2
Partially compensated	↓ 7.30	↓ 30	↓ 22	↓ −2
Compensated	7.30–7.40	↓ 30	↓ 22	↓ −2
METABOLIC ALKALOSIS				
Uncompensated	↑ 7.50	Normal	↑ 27	↑ +2
Partially compensated*	↑ 7.50	↑ 50	↑ 27	↑ +2
Compensated*	7.40–7.50	↑ 50	↑ 27	↑ +2
COMBINED VENTILATORY FAILURE AND				
METABOLIC ACIDOSIS	↓ 7.30	↑ 50	↓ 22	↓ −2
COMBINED ALVEOLAR HYPERVENTILATION				
AND METABOLIC ALKALOSIS	↑ 7.50	↓ 30	↑ 27	↑ +2

*In general, partially compensated or compensated metabolic alkalosis is rarely seen clinically because of the body's mechanism to prevent hypoventilation, as outlined in Chapter 5.

D. Approach to blood gas interpretation (classic method: see Table 12–1)
   1. Determine if the pH is within the normal range
      a. If normal, the blood gas is normal or compensated.
      b. If it is outside the normal range, it is uncompensated or partially compensated.
   2. Determine if the Pco₂ is normal or abnormal
      a. If the Pco₂ is normal and:
         (1) The pH is normal, the blood gas is normal.
         (2) The pH is decreased, an uncompensated metabolic acidosis exists.
         (3) The pH is increased, an uncompensated metabolic alkalosis exists.
      b. If the Pco₂ is higher than normal and:
         (1) The pH is decreased and the HCO₃⁻ is normal, an uncompensated respiratory acidosis exists.
         (2) The pH is decreased and the HCO₃⁻ is above normal, a partially compensated respiratory acidosis exists.
         (3) The pH is between 7.35 and 7.45 and the HCO₃⁻

is elevated, it is most probably a compensated respiratory acidosis.

(4) The pH is 7.40–7.45 and the HCO_3^- is elevated it *may be* a compensated metabolic alkalosis: However this acid-base state is rare, and usually a compensated respiratory acidosis with a mild metabolic alkalosis actually exists.

(5) The pH is increased with an elevated HCO_3^-, a partially compensated metabolic alkalosis exists.

c. If the P_{CO_2} is lower than normal and:

(1) The pH is increased and the HCO_3^- is normal, an uncompensated respiratory alkalosis exists.

(2) The pH is between 7.35 and 7.40 and the HCO_3^- is decreased, a compensated metabolic acidosis exists.

(3) The pH is between 7.40 and 7.45 and the HCO_3^- is decreased, a compensated respiratory alkalosis exists.

(4) The pH is increased and the HCO_3^- is decreased, a partially compensated respiratory alkalosis exists.

(5) The pH is decreased and the HCO_3^- is decreased, a partially compensated metabolic acidosis exists.

d. In addition, combined respiratory and metabolic acidosis or combined respiratory and metabolic alkalosis can occur.

(1) If the pH is markedly decreased, the P_{CO_2} is increased, and the HCO_3^- is decreased, an uncompensated respiratory and metabolic acidosis exists.

(2) If the pH is markedly increased, the P_{CO_2} is decreased, and the HCO_3^- is increased, an uncompensated respiratory and metabolic alkalosis exists.

e. The same guidelines can be used for the clinical method of interpretation, with the following variations:

(1) The acceptable pH range is 7.30–7.50.

(2) The acceptable P_{CO_2} range is 30–50 mm Hg.

(3) Replace "uncompensated" and "partially compensated" respiratory acidosis with "acute ventilatory failure."

(4) Replace "compensated" respiratory acidosis with "chronic ventilatory failure."

(5) Replace "uncompensated" and "partially compensated" respiratory alkalosis with "acute alveolar hyperventilation."

(6) Replace "compensated" respiratory alkalosis with "chronic alveolar hyperventilation."

XV. Assessment of Level of Hypoxemia
  A. For patients on 21% oxygen and under 60 years of age:
    1. Mild hypoxemia: Arterial P_{O_2} 60–79 mm Hg
    2. Moderate hypoxemia: Arterial P_{O_2} 40–59 mm Hg
    3. Severe hypoxemia: Arterial P_{O_2} < 40 mm Hg
  B. For individuals over age 60, 1 mm Hg should be subtracted from the lower limits of mild and moderate hypoxemia for each year over 60. At any age a P_{O_2} less than 40 mm Hg indicates severe hypoxemia and a P_{O_2} of less than 60–65 is always considered hypoxemic.
  C. More precisely, acceptable lower limits for P_{O_2} can be determined by the following (at sea level):
    1. For patients in the supine position, P_{O_2} = 103.5 − (.42 × age) ± 4 mm Hg.
    2. For patients in the sitting position, P_{O_2} = 104.2 − (.27 × age) mm Hg.
  D. Patients on $F_{I_{O_2}}$ greater than 0.21
    1. Uncorrected hypoxemia: Arterial P_{O_2} less than room air acceptable limit.
    2. Corrected hypoxemia: Arterial P_{O_2} between minimal acceptable room air limit and 100 mm Hg.
    3. Excessively corrected hypoxemia: Arterial P_{O_2} greater than 100 mm Hg.

XVI. Assessment of Tissue Hypoxia
  A. At present there is no direct method of assessing tissue hypoxia; it must be clinically assessed indirectly.
  B. Normally, adequate tissue oxygenation requires:
    1. Normal volume of oxygen must be carried by arterial blood
    2. Acid-base status must be relatively normal
    3. Tissue perfusion must be adequate
  C. The likelihood of tissue hypoxia existing is increased in the presence of the following:
    1. Severe hypoxemia
    2. Metabolic acidosis
    3. Decreased cardiac output or poor perfusion
  D. If tissue hypoxia has occurred, blood lactate levels are increased (see Chap. 11).

XVII. Clinical Causes of Acid-Base Abnormalities
  A. Ventilatory failure (respiratory acidosis): Primary causes:
    1. Cardiopulmonary disease, particularly end-stage chronic

obstructive pulmonary disease (COPD) or chronic restrictive pulmonary disease.

2. CNS depression by drugs, trauma, or lesion.

3. Neurologic or neuromuscular disease resulting in profound weakness of ventilatory muscles.

4. Fatigue following any acute pulmonary disease.

B. Alveolar hyperventilation (respiratory alkalosis): Primary causes:

1. Hypoxemia: Its primary effect on the respiratory system is hyperventilation.

2. Compensation for primary metabolic acidosis.

3. CNS stimulation by drugs, trauma, or lesion.

4. Emotional disorders (e.g., pain, anxiety, or fear).

C. Metabolic acidosis

1. Primary causes

   a. Lactic acidosis

   (1) In the absence of oxygen as final electron acceptor in the electron transport chain, aerobic metabolism is decreased.

   (2) An increase in anaerobic metabolism results which increases formation of lactic acid, a nonvolatile organic acid.

   (3) If the oxygenation state of the patient is improved, lactic acidosis is reversed.

   b. Ketoacidosis

   (1) Primary causes

      (a) Uncontrolled diabetes mellitus

      (b) Starvation

      (c) High fat content in the diet for extended periods

   (2) In all cases insufficient volumes of glucose enter the cell, resulting in an increase in metabolism of body fats.

   (3) The metabolic end products of fat metabolism are ketoacids (acetone and beta hydroxybutyric acid).

   (4) The patient in a diabetic acidosis is generally hyperventilating significantly and his/her breath has a sweet, acetone odor.

   (5) The patient needs glucose, and insulin.

   c. Renal failure (see Chap. 9)

   (1) Decreased renal function inhibits the body's primary mechanism for maintaining blood HCO_3^- levels and excretion of H^+.

(2) Thus free $[H^+]$ increases and free $[HCO_3^-]$ decreases.
  d. Ingestion of base-depleting drugs or acids
    (1) Aspirin
    (2) Alcohol
    (3) Ethylene glycol
    (4) Paraldehyde
D. Metabolic alkalosis
  1. Primary causes
    a. Hypokalemia (see Chap. 15)
    b. Hypochloremia (see Chap. 15)
    c. Gastric suction or vomiting
      (1) Since gastric contents are very acidic (pH of 1.0 to 2.0), excessive loss of gastric fluid results in alkalosis.
    d. Massive doses of steroids
      (1) Steroids increase reabsorption of Na^+ and accelerate excretion of H^+ and K^+.
    e. Diuretics
      (1) Diuretics cause an increase in the amount of K^+ excreted.
      (2) With excessive or uncontrolled use, hypokalemia may result.
    f. Ingestion of acid-depleting drugs or bases
      (1) $NaHCO_3$ (sodium bicarbonate)
XVIII. Estimation of Base Excess/Base Deficit
  A. Determine the pH predicted by an acute change in the P_{CO_2}.
    1. For every 10 mm Hg P_{CO_2} increase, the pH decreases by 0.05.
    2. For every 10 mm Hg P_{CO_2} decrease, the pH increases by 0.10.
  B. Determine the difference between the actual and predicted pH.
    Example:
    actual pH   7.50
    predicted pH   7.35
    difference   .15
  C. Eliminate the decimal and multiply by ⅔ to obtain BE/BD in mEq/L.
    Example:
    ⅔ of 15 = 10 mEq/L
  D. If the actual pH is less than the predicted pH, this is a base deficit.

E. If the actual pH is greater than the predicted pH, this is a base excess.

   Example:
   actual pH   7.50
   predicted pH   7.35
   base excess of 10 mEq/L

F. This is an excess of 10 mEq/L of base in all extracellular fluid.

XIX. Calculation of Bicarbonate Administration

   A. Normally HCO_3^- is administered only in the case of severe metabolic acidosis.

   B. Severe metabolic acidosis is defined as a base deficit of at least 10 mEq/L and one of the following:
      1. A pH of less than 7.20
      2. A pH between 7.20 and 7.25 with an unstable cardiovascular system.

   C. If the pH is greater than 7.25, HCO_3^- is normally not administered, even if the base deficit is 10 mEq/L.

   D. Extracellular fluid volume in liters can be estimated by taking ¼ the body weight in kilograms.

   E. By multiplying the extracellular fluid volume by the base deficit in mEq/L, the total body deficit in base is determined.

   F. One-half this estimated amount is normally administered.

   Example:
   Base deficit   15 mEq/L
   Weight   80 kg
   Extracellular fluid volume   80/4 = 20 L
   20 L × 15 mEq/L = 300 mEq total body deficit
   ½ of 300 mEq = 150 mEq administered

XX. Calculation of Ammonium Chloride (NH_3Cl) or Dilute Hydrochloric Acid (HCl) Administration

   A. In severe metabolic alkalosis, NH_3Cl or HCl can be administered to correct an acute base excess.

   B. The same calculations outlined in section XIX are used.

XXI. Typical Blood Gas Contaminants

   A. Heparin
      1. Sodium heparin is commonly used to prevent coagulation of arterial blood to be used for blood gas analysis.
      2. Ammonium heparin may affect pH even in small quantities.
      3. Normal pH of sodium heparin is 6.0–7.0.
      4. Concentration used is 1,000 units/cc.
      5. P_{CO_2} of sodium heparin is less than 2 mm Hg.

    6. Normally 0.05 ml heparin per 1 ml of blood should be used for anticoagulation.

    7. If the concentration or volume of heparin used is above this level:

      a. pH of blood may decrease or remain the same.

      b. P_{CO_2} of blood will decrease.

      c. P_{O_2} may be altered, depending on the blood's original P_{O_2} in relation to heparin's P_{O_2}.

      d. HbO_2% sat. may be altered, depending on the blood's original P_{O_2} and HbO_2% sat.

      e. HbCO% sat. will not be altered.

      f. Hb content will decrease.

      g. HCO_3^- will decrease.

      h. Base excess will decrease.

      i. Oxygen content may be altered.

    8. If insufficient heparin levels are used:

      a. Machine clotting is very likely.

      b. Results are questionable.

B. Saline and other intravenous solutions alter blood gas values in a manner similar to that of heparin except that the pH may also increase.

C. Air bubbles

    1. pH of blood normally will increase.

    2. P_{CO_2} of blood normally will decrease.

    3. P_{O_2} of blood may be altered, depending on blood's original P_{O_2} compared to atmospheric P_{O_2}.

    4. HbO_2% sat. may be altered, depending on blood's original P_{O_2} and HbO_2% sat.

    5. HbCO% sat. may increase.

    6. Hb content is unaltered.

    7. HCO_3^- may decrease.

    8. Base excess may decrease.

    9. Oxygen content may be altered.

BIBLIOGRAPHY

Bendixen H.H., et al.: *Respiratory Care*. St. Louis, C.V. Mosby Co., 1965.

Burton G.C., Hodgkin J.E.: *Respiratory Care: A Guide to Clinical Practice*, ed. 2. Philadelphia, J.B. Lippincott Co., 1984.

Carveth M.L., Schriver A.J., Peterson W.E., et al.: Acid-base assessment without journal peripheral venous blood. *Heart Lung* 13:48–54, 1984.

Clank L.C., Noyes L.K., Grooms T.A., et al.: Rapid micromeasurements of lactate in whole blood. *Crit. Care Med.* 12:461–464, 1984.

Cohen J.J., Kassiser J.P.: *Acid-Base*. Boston, Little, Brown & Co., 1982.

Comroe J.H.: *Physiology of Respiration,* ed. 2. Chicago, Year Book Medical Publishers, Inc., 1974.

Davenport H.W.: *The ABC's of Acid-Base Chemistry,* ed. 6. Chicago, University of Chicago Press, 1977.

Filey G.F.: *Acid-Base and Blood Gas Regulation.* Philadelphia, Lea & Febiger, 1972.

Guyton A.C.: *Textbook of Medical Physiology,* ed. 6. Philadelphia, W.B. Saunders Co., 1981.

Hodgkins J.E., Soeprono F.F., Chan D.M.: Incidence of metabolic alkalemia in hospitalized patients. *Crit. Care Med.* 8:725–728, 1980.

Jones N.L.: *Blood Gases and Acid-Base Physiology.* New York, Marcel Decker, Inc., 1980.

Levesque P.R.: Acid-base disorders: Application of total body carbon dioxide titration in anesthesia. *Anesth. Analg.* 54:299–307, 1975.

Masoro E.J., Siegel P.D.: *Acid-Base Regulation: Its Physiology, Pathophysiology and the Interpretation of Blood Gas Analysis,* ed. 2. Philadelphia, W.B. Saunders Co., 1977.

Masterton W.L., Slowinski E.J.: *Chemical Principles,* ed. 4. Philadelphia, W.B. Saunders Co., 1977.

Olszowka A.J., et al.: *Blood Gases, Hemoglobin, Base Excess and Maldistribution.* Philadelphia, Lea & Febiger, 1973.

Rooth G.: *Acid-Base and Electrolyte Balance.* Chicago, Year Book Medical Publishers, Inc., 1974.

Rose B.D.: *Clinical Physiology of Acid-Base and Electrolyte Disorders.* New York, McGraw-Hill Book Co., 1977.

Ryder K.W., Jay S.J.: Comparison of measured and calculated arterial bicarbonate concentrations: Potential application for prevention of random errors in blood gas results. *Respir. Care* 28:1268–1272, 1983.

Shapiro B.A., Harrison R.A., Walton J.R.: *Clinical Application of Blood Gases,* ed. 3. Chicago, Year Book Medical Publishers, Inc., 1982.

Spearman C.B., Sheldon R.L., Egan D.F.: *Egan's Fundamentals of Respiratory Therapy,* ed. 4. St. Louis, C.V. Mosby Co., 1982.

Walter R.M., Warsaw T.: Diabetic ketoacidosis: A treatment appraisal. *Heart Lung* 10:112–113, 1981.

Winters R.W., Dell R.B.: *Acid-Base Physiology in Medicine,* ed. 3. Boston, Little, Brown & Co., 1982.

13 / Intrapulmonary Shunting and Dead Space

I. Spectrum of Ventilation/Perfusion ($\dot{V}/\dot{Q}$) Abnormalities (Fig 13–1)
   A. Ideal alveolar-capillary unit: An alveolar-capillary unit in which perfusion and ventilation are normal. Theoretically a unit with a $\dot{V}/\dot{Q}$ ratio of 1.0.
   B. Deadspace unit: An alveolar-capillary unit in which ventilation is normal but perfusion is diminished or absent. A unit with a $\dot{V}/\dot{Q}$ ratio greater than 1.0.
   C. Shunt unit: An alveolar-capillary unit in which perfusion is normal but ventilation is diminished or absent. A unit with a $\dot{V}/\dot{Q}$ ratio less than 1.0.
   D. Silent unit: An alveolar-capillary unit without perfusion or ventilation and therefore a $\dot{V}/\dot{Q}$ ratio of 0.0.
   E. For greater detail on ventilation/perfusion relationships, see Chapter 4.
II. Intrapulmonary Shunting
   A. A pathophysiologic process in which blood enters the left side of the heart without having been oxygenated by the lungs. The mixing of venous blood with oxygenated blood from the pulmonary capillaries to form arterial blood.
   B. The total quantity of shunted blood is the *physiologic shunt*, which is composed of three subdivisions (Fig 13–2).
      1. Anatomic shunt: That portion of the total cardiac output which bypasses the pulmonary capillary bed.
         a. Normally about 2%–5% of the cardiac output bypasses the pulmonary capillaries because the following veins empty into the left side of the heart:
            (1) Bronchial
            (2) Pleural
            (3) Thebesian
         b. Increases in anatomic shunt may occur as a result of:
            (1) Vascular pulmonary tumors
            (2) Arterial venous anastomosis
            (3) Congenital cardiac anomalies (see Chap. 21)

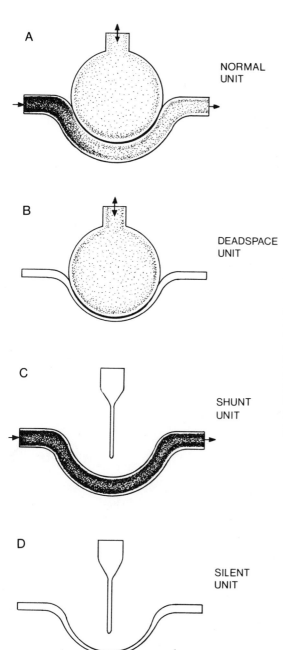

A

NORMAL
UNIT

B

DEADSPACE
UNIT

C

SHUNT
UNIT

D

SILENT
UNIT

Fig 13–1.—The theoretical respiratory unit. *A,* normal ventilation, normal perfusion; *B,* normal ventilation, no perfusion; *C,* no ventilation, normal perfusion; *D,* no ventilation, no perfusion. (From Shapiro B.A., Harrison R.A., Walton J.R.: *Clinical Application of Arterial Blood Gases,* ed. 3. Chicago, Year Book Medical Publishers, 1982. Reproduced by permission.)

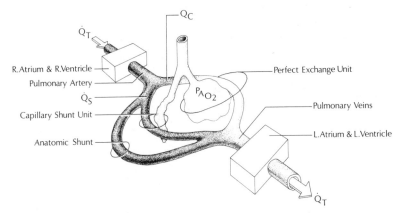

Fig 13–2.—Concept of physiologic shunting (see text). $\dot{Q}t$ is cardiac output per unit time; $\dot{Q}c$ is the portion of the cardiac output that exchanges perfectly with alveolar air; $\dot{Q}s$ is the portion of the cardiac output that does not exchange with alveolar air; $P_{A_{O_2}}$ is the alveolar oxygen tension. (From Shapiro B.A., Harrison R.A., Walton J.R.: *Clinical Application of Arterial Blood Gases*, ed. 3. Chicago, Year Book Medical Publishers, Inc., 1981. Reproduced by permission.)

2. Capillary shunt: That portion of the total cardiac output that perfuses nonventilated alveoli.
   a. Normally, capillary shunting does not exist.
   b. Capillary shunting is caused by:
      (1) Atelectasis
      (2) Consolidating pneumonia
      (3) Complete airway obstruction
      (4) Pneumothorax
      (5) Any pathophysiologic process that eliminates ventilation to perfused alveoli.
3. Shunt effect (ventilation/perfusion inequality, venous admixture): Any pathophysiologic process in which perfusion is in excess of ventilation; however, some ventilation is still present.
   a. Under normal conditions, shunt effect occurs in the bases of the lung where $\dot{V}/\dot{Q}$ ratios are less than 1.0.
   b. Shunt effect may be increased by:
      (1) Retained secretions
      (2) Bronchospasm
      (3) Partial airway obstruction
      (4) Regional increases in fibrotic tissue
      (5) Decreased tidal volumes
      (6) Mucosal edema at the bronchiolar level

III. Derivation of Classic Shunt Equation
  A. Definition of abbreviations
     1. $\dot{V}_{O_2}$: Volume of oxygen consumed per minute
     2. $\dot{Q}s$: Shunted cardiac output
     3. $\dot{Q}c$: Capillary cardiac output
     4. $\dot{Q}t$: Total cardiac output
     5. Cc_{O_2}: Capillary oxygen content
     6. Ca_{O_2}: Arterial oxygen content
     7. $C\bar{v}_{O_2}$: Mixed venous oxygen content
     8. $P_{A_{O_2}}$: Alveolar oxygen partial pressure
     9. Pa_{O_2}: Arterial oxygen partial pressure
  B. The shunt equation is based on the Fick equation, which normally is used to calculate oxygen consumption or cardiac output:

$$\dot{V}_{O_2} = \dot{Q}t(Ca_{O_2} - C\bar{v}_{O_2}). \tag{1}$$

  C. Since $\dot{Q}c$ represents that portion of the cardiac output that actually perfuses ventilated alveoli and Cc_{O_2} is the oxygen content of blood leaving those perfused and ventilated alveoli, this equation may be rewritten as:

$$\dot{V}_{O_2} = \dot{Q}c(Cc_{O_2} - C\bar{v}_{O_2}) \tag{2}$$

  D. Thus, total cardiac output is equal to shunted cardiac output plus capillary cardiac output:

$$\dot{Q}t = \dot{Q}s + \dot{Q}c \tag{3}$$

  E. Solving equation 3 for $\dot{Q}c$:

$$\dot{Q}c = \dot{Q}t - \dot{Q}s \tag{4}$$

  F. Substituting into equation 2 the equivalent of $\dot{V}_{O_2}$ from equation 1:

$$\dot{Q}t(Ca_{O_2} - C\bar{v}_{O_2}) = \dot{Q}c(Cc_{O_2} - C\bar{v}_{O_2}) \tag{5}$$

  G. Substituting into equation 5 the equivalent of $\dot{Q}c$ from equation 4:

$$\dot{Q}t(Ca_{O_2} - C\bar{v}_{O_2}) = (\dot{Q}t - \dot{Q}s)(Cc_{O_2} - C\bar{v}_{O_2}) \tag{6}$$

  H. Rearranging equation 6:

$$\dot{Q}tCa_{O_2} - \dot{Q}tC\bar{v}_{O_2} = \dot{Q}tCc_{O_2} - \dot{Q}tC\bar{v}_{O_2} - \dot{Q}sCc_{O_2} + \dot{Q}sC\bar{v}_{O_2} \tag{7}$$

  I. Eliminating $-\dot{Q}tC\bar{v}_{O_2}$ from both sides of equation 7:

$$\dot{Q}tCa_{O_2} = \dot{Q}tCc_{O_2} - \dot{Q}sCc_{O_2} + \dot{Q}sC\bar{v}_{O_2} \tag{8}$$

J. Rearranging equation 8:

$$\dot{Q}sCc_{O_2} - \dot{Q}sC\bar{v}_{O_2} = \dot{Q}tCc_{O_2} - \dot{Q}tCa_{O_2} \qquad (9)$$

K. Simplifying equation 9:

$$\dot{Q}s(Cc_{O_2} - C\bar{v}_{O_2}) = \dot{Q}t(Cc_{O_2} - Ca_{O_2}) \qquad (10)$$

L. Rearranging equation 10:

$$\dot{Q}s/\dot{Q}t = \frac{Cc_{O_2} - Ca_{O_2}}{Cc_{O_2} - C\bar{v}_{O_2}} \qquad (11)$$

M. Equation 11 is the classic shunt equation, which states that the difference between the capillary oxygen content and arterial oxygen content divided by the difference between the capillary oxygen content and the mixed venous oxygen content equals the intrapulmonary shunt fraction.

N. This equation is used to calculate the total physiologic shunt.

IV. Calculating the Total Physiologic Shunt

  A. In order to calculate the intrapulmonary shunt, the capillary oxygen content, arterial oxygen content, and mixed venous oxygen content must be calculated.

  B. All oxygen content determinations are based on the following equation (see Chap. 11 for details):

O_2 content (vol%) =
$$\text{(Hb cont) } (HbO_2\% \text{ sat}) (1.34) + (.003) (Po_2) \qquad (12)$$

  C. Calculation of the arterial oxygen content requires data from an arterial blood gas.

  D. Calculation of the mixed venous oxygen content requires data from a pulmonary artery blood gas.

  E. Capillary oxygen content

    1. Since a blood sample from an *ideally functioning alveolar-capillary* unit is impossible to obtain, this calculation is based on the assumption that the end pulmonary capillary oxygen tension (Pc_{O_2}) is equal to the alveolar oxygen tension (PA_{O_2}) in an ideally ventilated and perfused alveolar-capillary unit.

    2. The PA_{O_2} is obtained by calculation, using the ideal alveolar gas equation (see Chap. 4 for details).

$PA_{O_2} =$
$$(P_B - P_{H_2O}) (F_{I_{O_2}}) - (Pa_{CO_2}) \left(F_{I_{O_2}} + \frac{1 - F_{I_{O_2}}}{R} \right) \qquad (13)$$

3. Hemoglobin content is the same as that measured in arterial blood or mixed venous blood.
4. Oxyhemoglobin percent saturation (HbO_2% sat)
   a. If the $P_{A_{O_2}}$ is 150 mm Hg or greater, it is assumed that the HbO_2% sat is 100%.
   b. For $P_{A_{O_2}}$ values of less than 150 mm Hg, an oxyhemoglobin dissociation curve is used to estimate the HbO_2% sat.
   c. The capillary HbO_2% sat is also corrected for the HbCO% sat present in the arterial blood.

F. *Example:*

$$C_{a_{O_2}} = 17.5 \text{ vol}\%$$
$$C_{c_{O_2}} = 19.5 \text{ vol}\%$$
$$C\bar{v}_{O_2} = 13.0 \text{ vol}\%$$

$$\frac{\dot{Q}s}{\dot{Q}t} = \frac{C_{c_{O_2}} - C_{a_{O_2}}}{C_{c_{O_2}} - C\bar{v}_{O_2}}$$

$$\frac{\dot{Q}s}{\dot{Q}t} = \frac{19.5 - 17.5}{19.5 - 13.0} = 0.31$$

or 31% intrapulmonary shunt

V. Estimated Intrapulmonary Shunt Calculation
   A. In patients without a pulmonary artery catheter, it is impossible to measure the $C\bar{v}_{O_2}$.
   B. However, in the majority of critically ill patients with cardiovascular stability, it has been determined that the $C_{a_{O_2}} - C\bar{v}_{O_2}$ is approximately 3.5 vol%.
   C. Thus, in these patients 3.5 vol% may be used as an estimate of $C_{a_{O_2}} - C\bar{v}_{O_2}$.
   D. The denominator of the classic shunt equation may be expressed as follows:

$$C_{c_{O_2}} - C\bar{v}_{O_2} = (C_{c_{O_2}} - C_{a_{O_2}}) + (C_{a_{O_2}} - C\bar{v}_{O_2}) \quad (14)$$

   E. Since $C_{a_{O_2}} - C\bar{v}_{O_2}$ is estimated at 3.5 vol%, the denominator in equation 11 can be expressed as:

$$(C_{c_{O_2}} - C_{a_{O_2}}) + 3.5 \quad (15)$$

   F. The modified shunt equation used to estimate intrapulmonary shunt is:

$$\frac{\dot{Q}s}{\dot{Q}t} = \frac{C_{c_{O_2}} - C_{a_{O_2}}}{(C_{c_{O_2}} - C_{a_{O_2}}) + 3.5} \quad (16)$$

G. Equation 16 should only be used if pulmonary artery blood is unavailable and the patient is cardiovascularly stable.

VI. Alveolar-Arterial P_{O_2} Difference (A-aDO_2)

    A. The (A-aDO_2) gradient has been used to estimate the percent intrapulmonary shunt.

    B. If the patient is receiving 100% O_2, for every 10–15 mm Hg gradient the shunt is approximately 1%.

    C. However, it has been demonstrated that a negative correlation exists between the A-aDO_2 and the percent shunt.

    D. Thus even though this procedure is used in some centers, it cannot be recommended as a reliable method of estimating percent shunt.

VII. $F_{I_{O_2}}$ Used to Calculate Percent Intrapulmonary Shunt

    A. Historically, shunt fractions were determined at an $F_{I_{O_2}}$ of 1.0.

    B. However, it has been demonstrated that the shunt fraction is increased at an $F_{I_{O_2}}$ of 1.0.

    C. This occurs secondary to:

        1. Nitrogen washout atelectasis

           a. Areas of the lung that are ventilated poorly tend to collapse if the nitrogen is removed.

           b. Nitrogen normally maintains alveolar stability. When nitrogen is removed and replaced by oxygen, the oxygen is absorbed by the blood faster than it can be replaced because of the poor ventilation.

           c. As a result, alveolar size decreases, eventually falling below its critical volume, and collapse occurs (Fig 13–3).

        2. Redistribution of pulmonary blood flow

           a. If an area of lung is poorly ventilated or not ventilated at all, the decreased P_{O_2} in the area causes the pulmonary vasculature surrounding the alveoli to constrict.

           b. This decreases blood flow to poorly ventilated areas and increases blood flow to areas more appropriately ventilated.

           c. When a high $F_{I_{O_2}}$ is administered, this autoregulatory mechanism is abated, because the P_{O_2} throughout the

$\rightarrow$

Fig 13–3.—Schematic representation of primary mechanisms causing denitrogenation absorption atelectasis. *Top drawings* represent alveolocapillary units shortly after administration of 100% inspired oxygen. *White circles* represent oxygen molecules that have increased in concentration in both units *A* and *B*. The ablation of alveolar hypoxia in unit *A* results in loss of vasoconstriction with considerably increased blood flow. The increased blood flow to this still poorly ven-

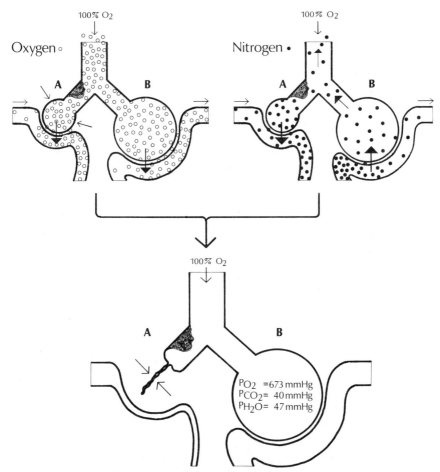

$$P_{O_2} = 673 \text{ mmHg}$$
$$P_{CO_2} = 40 \text{ mmHg}$$
$$P_{H_2O} = 47 \text{ mmHg}$$

tilated alveolus results in significantly increased oxygen extraction, which results in diminished gas volume. *Black circles* represent nitrogen, which is rapidly depleted from all units secondary to the fact that inspired nitrogen concentration is now zero. Initially, more nitrogen leaves the blood and the body via unit *B* because it is better ventilated. However, as the blood P_{N_2} level progressively decreases, nitrogen will start to leave alveolus *A* via the blood. This results in further loss of gas volume from alveolus *A* since it remains poorly ventilated but well perfused. Thus, nitrogen is depleted from all units within 5–15 minutes. *Bottom drawing* represents the final steady state, in which increased oxygen and nitrogen extraction has caused the alveolus to collapse. Thus, a poorly ventilated, poorly perfused unit *A* becomes a nonventilated, poorly perfused unit after administration of 100% inspired oxygen. (From Shapiro B.A., Harrison R.A., Walton J.R.: *Clinical Application of Blood Gases*, ed. 3. Chicago, Year Book Medical Publishers, Inc., 1982. Reproduced by permission.)

lung is elevated and capillaries that were previously con-
stricted are now dilated.

    d. This results in increased blood being shunted past non-
ventilated and poorly ventilated alveoli.

  D. Figure 13–4 represents the relationship between F_{IO_2} and percent shunt. Clinically it appears that the lowest measured shunt
occurs at about 50% oxygen.

    1. The percent shunt increases as the F_{IO_2} decreases below 0.5
because of the effect of venous admixture.

    2. The percent shunt increases as the F_{IO_2} increases above 0.5
because of nitrogen washout atelectasis and redistribution of
pulmonary blood flow.

  E. Percent intrapulmonary shunts should be calculated at the F_{IO_2}
at which the patient is maintained.

  F. If a determination at a comparable F_{IO_2} is desired, an F_{IO_2} of
0.5 is recommended.

VIII. Clinical Use of the Shunt Calculation

  A. Differentiating causes of hypoxemia

    1. Hypoxemia is caused by:

      a. True shunting: a combination of anatomic and capillary
shunting

      b. Shunt effect: a decrease in alveolar oxygen tension

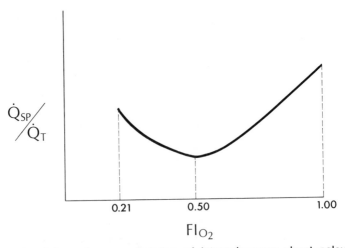

Fig 13–4.—Schematic representation of intrapulmonary shunt calculations
($\dot{Q}s/\dot{Q}t$) versus inspired oxygen concentration (F_{IO_2}) in both normal and diseased
lungs. (From Shapiro B.A., Harrison R.A., Walton J.R.: *Clinical Application of
Blood Gases*, ed. 3. Chicago, Year Book Medical Publishers, Inc., 1982. Reproduced by permission.)

  c. Decreased mixed venous oxygen content
    (1) This only causes hypoxemia or an increase in hypoxemia if intrapulmonary shunting also exists.
    (2) Essentially it accentuates the effect of a preexisting shunt, because the blood that is shunted is now more deoxygenated than normal.
  2. The numerator of the shunt equation, $Cc_{O_2} - Ca_{O_2}$, can be considered a reflection of intrapulmonary pathology. That is, hypoxemia of pulmonary origin will increase the $Cc_{O_2} - Ca_{O_2}$ value, increasing the calculated shunt fraction.
  3. The denominator in the shunt equation, $Cc_{O_2} - C\bar{v}_{O_2}$, can be considered a reflection of the relationship of cardiac output to oxygen demand.
    a. This is true because $Ca_{O_2} - C\bar{v}_{O_2}$ is contained in the denominator.
    b. If hypoxemia is a result of cardiovascular pathology, it is primarily reflected in a widening of the $Cc_{O_2} - C\bar{v}_{O_2}$, but may not be accompanied by a proportional widening of the numerator.
  4. Hypoxemia accompanied by an increased shunt measurement generally denotes an increase in intrapulmonary pathology.
  5. Hypoxemia without a major increase in shunt fraction usually denotes cardiovascular causes of hypoxemia.
B. Monitoring oxygen and PEEP therapy
  1. If the hypoxemia is of pulmonary origin and primarily caused by shunt effect, the appropriate application of oxygen therapy should demonstrate a decrease in intrapulmonary shunt (see Chap. 24).
  2. If the hypoxemia is of pulmonary origin and primarily caused by capillary shunting of a generalized diffuse nature (ARDS), the effectiveness of PEEP therapy may be evaluated by serial shunt measurements (see Chap. 33).
C. Assessment of spontaneous ventilatory capabilities in patients being mechanically ventilated
  1. An intrapulmonary shunt determination of less than 10% is clinically comparable to normal lungs.
  2. An intrapulmonary shunt determination of 10%–19% should not represent sufficient pulmonary disease to interfere with spontaneous ventilation.
  3. An intrapulmonary shunt of 20%–30% may result in ventilatory failure in patients with CNS or cardiovascular dysfunction if spontaneous ventilation is attempted. However, many

patients are able to sustain spontaneous ventilation with this level of shunt.

4. An intrapulmonary shunt of greater than 30% represents a degree of pulmonary disease that normally requires aggressive cardiopulmonary support.

D. Assessment of specific cardiopulmonary abnormalities

1. Performance of intrapulmonary shunt studies while a patient is in different positions may delineate the locale and extent of certain pulmonary pathology.

   a. This is true because of the effects of gravity on pulmonary blood flow.

   b. If the diseased area is gravity dependent, the percent intrapulmonary shunt is increased.

2. In the neonate the extent of right-to-left shunting in the presence of the following congenital anomalies can be determined:

   a. Ventricular septal defects

   b. Atrial septal defects

   c. Patent ductus arteriosus

IX. Pulmonary Deadspace

A. That portion of the total ventilation that does not undergo external respiration.

B. The total quantity of pulmonary deadspace is the *physiologic deadspace* and is composed of three subdivisions:

1. Anatomic deadspace: That portion of the total ventilation that does not contact the alveolar epithelium.

   a. Normally the anatomic deadspace is equal to about 1.0 ml/lb of ideal body weight.

   b. The relationship between anatomical deadspace and tidal volume is increased by small tidal volumes and rapid rates.

   c. The absolute quantity of anatomical deadspace is increased by:

      (1) Positive pressure ventilation

      (2) The use of mechanical deadspace

   d. Anatomical deadspace is decreased by:

      (1) Tracheostomy/endotracheal tubes

      (2) Pneumothorax

2. Alveolar deadspace: That portion of the total ventilation that contacts the alveolar epithelium but does not participate in gas exchange due to a lack of pulmonary capillary blood flow.

   a. Alveolar deadspace accounts for a very small amount of the total physiologic deadspace in the healthy individual.

    b. Alveolar deadspace is increased by:
      (1) Pulmonary emboli
      (2) Vascular tumors
  3. Deadspace effect (ventilation/perfusion inequality): Any pathophysiologic process in which ventilation is in excess of perfusion but some perfusion does exist; i.e., $\dot{V}/\dot{Q}$ ratio greater than 1.0.
    a. In the standing individual, deadspace effect occurs in the apices of the lungs since blood flow to this region is greatly diminished.
    b. Deadspace effect is increased by:
      (1) Positive pressure ventilation
      (2) Decreased cardiac output
      (3) Alveolar septal wall destruction

X. Derivation of the Deadspace Equation
  A. Definition of abbreviations
    1. TV: Tidal volume
    2. V_D: Deadspace volume
    3. V_A: Alveolar volume
    4. $F_{A_{CO_2}}$: Fractional concentration of CO_2 in alveolar gas
    5. $F\overline{E}_{CO_2}$: Mean fractional concentration of CO_2 in mixed expired gas
    6. Pa_{CO_2}: Partial pressure of arterial CO_2
    7. $P\overline{E}_{CO_2}$: Partial pressure of mean expired CO_2
    8. $F_{D_{CO_2}}$: Fractional concentration of deadspace CO_2
  B. Tidal volume is equal to deadspace volume plus alveolar volume.

$$TV = V_D + V_A \qquad (17)$$

  C. The total volume of CO_2 in exhaled gas is equal to TV times the fractional concentration of CO_2 in the exhaled gas.

$$(TV)(F\overline{E}_{CO_2}) = \text{total } CO_2 \text{ exhaled} \qquad (18)$$

  D. This volume can be subdivided into the amount of CO_2 exhaled from deadspace and alveoli:

$$(TV)(F\overline{E}_{CO_2}) = (V_A)(F_{A_{CO_2}}) + (V_D)(F_{D_{CO_2}}) \qquad (19)$$

  E. Since the concentration of CO_2 in exhaled deadspace gas is about zero, equation 19 can be rewritten as:

$$(TV)(F\overline{E}_{CO_2}) = (V_A)(F_{A_{CO_2}}) \qquad (20)$$

  F. And since $V_A = TV - V_D$, equation 20 may be rewritten as:

$$(TV)(F\overline{E}_{CO_2}) = (TV)(F_{A_{CO_2}}) - (V_D)(F_{A_{CO_2}}) \qquad (21)$$

G. By rearranging and simplifying equation 21, the Bohr equation for the determination of the deadspace to tidal volume ratio (V_D/TV ratio) is generated.

$$V_D/TV = \frac{F_{A_{CO_2}} - F\overline{E}_{CO_2}}{F_{A_{CO_2}}} \qquad (22)$$

H. Since the concentration of CO_2 in the alveoli is equal to the concentration of CO_2 in the arterial blood and since the partial pressures of gases are proportional to their concentration, equation 22 may be rewritten as the Enghoff modification of the Bohr equation:

$$V_D/TV = \frac{Pa_{CO_2} - P\overline{E}_{CO_2}}{Pa_{CO_2}} \qquad (23)$$

I. In all circumstances, as the deadspace increases there is a widening of the $Pa_{CO_2} - P\overline{E}_{CO_2}$ gradient.

J. Normal V_D/TV ratios are about 20%–40%.

XI. Calculating the Deadspace to Tidal Volume Ratio
A. A *simultaneous* sampling of arterial blood and exhaled gas is obtained.
   1. The exhaled gas sample must be large enough to reflect a mean exhaled P_{CO_2} value.
   2. In spontaneously breathing patients, about 40 L of exhaled gas is collected. This is done to compensate for tidal volume variations.
   3. If a patient is being ventilated in the control mode with consistent tidal volumes, a 5L sample is sufficient.
B. The patient should be stable and quiet at the time the sample is obtained.
   Example:

$$V_D/TV = \frac{Pa_{CO_2} - P\overline{E}_{CO_2}}{Pa_{CO_2}}$$

$$0.52 = \frac{42 - 20}{42}$$

XII. Minute Volume—Pa_{CO_2} Relationship
A. Since the physiologic adequacy of ventilation is clinically defined by the arterial Pa_{CO_2} level, a relationship between total minute volume and arterial Pa_{CO_2} must exist.
B. In the average adult a minute volume of 4–6 L maintains a Pa_{CO_2} of 40 mm Hg.
C. If the minute volume increases the Pa_{CO_2} should decrease, and if the minute volume decreases the Pa_{CO_2} should increase.

D. It is generally accepted that with each doubling of the minute volume, the Pa_{CO_2} decreases by 10 mm Hg (Table 13–1).

E. If there is a disparity between the minute volume and the expected Pa_{CO_2}, deadspace is increased.

Example:

If the Pa_{CO_2} is 42 mm Hg while the minute volume is 20 L, deadspace ventilation is increased. A Pa_{CO_2} of about 20 mm Hg would be expected with a minute ventilation of 20 L.

XIII. Clinical Use of the Deadspace to Tidal Volume Ratios

A. Assessment of spontaneous ventilatory capabilities in patients being mechanically ventilated.

1. The V_D/TV ratio is typically increased during mechanical ventilation and is considered normal up to 0.50.

2. A V_D/TV ratio less than 0.60 normally does not represent pulmonary pathology of sufficient magnitude to interfere with spontaneous ventilation.

3. A V_D/TV ratio of 0.60 to 0.80 represents significant disease and frequently interferes with an individual's ability to maintain prolonged spontaneous ventilation.

4. A V_D/TV ratio greater than 0.80 normally requires mechanical ventilatory support.

B. Evaluation of the presence of pulmonary embolism

1. An increase in deadspace supports the diagnosis of pulmonary embolism.

2. However, a definitive diagnosis cannot be made by deadspace studies alone.

C. Because of the difficulty in securing an ideal sample of exhaled gas, the determination of V_D/TV ratio is infrequently performed outside of the pulmonary function laboratory.

XIV. Guidelines for Differentiating Shunt-Producing From Deadspace-Producing Diseases

A. Deadspace-producing diseases

1. Minute volume greatly increased with little or no decrease in Pa_{CO_2}.

TABLE 13–1.—NORMAL MINUTE
VOLUME-Pa_{CO_2} RELATIONSHIPS

V_A (L/min)	Pa_{CO_2} (mm Hg)
1.25	60
2.50	50
5.00	40
10.00	30
20.00	20

    2. Even though hypoxemia is present and correctable by oxygen therapy, minute ventilation changes are minimal when hypoxemia is corrected.

  B. Shunt-producing diseases

    1. Pa_{CO_2} decreases as minute volume increases.

    2. Assuming the hypoxemia is responsive, oxygen therapy will decrease myocardial and ventilatory work and relieve hypoxemia. Thus, minute volume and Pa_{CO_2} return to normal.

    3. If hypoxemia is refractory, the application of PEEP is necessary to reverse the hypoxemia.

BIBLIOGRAPHY

Burton G.G., Hodgkin J.E.: *Respiratory Care, A Guide to Clinical Practice*, ed. 2. Philadelphia, J.B. Lippincott, 1984.

Cane R.D., Shapiro B.A., Harrison R.A., et al.: Minimizing errors in intrapulmonary shunt calculation. *Crit. Care Med.* 8:294–297, 1980.

Cohen J.J., Kassirer J.P.: *Acid/Base*. Boston, Little, Brown & Co., 1982.

Comroe J.H.: *Physiology of Respiration*, ed. 2. Chicago, Year Book Medical Publishers, Inc., 1974.

Comroe J.H., Forster R.E. II, Dubois A.B., et al.: *The Lung: Clinical Physiology and Pulmonary Function Tests*, ed. 2. Chicago, Year Book Medical Publishers, Inc., 1962.

Dimas S., Kacmarek R.M.: Intrapulmonary shunting: Part I. Basic concepts and derivation of equation. *Curr. Rev. Respir. Ther.* 1:35–39, 1981.

Dimas S., Kacmarek R.M.: Intrapulmonary shunting: Part II. Clinical application. *Curr. Rev. Respir. Ther.* 1:43–47, 1981.

Duranceau A., et al.: Ventilatory deadspace in diagnosis of acute pulmonary embolism. *Surg. Forum* 25:229–233, 1974.

Fisher S.R., et al.: Comparative changes in ventilatory deadspace following micro and massive pulmonary emboli. *J. Surg. Res.* 29:195–199, 1976.

Gilbert R., Auchinloss J.H. Jr., Kuppinger M., et al.: Stability of the arterial-alveolar oxygen partial pressure ratio. *Crit. Care Med.* 7:267–272, 1979.

Kacmarek R.M., Dimas S.: Pulmonary deadspace: Concepts and clinical application. *Curr. Rev. Respir. Ther.* 1:147–150, 1981.

Murray J.F.: *The Normal Lung: The Basis for Diagnosis and Treatment of Pulmonary Disease*. Philadelphia, W.B. Saunders Co., 1976.

Shapiro B.A., Cane R.D., Harrison R.A., et al.: Changes in intrapulmonary shunting with administration of 100 percent oxygen. *Chest* 77:138–141, 1980.

Shapiro B.A., Harrison R.A., Walton J.R.: *Clinical Application of Blood Gases*, ed. 3. Chicago, Year Book Medical Publishers, Inc., 1982.

Shapiro B.A., Harrison R.A., Kacmarek R.M., et al.: *Clinical Application of Respiratory Care*, ed. 3. Chicago, Year Book Medical Publishers, Inc., 1985.

Spearman C.B., Sheldon R.L., Egan D.F.: *Egan's Fundamentals of Respiratory Therapy*, ed. 4. St. Louis, C.V. Mosby Co., 1982.

14 / Hemodynamic Monitoring

I. Systemic Arterial Blood Pressure

Systemic arterial blood pressure is expressed as a systolic pressure divided by a diastolic pressure (Fig 14–1).

A. Systolic pressure is the highest pressure attained in the artery and is determined by three major factors:
1. Stroke volume
a. Increased stroke volume generally causes an increased systolic pressure.
b. Decreased stroke volume generally causes a decreased systolic pressure.
2. Rate of blood ejection from left ventricle
a. An increased rate of left ventricular ejection generally results in increased systolic pressure.
b. A decrease in the rate of ejection generally results in decreased systolic pressure.
3. Elasticity of the arterial tree
a. Increased arterial elasticity generally results in an increased systolic pressure.
b. Decreased arterial elasticity generally results in a decreased systolic pressure.

B. Diastolic pressure is the lowest pressure attained in the artery and is determined by three major factors:
1. Magnitude of preceding systolic pressure
a. In general, the higher the preceding systolic pressure, the higher the resulting diastolic pressure.
b. The lower the preceding systolic pressure, the lower the resulting diastolic pressure.
2. Length of ventricular diastolic interval
a. The longer the diastolic interval, the greater the time available for blood to leave the arterial system and the lower the resultant diastolic pressure.
b. The shorter the diastolic interval, the higher the diastolic pressure by the opposite mechanism.
3. State of peripheral resistance

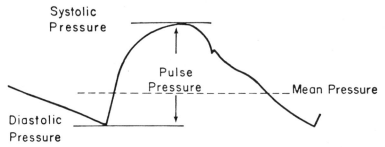

Fig 14–1.—Graphic representation of arterial pressure tracing depicting systolic, diastolic, mean, and pulse pressures (see text). (From Little R.C.: *Physiology of the Heart and Circulation.* ed. 2. Chicago, Year Book Medical Publishers, Inc., 1981. Reproduced by permission.)

    a. The greater the peripheral resistance, the lower the rate of arterial runoff and the higher the resultant diastolic pressure.

    b. The lower the peripheral resistance, the higher the rate of arterial runoff and the lower the resultant diastolic pressure.

C. In general, measurement of arterial blood pressure assesses left ventricular function by systolic pressure and peripheral resistance by diastolic pressure. It should be recalled that one factor responsible for systolic pressure is stroke volume and a factor responsible for diastolic pressure is the state of peripheral resistance.

D. Thus it is assumed that the greater the difference between systolic and diastolic pressures the greater the resultant flow. The difference between systolic and diastolic pressures is called the pulse pressure.

    1. By the equation

$$\dot{Q} = P \times \frac{1}{R} \tag{1}$$

increases in systolic pressure indicate increases in the pressure gradient (P) across the systemic circulation, and decreases in diastolic pressure indicate decreases in peripheral resistance (R).

    2. Therefore, widening of pulse pressure is generally thought to indicate increased blood flow ($\dot{Q}$).

    3. By the opposite mechanism, narrowing of pulse pressure is generally thought to indicate decreased flow.

    4. It should be noted that a widening of pulse pressure can occur without increased blood flow. Also, normal blood flow can exist

with a narrow pulse pressure. These phenomena occur by alterations in the other factors (i.e., diastolic interval, arterial elasticity) that determine systolic and diastolic pressure. Therefore it is imperative to assess all factors responsible for systolic and diastolic pressure before blindly stating that an increased or decreased pulse pressure represents increased or decreased blood flow in a given patient.

E. The mean arterial pressure (MAP) represents the average pressure over one complete systolic and diastolic interval.

   1. The MAP can be directly measured or estimated by the formula:

$$\text{MAP} = \frac{(2 \times \text{diastolic pressure}) + (\text{systolic pressure})}{3} \quad (2)$$

   2. The MAP is the average pressure in the arterial tree over a given time and therefore generally is used as an assessment of the average pressure to which the arterial system is exposed.

   3. The pressure gradient across the systemic circulation is generally expressed as MAP − CVP, where CVP equals central venous pressure (see II, below).

   4. The MAP is also commonly used as an indicator of left ventricular afterload, thus representing the resistance (in terms of pressure) that the left ventricle must pump against.

F. Both arterial blood pressure and mean arterial blood pressure can be directly measured by an intra-arterial line (catheter). Arterial blood pressure can be indirectly measured by use of a sphygmomanometer and the MAP calculated from the obtained values.

G. Normal values for arterial blood pressure in the adult are as follows:

> Systolic: 140–90 mm Hg
> Diastolic: 90–60 mm Hg
> Mean: 70–105 mm Hg

II. Central Venous Pressure (CVP)

The CVP usually is expressed as a single number representing the mean right atrial pressure ($\overline{\text{RAP}}$).

A. The numerical pressure value of CVP will be the result of the following factors:

   1. The pump capabilities of the right side of the heart in part determine the CVP. If the right ventricle pumps what it receives, blood will not back up in the atrium and the CVP

should be normal. If the right side of the heart is not pumping adequately, there will be a backup of blood in the atrium that will be reflected in an elevated CVP.

2. The venous tone determines CVP in that venous tone is responsible for determining the venous vascular space. It thus has major implications in venous return and filling pressure of the right atrium.

3. Blood volume, which in part determines CVP, must be adequate to fill the venous vascular space, or venous return to the heart will be impeded.

4. If the pump capabilities of the right side of the heart are adequate, the CVP will directly reflect the venous vascular volume (blood volume) to venous vascular space relationship. Fluid therapy and diuresis are frequently gauged in terms of the CVP's reflection of this relationship.

B. The CVP is commonly used as an indicator of right ventricular preload when measured as right ventricular end-diastolic pressure (RVEDP).

1. RVEDP represents compliance of the right ventricle.

2. RVEDP also represents the filling pressure necessary for adequate right ventricular function.

C. The CVP is measured directly through a catheter inserted in a peripheral vein, its tip resting in the right atrium (Fig 14–2).

D. Normal values for CVP in the adult are 0–8 mm Hg.

III. Pulmonary Artery Pressure

Pulmonary artery pressure (PAP) is expressed as a systolic pressure divided by a diastolic pressure.

A. Systolic pressure is the highest pressure attained in the pulmonary artery and is determined by the same three factors that determine systolic pressure in the systemic arterial system:

1. Size of stroke volume

2. Rate of blood ejection from right ventricle

3. Elasticity of pulmonary arterial tree

B. Diastolic pressure is the lowest pressure attained in the pulmonary artery and is determined by the same three factors that determine diastolic pressure in the systemic arterial system:

1. Magnitude of preceding systolic pressure

2. Length of right ventricular diastolic interval

3. State of peripheral resistance of pulmonary arterial tree

C. In general, measurement of PAP assesses right ventricular function by systolic pressure, and pulmonary arterial resistance by diastolic pressure. Thus PAP is used in precisely the same fashion

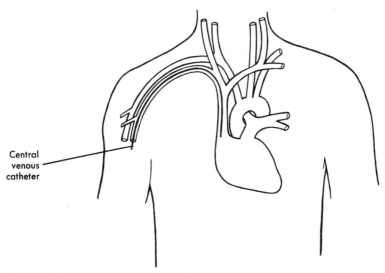

Central venous catheter

Fig 14–2.—Location of a central venous catheter. (From Spearman C.B., Sheldon R.L., Egan D.F.: *Egan's Fundamentals of Respiratory Therapy,* ed. 4. St. Louis, C.V. Mosby Co., 1982. Reproduced by permission.)

as systemic arterial pressure. In this light, it should be noted that all factors contributing to systolic and diastolic PAP should be fully assessed before inferences concerning blood flow are made from these values.

D. The mean pulmonary artery pressure ($\overline{\text{PAP}}$) represents the average pressure over one complete systolic and diastolic interval.

   1. $\overline{\text{PAP}}$ is the average pressure in the pulmonary artery over a given time and is used as an assessment of the average pressure head (or front) that the pulmonary arterial system is exposed to.

   2. Thus the pressure gradient across the pulmonary circulation is generally represented by the expression $\overline{\text{PAP}}$ − PWP, where PWP equals the mean left atrial or pulmonary wedge pressure (see IV, below).

   3. $\overline{\text{PAP}}$ is commonly used as an assessment of right ventricular afterload, thus representing the resistance (in terms of pressure) that the right ventricle must pump against.

E. Both PAP and $\overline{\text{PAP}}$ are directly measured by use of a pulmonary artery catheter. The pulmonary artery catheter is inserted through a peripheral vein and traverses the right atrium and ventricle, its tip resting in the pulmonary artery (Fig 14–3).

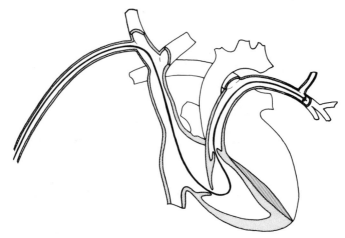

Fig 14–3.—Location of a pulmonary artery catheter. (From Spearman C.B., Sheldon R.L., Egan D.F.: *Egan's Fundamentals of Respiratory Therapy,* ed. 4. St. Louis, C.V. Mosby Co., 1982. Reproduced by permission.)

    F. Normal values for pulmonary arterial blood pressure in the adult are as follows:

Systolic:	15–28 mm Hg
Diastolic:	5–16 mm Hg
Mean:	10–22 mm Hg

IV. Pulmonary Wedge Pressure

    Pulmonary wedge pressure (PWP) is expressed as a single number representing the mean left atrial pressure ($\overline{\text{LAP}}$).

    A. The numerical pressure value of PWP will be the result of the following factors.

        1. The pump capabilities of the left side of the heart in part determine PWP. If the left ventricle pumps what it receives, blood will not back up into the atrium and PWP should be normal. If the left ventricle is not pumping adequately, there will be a backup of blood into the atrium that will be reflected as an elevated PWP.

        2. Blood return to the left atrium is due largely to an adequate blood volume to pulmonary venous (venomotor tone) vascular space relationship.

        3. If the left ventricle is pumping adequately, PWP is dependent on the forementioned vascular volume to vascular space relationship.

B. The PWP is commonly used as an indicator of left ventricular pre-load when measured as the left ventricular end-diastolic pressure (LVEDP).
   1. LVEDP represents compliance of the left ventricle.
   2. LVEDP also represents the filling pressure necessary for adequate left ventricular function.
C. PWP is measured directly through a pulmonary artery catheter by inflation of a balloon that occludes that branch of the pulmonary artery. Pressure readings are taken from the tip of the catheter, which is distal to the balloon. The pressure reflects backpressure from the left atrium.
D. Normal values for PWP in the adult are 2–12 mm Hg.

V. Calculating and Comparing Systemic and Pulmonary Vascular Resistance

A.
$$R = \frac{\Delta P}{\dot{Q}} \tag{3}$$

where R = vascular resistance expressed in mm Hg/L/min
ΔP = change in pressure across the circulation or pressure gradient, expressed in mm Hg
$\dot{Q}$ = cardiac output or flow expressed in L/min

B. Systemic vascular resistance equals
   1.
$$R = \frac{MAP - \overline{RAP}}{\dot{Q}} \tag{4}$$

where $\underline{MAP}$ = mean arterial pressure
$\overline{RAP}$ = mean right atrial pressure (CVP)
$\dot{Q}$ = cardiac output

   2. Replacing the factors with representative normal values results in:

$$R = \frac{(90 - 5) \text{ mm Hg}}{5 \text{ L/min}} = 17 \text{ mm Hg/L/min} \tag{5}$$

C. Pulmonary vascular resistance equals:
   1.
$$R = \frac{\overline{PAP} - \overline{LAP}}{\dot{Q}} \tag{6}$$

where $\overline{PAP}$ = mean pulmonary arterial pressure
$\overline{LAP}$ = mean left atrial pressure (PWP)
$\dot{Q}$ = cardiac output

2. Replacing the factors with representative normal values results in:

$$R = \frac{(16 - 6) \text{ mm Hg}}{5 \text{ L/min}} = 2 \text{ mm Hg/L/min} \qquad (7)$$

D. By these calculations, systemic vascular resistance equals 17 mm Hg/L/min and pulmonary vascular resistance equals 2 mm Hg/L/min. This relationship results in systemic vascular resistance being about 8½ times the pulmonary vascular resistance.

VI. Techniques of Measuring Cardiac Output

A. Fick method

1. The total amount of oxygen available for tissue utilization must be equal to arterial oxygen content (Ca_{O_2}), expressed in vol%, times the volume of blood presented to the tissues per unit time ($\dot{Q}$ or cardiac output), expressed in L/min:

$$\text{Total } O_2 \text{ available} = (\dot{Q}) \times (Ca_{O_2}) \qquad (8)$$

2. The total amount of oxygen returned to the lung from the tissues must be equal to the mixed venous oxygen content ($C\bar{v}_{O_2}$) times the volume of blood presented to the lung per unit time ($\dot{Q}$ or cardiac output):

$$\text{Total } O_2 \text{ returned} = (\dot{Q}) \times (C\bar{v}_{O_2}) \qquad (9)$$

3. Therefore, total tissue extraction of oxygen per unit time ($\dot{V}_{O_2}$) must be equal to the total oxygen available minus the total oxygen returned:

$$\dot{V}_{O_2} = [(\dot{Q}) \times (Ca_{O_2})] - [(\dot{Q}) \times (C\bar{v}_{O_2})] \qquad (10)$$

4. Equation 10 may be simplified by extracting the common factor of ($\dot{Q}$) and rewriting it as follows:

$$\dot{V}_{O_2} = (\dot{Q}) \times (Ca_{O_2} - C\bar{v}_{O_2}) \qquad (11)$$

5. Equation 11 is called the Fick equation and, by solving for cardiac output ($\dot{Q}$), it becomes

$$\dot{Q} = \frac{\dot{V}_{O_2}}{Ca_{O_2} - C\bar{v}_{O_2}} \qquad (12)$$

6. Thus, by measuring total oxygen consumption per minute and arterial and mixed venous oxygen content in vol%, the cardiac output can be easily calculated by equation 12.

(1) Total oxygen consumption generally is calculated by analysis of exhaled gases.

(2) Arterial oxygen content requires systemic arterial blood sampling.

(3) Mixed venous oxygen content requires pulmonary arterial blood sampling.

7. *Example:* Given the following values:

$$\dot{V}_{O_2} = \frac{280 \text{ cc of } O_2}{\text{min}}$$

$$C_{aO_2} = \frac{20 \text{ cc of } O_2}{100 \text{ cc blood}} \text{ or } 20 \text{ vol}\%$$

$$C\bar{v}_{O_2} = \frac{15 \text{ cc of } O_2}{100 \text{ cc blood}} \text{ or } 15 \text{ vol}\%$$

then the cardiac output must equal 5.6 L/min by the following calculation:

$$\dot{Q} = \frac{\dfrac{280 \text{ cc of } O_2}{\text{min}}}{\dfrac{20 \text{ cc of } O_2}{100 \text{ cc blood}} - \dfrac{15 \text{ cc of } O_2}{100 \text{ cc blood}}}$$

$$\dot{Q} = \frac{5600 \text{ cc of blood}}{\text{min}} \text{ or } \frac{5.6 \text{ L of blood}}{\text{min}}$$

8. The cardiac output determination obtained by using the Fick equation is considered the most accurate. The Fick method is therefore the standard by which other methods of cardiac output determinations are compared for accuracy.

B. Dye dilution method

1. A dye (typically indocyanine green) that can be analyzed by a spectrophotometer is used as an indicator.

2. A known amount (mg) of dye is injected rapidly into the right atrium or pulmonary artery.

3. The dye is allowed to mix in the pulmonary circulation, and a continuous representative sampling of blood is drawn from the sampling catheter located in a major systemic artery.

4. Blood samples are analyzed by spectrophotometry for concentration of dye, and the concentrations are plotted on a graph against time.

5. Knowing the number of milligrams of dye injected and plotting

the measured concentrations against time allow calculation of the cardiac output ($\dot{Q}$) by the following equation:

$$\dot{Q} = \frac{d_o}{\overline{d_c} \times t} \tag{13}$$

where $\dot{Q}$ = cardiac output
d_o = mg of dye injected
$\overline{d_c}$ = mean concentration of dye
t = time from appearance to disappearance of dye at sampling site

C. Thermal dilution method
1. This technique uses a four-lumen pulmonary artery catheter (Swan-Ganz catheter) with a port about 30 cm proximal from the end of the catheter (Fig 14–4).
2. This proximal port usually lies in the right atrium and is used for injection of a known volume (usually 10 cc) of fluid (D_5W) at a known temperature (usually 0° C).
3. At the distal end of the catheter is a device, a thermistor, which senses changes in temperature. This device normally resides in a branch of the pulmonary artery.
4. The bolus of cold solution is injected into the right atrium. The

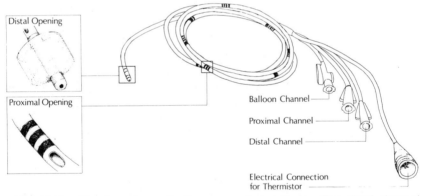

Fig 14–4.—The four-channel pulmonary artery catheter. The distal channel and balloon channel comprise the basic two-channel catheter. Addition of the proximal channel that opens in the right atrium results in the triple-channel catheter, usually 7 French in diameter. Addition of the thermistor channel results in the four-channel catheter used for thermodilution cardiac output measurements, usually 7 French in diameter. (From Shapiro B.A., Harrison R.A., Walton J.R.: *Clinical Application of Blood Gases,* [ed. 3. Chicago, Year Book Medical Publishers, 1982]).

right ventricle is used as the mixing chamber, and the blood is continually sampled by the thermistor for changes in temperature.

5. The changes in blood temperature can be plotted on a graph against time.
6. The principle underlying cardiac output determination by thermal dilution is identical to that previously described for dye dilution.
7. Knowing the volume of the injected solution and the blood and solution temperatures and plotting the changes in blood temperature against time allow calculation of the cardiac output by the following equation:

$$\dot{Q} = \frac{V \times (T_b - T_s)}{\overline{T_b} \times t} \tag{14}$$

where $\dot{Q}$ = cardiac output
   V = volume of solution injected
   T_b = temperature of blood
   T_s = temperature of solution injected
   $\overline{T_b}$ = mean change in temperature of blood
   t = time from appearance to disappearance of temperature change at sampling site

D. The cardiac output of different individuals varies greatly according to body size. Therefore, cardiac output is frequently expressed in terms of body size and is then called the cardiac index.
   1. The cardiac index is equal to the cardiac output in liters per minute per body surface area in square meters.
   2. The cardiac index becomes a more meaningful value when comparing cardiac outputs of different individuals.
   3. Since cardiac index is a more consistent value among different individuals, it has a narrower normal range of 2.5–4 L/min/sq m.

BIBLIOGRAPHY

Guton A.C.: *Textbook of Medical Physiology,* ed. 5. Philadelphia, W.B. Saunders Co., 1976.
Little R.C.: *Physiology of the Heart and Circulation.* Chicago, Year Book Medical Publishers, Inc., 1977.
McLaughlin A.J.: *Essentials of Physiology for Advanced Respiratory Therapy.* St. Louis, C.V. Mosby Co., 1977.
Mountcastle V.B.: *Medical Physiology,* ed. 14. St. Louis, C.V. Mosby Co., 1980.
Ross G.: *Essentials of Human Physiology.* Chicago, Year Book Medical Publishers, Inc., 1978.

Ruch T.C., Patton H.D.: *Physiology and Biophysics*, ed. 20. Philadelphia, W.B. Saunders Co., 1974.

Rushmer R.F.: *Cardiovascular Dynamics*, ed. 3. Philadelphia, W.B. Saunders Co., 1970.

Schroeder J.S., Daily E.K.: *Techniques in Bedside Hemodynamic Monitoring*, ed. 2. St. Louis, C.V. Mosby Co., 1981.

Shapiro B.A., Harrison R.A., Kacmarek R.M., et al.: *Clinical Applications of Respiratory Care*, ed. 3. Chicago, Year Book Medical Publishers, Inc., 1985.

Spearman C.B., Sheldon R.L., Egan D.F.: *Egan's Fundamentals of Respiratory Therapy*, ed. 4. St. Louis, C.V. Mosby Co., 1982.

15 / Fluid and Electrolyte Balance

I. Distribution of Body Fluids
   A. Percent of body weight made up by water:
      1. Adult men, 60%
      2. Adult women, 55%
      3. Newborn, 75%
      4. Obese persons, 45% or less. Fat is much less vascular than muscle, thus the greater the fat content the lower the water content.
   B. In the average adult, total body fluid volume is about 40 L.
      1. 25 L is intracellular:
         a. 2 L RBC volume
         b. 23 L other cellular compartments
      2. 15 L is extracellular:
         a. 3 L plasma volume
         b. 12 L other extracellular fluid
II. Normal Intake and Output of Fluids
   A. In the healthy individual, intake and output should be in complete balance.
   B. Normal intake:
      1. Drink   1,200 ml/day
      2. Food   1,000 ml/day
      3. Metabolically produced   350 ml/day
      4. Total intake   2,550 ml/day
   C. Normal output
      1. Evaporation (lung and skin)   900 ml/day
      2. Sweat (on hot, humid days this can increase markedly)   50 ml/day
      3. Feces   100 ml/day
      4. Urine   1,500 ml/day
      5. Total output   2,550 ml/day
III. Composition of the Intravascular Space
   A. Normally, all compartments are in electrostatic balance; that is, cation and anion concentrations are equal.

241

1. Cation mean values (mEq/L):

Na^+	142
K^+	5
Ca^{+2}	5
Mg^{+2}	3
Total	155

2. Anion mean values (mEq/L):

HCO_3^-	27
Cl^-	103
Protein	16
Organic acids	6
PO_4^{-3}	2
SO_4^{-2}	1
Total	155

B. Plasma protein concentrations can be subdivided into:

	(mean values)
Albumin	4.8 gm/100 ml
Globulin	2.5 gm/100 ml
Fibrinogen	300 mg/100 ml

C. Additionally, the following substances are present in vascular fluid:

	(mean values)
Glucose	90 mg/100 ml
Lipids	600 mg/100 ml

D. Anion gap: The difference between the commonly measured anions and cations, reflecting the quantity of unmeasured anions:

$$\text{Anion gap} = [[Na^+] + [K^+]] - [[Cl^-] + [HCO_3^-]] \quad (1)$$
$$17 \text{ mEq/L} = [142 + 5] - [103 + 27]$$

Normally, the anion gap ranges from about 15 to 20 mEq/L.

IV. Composition of Extravascular (Interstitial) Fluid
   A. The extravascular concentrations of most substances are about the same as their intravascular concentrations.
   B. The major exception is protein. Since protein is not freely diffusible across the capillary membrane extravascular protein concentrations are less than one third intravascular concentrations.
   C. As with all other compartments, electrostatic balance is maintained.

V. Composition of the Intracellular Compartment
    A. Electrostatic balance is maintained within the intracellular space.
    B. However, the composition of anions and cations differs considerably from intravascular levels.
    C. 1. Cations, mean values (mEq/L):

Na^+	10
K^+	140
Ca^{+2}	0
Mg^{+2}	30
Total	180

      2. Anions, mean values (mEq/L):

HCO_3^-	10
Cl^-	4
Protein	61
PO_4^{-3}	11
SO_4^{-2}	2
Other anions	92
Total	180

VI. Movement Across Membranes
    A. The following mechanisms are responsible for the movement of fluid and dissolved substances across membranes:
      1. Simple diffusion (see Chap. 2)
      2. Osmosis (see Chap. 2)
      3. Facilitated diffusion
      4. Active transport
    B. Facilitated diffusion (Fig 15–1) occurs from an area of high con-

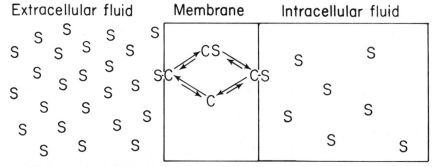

Fig 15–1.—Facilitated diffusion. *S,* substance diffusing; *C,* carrier substance. (From Sullivan L.P.: *Physiology of the Kidney.* Philadelphia, Lea & Febiger, 1975. Reproduced by permission.)

centration of the diffusing substance to an area of low concentration. However, a carrier substance is necessary for movement to occur across the membrane.

    1. No energy is expended, in comparison to active transport.

    2. Glucose moves across cell membranes by facilitated diffusion. Insulin allows a rapid attachment of glucose to the intramembrane carrier substance.

C. Active transport is the movement of a substance from an area of low concentration to an area of high concentration.

    1. Movement is always uphill—low concentration to high concentration.

    2. Energy in the form of adenosine triphosphate (ATP) is necessary for transport to occur.

    3. The movement of many substances is controlled by active transport. Figure 15–2 depicts the most common active transport mechanism, the movement of Na^+ out of the cell and the movement of K^+ into the cell.

VII. Starling Law of Fluid Exchange

A. The interrelationship among factors that determine the quantity and the direction of fluid movement across membranes.

B. The relationship is expressed as:

$$J = k\,[(P_{cap} - P_{is}) - (\pi_{pl} - \pi_{is})] \qquad (2)$$

where J = net fluid movement
k = capillary membrane permeability
P_{cap} = capillary hydrostatic pressure
P_{is} = interstitial hydrostatic pressure
π_{pl} = plasma colloid osmotic pressure
π_{is} = interstitial colloid osmotic pressure

C. Theoretically, there are two pressures on each side of a capillary membrane.

    1. Hydrostatic pressure: Blood pressure or interstitial fluid pressure.

    2. Colloid osmotic pressure:

        a. The osmotic pressure caused by nondiffusible protein.

        b. Since all dissolved substances except protein are readily diffusible, the effective osmotic pressure of either plasma or interstitial fluid is established by protein.

        c. The quantity of protein is about three times greater in the plasma than in the interstitial fluid.

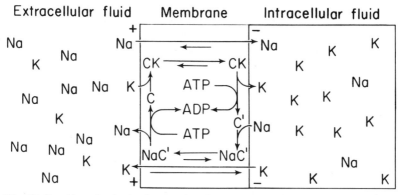

Fig 15–2.—Hypothetical scheme of active transport of sodium (Na) and potassium (K) across cellular membrane. *C*, carrier substance; *ATP*, adenosine triphosphate; *ADP*, adenosine diphosphate. (From Sullivan L.P.: *Physiology of the Kidney.* Philadelphia, Lea & Febiger, 1975. Reproduced by permission.)

   D. Capillary membrane permeability can be altered by many forms of physiologic stress, resulting in alterations in net fluid movement, given fixed hydrostatic and colloid osmotic pressures.

   E. The pressures across the *pulmonary* capillary membrane are depicted in Figure 15–3.

      1. Forces tending to move fluid *out* of the pulmonary capillary, mean values:

Capillary hydrostatic pressure	7 mm Hg
Interstitial hydrostatic pressure*	6 mm Hg
Interstitial colloid osmotic pressure	16 mm Hg
Total force moving fluid out of capillary	29 mm Hg

      2. Forces tending to *maintain fluid in* the pulmonary capillary, mean values:

Plasma colloid osmotic pressure	28 mm Hg
Total force maintaining fluid inside the pulmonary capillaries	28 mm Hg

      3. Net force causing fluid to leave pulmonary capillaries is 1 mm Hg (29–28 mm Hg).

      4. The amount of fluid leaving the capillary as a result of the 1 mm Hg pressure gradient is dependent on the permeability of the pulmonary capillary membrane.

      5. The negative interstitial hydrostatic pressure not only assists in moving fluid out of pulmonary capillaries but also main-

---

*This value is negative; however, with respect to direction of fluid movement it is a force moving fluid out of the capillary; thus, a positive value is listed.

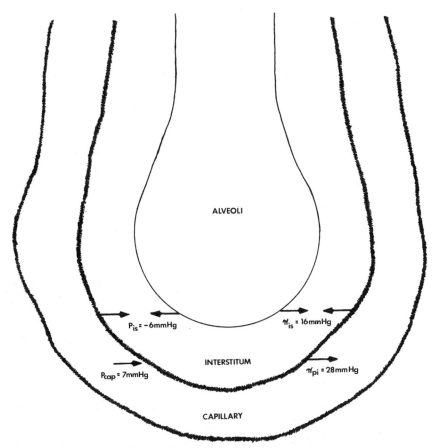

Fig 15–3.—Pressures affecting fluid exchange at the pulmonary capillaries. *Arrows* indicate direction individual pressures cause fluid movement. P_{is}, interstitial hydrostatic pressure; P_{cap}, interstitial hydrostatic pressure; π_{is}, interstitial colloid osmotic pressure; π_{pi}, plasma colloid osmotic pressure.

tains the alveoli "dry." This force, along with the interstitial colloid osmotic pressure, moves fluid from the lung into the interstitial space.

6. The pulmonary interstitial colloid osmotic pressure is much higher than the systemic interstitial colloid osmotic pressure because the pulmonary capillaries are much more permeable than the systemic capillaries.

7. Any alteration in the pressures listed can result in increased fluid movement into the interstitium or the alveoli.

8. The most common causes of increased fluid movement are:
   a. Increased capillary hydrostatic pressure
      (1) Left heart failure
      (2) Fluid overload
   b. Increased capillary permeability—any form of significant physiologic stress
      (1) ARDS
      (2) Noxious gas inhalation
      (3) Pulmonary burns
   c. Decreased capillary colloid osmotic pressure
      (1) Hypermetabolic state
      (2) Starvation
      (3) Fluid overload

F. Forces affecting *systemic* capillary fluid movement, mean values:
   1. Forces moving fluid *out* of the capillary:

Capillary hydrostatic pressure	16.0 mm Hg
Interstitial hydrostatic pressure	6.3 mm Hg
Interstitial colloid osmotic pressure	6.0 mm Hg
Total force moving fluid out of the capillary	28.3 mm Hg

   2. Forces moving fluid *into* the capillary:

Capillary colloid osmotic pressure	28 mm Hg
Total force moving fluid into the capillary	28 mm Hg

   3. Net force causing fluid movement out of the capillary is 0.3 mm Hg (28.3–28 mm Hg).
   4. The amount of fluid leaving the capillary as a result of the 0.3 mm Hg pressure gradient is dependent on the permeability of the capillary membrane.
   5. Any alteration in the pressures listed can cause fluid to move into the interstitium.
   6. The most common causes of increased fluid movement are:
      a. Increased capillary hydrostatic pressure
         (1) Right heart failure
         (2) Fluid overload
      b. Increased capillary permeability—any significant physiologic stress
         (1) Bacteremia
         (2) Septicemia
         (3) Trauma
      c. Decreased capillary colloid osmotic pressure
         (1) Hypermetabolic state
         (2) Starvation
         (3) Fluid overload

VIII. Sodium
    A. Normal serum levels range from about 135 to 144 mEq/L.
    B. Na^+ concentration is normally a reflection of extracellular fluid volume.
    C. Approximately 70–100 mEq of sodium is excreted daily:
        1. 5–10 mEq in feces and skin
        2. 25 mEq in sweat
        3. About 40 mEq in urine
    D. Hyponatremia (decreased serum Na^+ concentration) may reflect:
        1. Decreased extracellular fluid volume
            a. Excessive Na^+ loss
            b. Decreased Na^+ intake
        2. Normal extracellular fluid volume
            a. Excessive ADH
            b. Glucocorticoid deficiency, Addison's disease
            c. Severe hypothyroidism
            d. Fluid overload with normal renal function
        3. Increased extracellular fluid volume
            a. Cardiac failure
            b. Renal failure
            c. Nephrotic syndrome
            d. Hepatic insufficiency
            e. Trauma
    E. Clinical signs of hyponatremia:
        1. Headache
        2. Muscle cramps and weakness
        3. Thirst
        4. Nausea
        5. Agitation
        6. Anorexia
        7. Disorientation
        8. Apathy
        9. Lethargy
    F. Hypernatremia (increase in serum Na^+ concentration) always reflects a deficiency of water compared to total body solute volume.
IX. Chloride
    A. Chloride balance is very similar to Na^+ balance.
    B. Normal serum levels range from about 95 to 105 mEq/L.
    C. Hypochloremia (decreased serum Cl^- concentration) may be caused by:
        1. Increased secretion and loss of gastric juices

2. Increased renal excretion
3. Aldosteronism
4. Dilution
5. Actual hyponatremia
6. Bicarbonate ion retention

D. Hyperchloremia (increased serum Cl^- concentration) may be caused by:
   1. Increased intake
   2. Decreased bicarbonate ion concentration
   3. Respiratory alkalosis
   4. Decreased renal excretion
   5. Dehydration

E. Because of the exchange of Cl^- and HCO_3^- by the kidney, serum concentrations of these electrolytes are indirectly related. In addition, the pH of the urine and the plasma change in opposite direction as Cl^- levels change.
   1. Hypochloremia
      a. Increased serum HCO_3^-, alkalosis
      b. Decreased urine HCO_3^-, acidosis
   2. Hyperchloremia
      a. Decreased serum HCO_3^-, acidosis
      b. Increased urine HCO_3^-, alkalosis

F. In chronic CO_2 retention with increased HCO_3^-, Cl^- is decreased.

X. Potassium
A. Normal serum potassium concentrations are about 3.5–5.5 mEq/L.
B. Normal potassium loss
   1. 15–30 mEq/L via skin and feces
   2. 10–30 mEq/L via urine
C. Normal potassium ingestion, 50–100 mEq
D. Minimum potassium ingestion, 40 mEq
E. Hypokalemia (decreased serum potassium concentration) may be caused by:
   1. Diuretics
   2. Vomiting or nasogastric suction
   3. Malabsorption
   4. Laxative abuse
   5. Diarrhea
   6. Decreased intake
   7. Excessive output

F. Clinical signs and symptoms of hypokalemia:
   1. Metabolic alkalosis
   2. Acidic urine (because of exchange with H^+, as K^+ excretion decreases, H^+ excretion increases)
   3. Muscle weakness
   4. Fatigue
   5. Hypotension
   6. Confusion
   7. Cardiac arrhythmias (cardiac arrest)
   8. On ECG, flat or inverted T waves
G. Hyperkalemia (increased serum potassium concentration) may be caused by:
   1. Increased intake
   2. Decreased excretion
   3. Redistribution from the intracellular space (a result of severe tissue trauma: burns, muscle trauma, spinal cord injuries, renal failure)
   4. Clinical signs and symptoms
      a. Metabolic acidosis
      b. Alkaline urine
      c. Muscle weakness
      d. Confusion
      e. Paresthesia
      f. Cardiac arrhythmias (cardiac arrest)
      g. On ECG, spiked T wave
XI. Calcium
   A. Normal serum calcium concentrations are about 5–10 mEq/L.
   B. About 50% of the calcium in the blood is bound to protein. The amount of Ca^{+2} bound to protein is affected by plasma pH.
      1. If plasma pH increases, more Ca^{+2} is bound to protein.
      2. If plasma pH decreases, less Ca^{+2} is bound to protein.
   C. Hypercalcemia (increased serum Ca^{+2} concentration) may be caused by:
      1. Malignancy
      2. Primary hyperparathyroidism
      3. Acute renal failure
      4. Vitamin D intoxication
      5. Hyperthyroidism
   D. Clinical signs and symptoms of hypercalcemia:
      1. Tiredness, muscle weakness, neuromuscular paralysis
      2. Cardiac arrhythmias
      3. Anorexia, nausea and vomiting

      4. Weight loss

      5. Peptic ulcer, abdominal pain

  E. Hypocalcemia (decreased serum calcium concentration) may be caused by:

      1. Hyperthyroidism

      2. Vitamin D deficiency

      3. Magnesium deficiency

      4. Renal failure

  F. Clinical signs and symptoms of hypocalcemia:

      1. Impaired neuromuscular function

         a. Paresthesia

         b. Muscle cramps

         c. Tetany

      2. Tingling, numbness

      3. Cardiac arrhythmias

XII. Magnesium

  A. Normal serum concentration is 2.5–3.5 mEq/L.

  B. Hypermagnesemia (increased serum Mg^{+2} concentration) may be caused by:

      1. Acute or chronic renal failure

      2. Uncontrolled diabetes mellitus

      3. Adrenocortical insufficiency

      4. Metabolic acidosis

      5. Increased ingestion

  C. Clinical signs and symptoms of hypermagnesemia:

      1. Muscle weakness

      2. Loss of deep tendon reflexes

      3. Impaired autonomic nerve transmission

      4. Vasodilation

      5. Drowsiness

      6. Cardiac arrhythmias

  D. Hypomagnesemia (decreased serum Mg^{+2} concentration) may be caused by:

      1. Decreased intake

      2. Gastrointestinal disturbances

      3. Endocrine disturbances

      4. Renal disease

      5. Alcoholism

  E. Clinical signs and symptoms of hypomagnesemia:

      1. Muscle weakness

      2. Nausea and vomiting, abdominal pain

      3. Neuromuscular excitability

4. CNS depression, irritability
5. Tachycardia

XIII. Phosphate
  A. Normal serum phosphate levels (PO_4^{-3}) are 1.5–2.5 mEq/L.
  B. Hyperphosphatemia (increased serum phosphate concentration) may be caused by:
    1. Hypoparathyroidism
    2. Vitamin D toxicity
    3. Renal failure
    4. High intake
    5. Acidosis
  C. Clinical signs and symptoms of hyperphosphatemia:
    1. Ectopic calcification
    2. Secondary hyperparathyroidism
  D. Hypophosphatemia (decreased serum phosphate concentration) may be caused by:
    1. Primary hyperparathyroidism
    2. Alkalosis
    3. Low intake
    4. Chronic alcoholism
    5. Beriberi
    6. Septicemia
  E. Clinical signs and symptoms of hypophosphatemia:
    1. Muscle weakness
    2. Paresthesia
    3. Rickets
    4. Impaired metabolism
    5. Seizures

XIV. Fluid Balance
  A. The venous system is referred to as the capacitance system, since it has the ability to store large quantities of blood.
  B. The storage capabilities of the venous system are depicted in Figure 15–4.
    1. Below minimum capacitance, large volume changes result in small pressure changes.
    2. Within the normal capacitance range, a volume change results in a small pressure change.
    3. Beyond the maximum capacitance level, a small volume change results in a large pressure change.
  C. Venous conductance is the ability of the venous system to conduct flow.

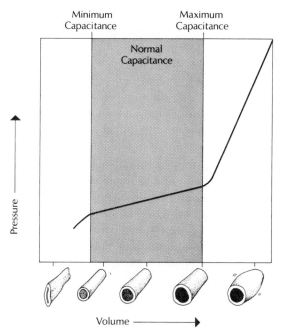

Fig 15–4.—Capacitance of the venous system (see text). (From Shapiro B.A., Harrison R.A., Kacmarek R.M., et al.: *Clinical Application of Respiratory Care,* ed. 3. Chicago, Year Book Medical Publishers, Inc., 1985. Reproduced by permission.)

    D. Conductance is a reciprocal of resistance and is equal to flow divided by change in pressure.

    E. The greater the conductance, the greater the ability of the vessel to conduct flow.

    F. Venous return can be increased by either increasing driving pressure or increasing conductance.

        1. Physiologically the organism increases venotone to increase driving pressure, thus increasing venous return.

        2. Clinically, increasing conductance is the most common method of increasing venous return.

        3. Conductance can be increased by optimizing the vascular volume to vascular space relationship.

        4. This is achieved by maintaining a vascular volume that moves the venous system to a capacitance level that is near its maximum capacitance.

G. Fluid administration (fluid challenge principle):
   1. This is an approach to fluid administration that results in optimization of the vascular volume to vascular space relationship.
   2. A general clinical and hemodynamic assessment of the patient is performed to establish baseline values. Specifically, the pulmonary wedge pressure (PWP) is determined.
   3. Approximately 50–200 ml of fluid is rapidly (over 10 minutes) administered. The volume used depends on the patient's clinical status.
   4. The patient is then assessed clinically for improvements in:
      a. Blood pressure
      b. Presence of crackles or wheezes
      c. Peripheral perfusion
      d. Urinary output
   5. The PWP is reassessed if:
      a. The PWP increases less than 3 mm Hg: This indicates that the capacitance is in the minimal range and the process should be repeated until:
         (1) Clinical improvement in circulation is noted
         (2) Abnormal breath sounds develop (crackles or wheezes)
      b. The PWP increase is between 3 and 7 mm Hg, wait 10 minutes and reassess PWP.
         (1) If the increase is now less than 3 mm Hg, repeat entire process.
         (2) If the increase is still between 3 and 7 mm Hg, repeat with one half the original fluid volume used.
      c. If the increase is greater than 7 mm Hg, the capacitance is at or above the maximum level and additional fluid may be poorly tolerated.
   6. The same guidelines may be applied to central venous pressure reading; however, a 2–5 cm H_2O pressure change is used as the guide.

BIBLIOGRAPHY
Ellerbe S.: *Fluid and Blood Component Therapy in the Critically Ill and Injured.* New York, Churchill Livingstone, 1981.
Gabow P.A.: *Fluids and Electrolytes: Clinical Problems and Their Solution.* Boston, Little, Brown & Co., 1983.
Guyton A.C.: *Textbook of Medical Physiology,* ed. 6. Philadelphia, Lea & Febiger, 1981.
Rose B.D.: *Clinical Physiology of Acid-Base and Electrolyte Disorders.* New York, McGraw-Hill Book Co., 1977.

Schrier R.W. (ed.): *Renal and Electrolyte Disorders,* ed. 2. Boston, Little, Brown & Co., 1980.

Smith K.: *Fluids and Electrolytes: A Conceptual Approach.* New York, Churchill Livingstone, 1980.

Sullivan L.P.: *Physiology of the Kidney.* Philadelphia, Lea & Febiger, 1975.

Tepperman J.: *Metabolic and Endocrine Physiology: An Introductory Text,* ed. 3. Chicago, Year Book Medical Publishers, Inc., 1976.

Vanatta J.C., Fogelman M.J.: *Moyer's Fluid Balance: A Clinical Manual,* ed. 2. Chicago, Year Book Medical Publishers, Inc., 1976.

Vander A.J.: *Renal Physiology,* ed. 2. New York, McGraw-Hill Book Co., 1980.

Weldy N.J.: *Body Fluids and Electrolytes: A Programmed Presentation,* ed. 3. St. Louis, C.V. Mosby Co., 1980.

16 / Cardiac Electrophysiology and ECG Interpretation

I. The electric conduction system of the heart functions in the:
   A. Provision of electric excitation of the myocardial fibers without extrinsic stimuli (automaticity).
   B. Conduction of electric impulses through the myocardium.
   C. Organized distribution of the electric impulses to the myocardium in a repetitive, sequential fashion.
II. Electroconduction System of the Heart (Fig 16–1)
   A. Sinoatrial (SA) node
      1. The SA node is located in the right atrium just inferior and posterior to the entrance of the superior vena cava.
      2. It is commonly referred to as the pacemaker of the heart, its *primary function*.
      3. The SA node has an intrinsic rate of depolarization of 60–100 per minute.
      4. The rate of depolarization ordinarily is under the control of the sympathetic and parasympathetic nervous systems.
         a. Sympathetic stimulation of the SA node increases the rate of depolarization–positive chronotropism.
         b. Parasympathetic stimulation of the SA node decreases the rate of depolarization–negative chronotropism.
      5. The wave of depolarization initiated from the SA node travels outwardly through the atrial musculature in concentric circles, thus depolarizing the atria and ultimately the atrioventricular node.
      6. For all practical purposes, the left and right atria depolarize simultaneously.
   B. Atrioventricular (AV) node
      1. The AV node is located in the right atrium between the opening of the coronary sinus and interatrial septum.
      2. Histologically it is comprised of cells identical to those of the SA node.
      3. The *function* of the AV node is threefold:
         a. Backup cardiac pacemaker because of its intrinsic depolarization rate of 40–60 per minute.

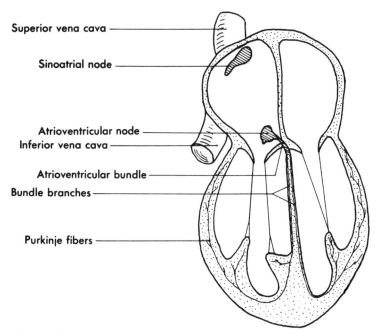

Fig 16–1.—The electrical conduction system of the heart (see text). (From Spearman C.B., Sheldon R.L., Egan D.F.: *Egan's Fundamentals of Respiratory Therapy,* ed. 4. St. Louis, C.V. Mosby Co., 1982. Reproduced by permission.)

     b. The only electrical bridge between atria and ventricles.

     c. Responsible for delaying impulses from atria to ventricles.

   4. The AV node becomes continuous with the common bundle branch (bundle of His) and is the only normal pathway for electric conduction between atria and ventricles. The fibroskeleton of the heart electrically separates atrial from ventricular muscle. The AV node and common bundle penetrate the cardiac fibroskeleton.

   5. That the tissue of the AV node slows the rate of electrical conduction accounts for the time delay between atrial and ventricular depolarization. This time delay also allows optimal ventricular filling prior to ventricular contraction (systole).

   6. The rate of conduction of electrical impulses through the AV node is under the control of the sympathetic and parasympathetic nervous systems.

     a. Sympathetic stimulation decreases conduction time and allows overall increases in cardiac rate.

   b. Parasympathetic stimulation increases conduction time of
      the AV node. Strong parasympathetic stimulation may ac-
      tually block all or a portion of the impulses originating from
      the atria.
C. Common bundle branch
   1. It is also known as the AV bundle or bundle of His.
   2. It is located on the right side of the interventricular septum
      and penetrates the right fibrous trigone.
   3. Its *function* is twofold:
      a. To conduct impulses from the AV node to the left and right
         bundle branches.
      b. To penetrate the fibroskeleton of the heart, electrically
         bridging the atrial conduction system to the ventricular con-
         duction system.
   4. The common bundle branch travels inferiorly in the interven-
      tricular septum for about 10–12 mm and then divides into one
      right and two left bundle branches.
D. Right and left bundle branches
   1. The right bundle branch appears simply as a continuation of
      the common bundle branch and follows an inferior course to-
      ward the apex of the heart.
   2. The left bundle branch penetrates the interventricular septum
      and divides into an anterior and posterior left bundle branch.
      Both bundle branches course inferiorly on the left side of the
      interventricular septum.
   3. The *function* of the three major bundle branches is to conduct
      electric impulses from the common bundle branch to the Pur-
      kinje fibers.
E. Purkinje fibers
   1. The Purkinje fibers are very fine ramifications of the bundle
      branches which terminate on the endocardial layer of the
      heart.
   2. They are located throughout the entire endocardial layer of
      both ventricles and conduct the electrical impulses from the
      bundle branches to the ventricles. Depolarization of the ven-
      tricles begins when impulses leaving the Purkinje fibers invade
      the endocardial layer.
   3. The wave of depolarization travels from the endocardial layer
      outward toward the epicardium and also from the apex toward
      the base of the ventricles.
F. Summary of pathway of normal electrical conduction
   1. Impulses originate in right atrium by spontaneous depolariza-
      tion of SA node.

2. Impulses are conducted through atrial muscle, which results in depolarization of right and left atria and AV node.
3. The impulse is delayed at AV node and then conducted through the cardiac fibroskeleton by the AV node and common bundle branch.
4. The impulse is then conducted from the common bundle branch through right and left bundle branches to Purkinje fibers.
5. The impulses exit the Purkinje fibers and cause depolarization of the ventricle from inside out and from apex to base.
6. Design of the electrical conduction system of the heart allows simultaneous depolarization of right and left atria totally separate from simultaneous depolarization of the right and left ventricles. This fact has important implications for the mechanical function of the heart.

III. Electrocardiogram (ECG)
   A. The ECG is a graphic display of current generated by the heart at the surface of the body. It depicts depolarization and repolarization of atria and ventricles.
   B. The ECG is used in assessing the electrical activity of the heart, which should be clearly delineated from the mechanical activity of the heart.
   C. Each portion of the cardiac cycle generates a specific type of electrical impulse. These impulses are repetitious and produce characteristic patterns on an ECG recording.
   D. The four major electrical cardiac events are atrial depolarization, atrial repolarization, ventricular depolarization, and ventricular repolarization.
      1. The polarized state is the normal resting state of cardiac muscle fiber. The extracellular charge is positive with respect to the intracellular charge (Fig 16–2, panel *a*).
      2. Depolarization is the process of reversing the normal state of polarity. Depolarization thus causes the extracellular charge to be negative with respect to the intracellular charge. This is largely because inflow of extracellular sodium ions is faster than outflow of intracellular potassium ions. Reversal of the cellular membrane charge is thus transmitted along cardiac muscle fiber, depolarizing subsequent fibers. If muscle fibers are normal, this electrochemical stimulation results in mechanical activity (shortening of muscle fibers and cardiac contraction) (Fig 16–2, panel *b*).
      3. Repolarization is the process of reestablishing the normal state of polarity, i.e., reestablishing a positive extracellular charge

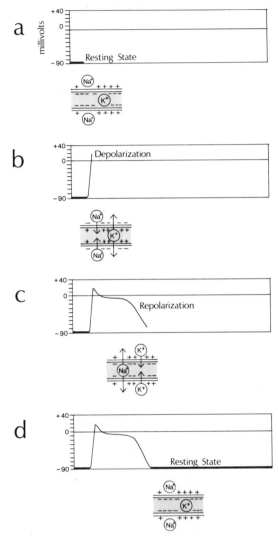

Fig 16–2.—Ion distribution and electric current (millivolt) generation in a myocardial cell: *a,* resting state; *b,* depolarization; *c,* repolarization; *d,* polarized (resting) state (see text). (From Shapiro B.A., Harrison R.A., Kacmarek R.M., et al.: *Clinical Application of Respiratory Care,* ed. 3. Chicago, Year Book Medical Publishers, Inc., 1985. Reproduced by permission.)

with respect to the intracellular charge. The reestablishment of the resting cellular membrane charge is transmitted along the cardiac muscle fiber, repolarizing subsequent fibers. If muscle fibers are normal, this electrochemical stimulation results in lengthening of muscle fibers and cardiac relaxation (Fig 16–2, panel *c*). (*Note:* It is a mistake to assume that the mechanical activity of the heart is normal simply because the electric activity—ECG—is normal.)

E. The electric deflections of ECG in normal sequence are: P wave, QRS complex, and T wave (Fig 16–3).

　　1. The P wave is produced by atrial depolarization and usually is 0.06–0.11 second in duration.

　　2. The QRS complex is produced by ventricular depolarization and usually is 0.03–0.12 second in duration. Repolarization of the atria occurs simultaneously with ventricular depolarization and is masked by the overwhelming electric event of the QRS complex.

　　3. The T wave is produced by ventricular repolarization and usually is 0.14–0.26 second in duration.

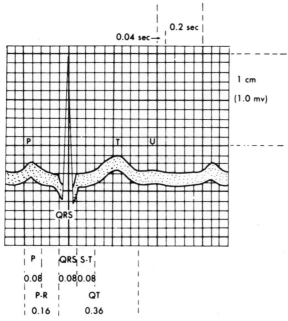

Fig 16–3.—Schematic representation of ECG tracing (see text). (From Spearman C.B., Sheldon R.L., Egan D.F.: *Egan's Fundamentals of Respiratory Therapy,* ed. 4. St. Louis, C.V. Mosby Co., 1982. Reproduced by permission.)

F. PR, RR, and PP intervals
  1. PR interval: Time from the beginning of atrial depolarization to the beginning of ventricular depolarization. The PR interval normally is 0.12–0.20 second in duration.
  2. RR interval: Time from the peak of one QRS complex to the next QRS complex. It is used to measure the total cardiac cycle and normally is 0.6–1.0 second in duration.
  3. PP interval: Time from the beginning of one P wave to the beginning of the next P wave. It can be used to measure the total cardiac cycle time and is normally equal to the RR interval (0.6–1.0 second in duration).
IV. ECG Interpretation
  A. The following system represents a simple organized approach to the evaluation of ECG tracings.
    1. P waves
      a. Should be present.
      b. Should have a configuration similar to that of other P waves.
      c. Should be related on a one-to-one basis to the QRS complex.
    2. PR intervals
      a. Should have a normal duration of 0.12–0.20 second.
      b. Should have consistent duration when compared with other PR intervals.
    3. QRS complexes
      a. Should have a duration of less than 0.12 second.
      b. Should have a similar configuration when compared with other QRS complexes.
    4. RR and PP intervals
      a. RR intervals should have a consistent duration when compared with other RR intervals.
      b. PP intervals should have a consistent duration when compared with other PP intervals.
      c. RR interval should be approximately equal to the PP interval in duration.
    5. Cardiac rate
      a. Should be 60–100/minute.
        (1) Rates less than 60/minute denote bradycardia.
        (2) Rates greater than 100/minute denote tachycardia.
      b. Atrial rate should be equal to the ventricular rate.
    6. After careful evaluation of the previous five steps, the underlying aberration, if any, should be revealed and the rhythm easily identified.

B. Normal sinus rhythm (Fig 16–4)
   1. P waves are present, have similar configurations, and are related to QRS complexes.
   2. PR interval is 0.12–0.20 second long and equal to other PR intervals.
   3. QRS complex is less than 0.12 second long and similar in configuration to other QRS complexes.
   4. RR intervals are regular and equal to PP intervals.
   5. Cardiac rate is 60–100/minute.

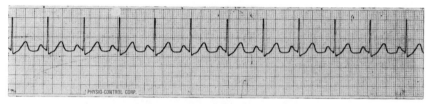

Fig 16–4.—Normal sinus rhythm.

C. Sinus arrhythmia (Fig 16–5)
   1. P waves are present, have similar configuration, and are related to QRS complexes.
   2. PR interval is normal in duration and equal to other PR intervals.
   3. QRS complex is normal in duration and similar in configuration to other QRS complexes.
   4. PP and RR intervals both vary; however, they are equal to one another for a given cardiac cycle.
   5. Cardiac rate varies; however, it generally averages 60–100/minute.

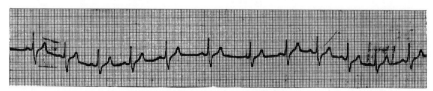

Fig 16–5.—Sinus arrhythmia.

D. Sinus bradycardia (Fig 16–6)
   1. P waves are present, have similar configuration, and are related to QRS complexes.
   2. PR interval is normal in duration and equal to other PR intervals.
   3. QRS complex is normal in duration and similar in configuration to other QRS complexes.

4. RR intervals are regular and equal to PP intervals.
5. Cardiac rate is less than 60/minute.

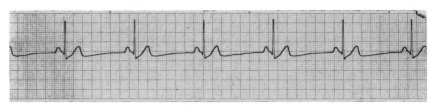

Fig 16–6.—Sinus bradycardia.

E. Sinus tachycardia (Fig 16–7)
   1. P waves are present, have similar configuration, and are related to QRS complexes.
   2. PR interval is normal in duration (lower limits of normal) and equal to other PR intervals.
   3. QRS complex is normal in duration and similar in configuration to other QRS complexes.
   4. RR intervals are regular and equal to PP intervals.
   5. Cardiac rate is greater than 100/minute.

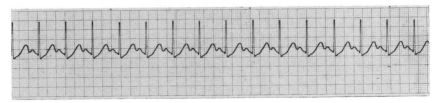

Fig 16–7.—Sinus tachycardia.

F. Premature atrial contraction (PAC) (Fig 16–8)
   1. P wave occurs earlier than expected and may have a normal or abnormal configuration.
   2. PR interval is usually normal and equal in duration to other PR intervals.
   3. QRS complex is usually normal in duration and similar in configuration to other QRS complexes; however, it may be absent if the P wave is not conducted through the AV node.
   4. PP and RR intervals vary with the PAC; however, they are equal to one another for a given cardiac cycle.

5. Cardiac rate: premature atrial contractions can occur at any rate.

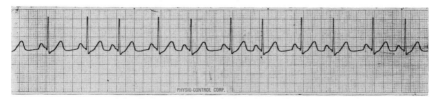

Fig 16–8.—Premature atrial contraction.

G. Atrial tachycardia (Fig 16–9)
   1. P waves are present; however, they may be superimposed on a preceding T wave.
   2. PR interval is usually normal in duration and equal to other PR intervals. However, with rapid rates it may be difficult to determine.
   3. QRS complex is usually normal in duration and similar in configuration to other QRS complexes.
   4. PP and RR intervals are regular and usually equal to each other.
   5. Rate: atrial rate is usually 160–220/minute and ventricular rate is 160–220/minute with 1:1 conduction; however, it may be 80–110/minute with 2:1 conduction.

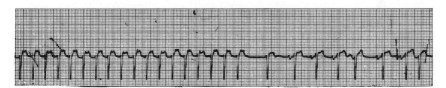

Fig 16–9.—Atrial tachycardia.

H. Atrial flutter (Fig 16–10)
   1. P waves are present, have similar configuration, and resemble a sawtooth or picket fence pattern.
   2. PR interval is usually normal and equal in duration to other PR intervals; however, it may be difficult to measure.
   3. QRS complex is usually normal in duration and similar in configuration to other QRS complexes.

   4. PP interval is regular and equal to other PP intervals; RR interval regular and equal to other RR intervals; PP interval is usually not equal to RR interval as a result of AV nodal block.
   5. Atrial rate typically 220–350/minute; ventricular rate is dependent on degree of conduction through AV node (i.e., 2:1, 3:1, 4:1 conduction).

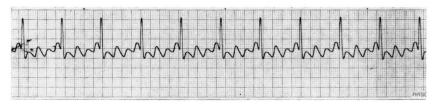

Fig 16–10.—Atrial flutter.

I. Atrial fibrillation (Fig 16–11)
   1. P waves are not truly present; rather, fine or coarse irregular rapid baseline undulations called fibrillatory waves (f waves) occur.
   2. PR interval is not present.
   3. QRS complex is usually normal in duration and similar in configuration to other QRS complexes.
   4. PP interval is not measurable. RR interval is irregular and not equal to other RR intervals.
   5. Atrial rate is approximately 350–700/minute; ventricular rate is 100–200/minute.

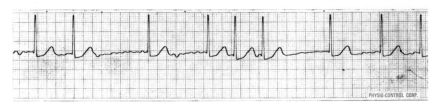

Fig 16–11.—Atrial fibrillation.

J. First-degree heart block (Fig 16–12)
   1. P waves are present, similar in configuration to other P waves, and are related to the QRS complex.
   2. PR interval is greater than 0.20 second and usually equal in duration to other PR intervals, but may vary.

3. QRS complex is normal in duration and similar in configuration to other QRS complexes.
4. RR intervals are regular and equal to PP intervals.
5. Rate: first-degree heart block can occur at any rate.

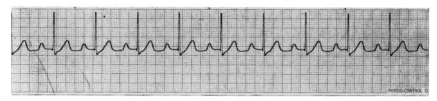

Fig 16–12.—First-degree heart block.

K. Type I second-degree heart block (Fig 16–13)
1. P waves are present, similar in configuration to other P waves, and are related to QRS complexes, except for the nonconducted P waves.
2. PR interval may begin with normal duration but lengthens progressively until one P wave is not conducted.
3. QRS complex is normal in duration and similar in configuration to other QRS complexes.
4. PP interval is regular and equal to other PP intervals. RR intervals vary, with absent QRS complexes.
5. Atrial rate is typically 60–100/minute. Ventricular rate varies with degree of block (i.e., 2:1, 3:2, 4:3 conduction).

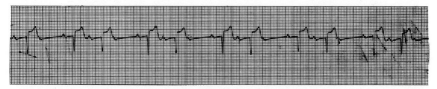

Fig 16–13.—Type I second-degree heart block.

L. Type II second-degree heart block (Fig 16–14)
1. P waves are present, similar in configuration to other P waves, and are related to QRS complexes, except for the nonconducted P waves.
2. PR interval may be normal or prolonged; however, it is equal in duration to other PR intervals.
3. QRS complex is usually normal in duration and similar in configuration to other QRS complexes.
4. PP interval is regular and equal to other PP intervals. RR in-

tervals vary, with absent QRS complexes; however, the PP and RR intervals are equal in cardiac cycles where the P wave is conducted.

5. Atrial rate is typically 60–100/minute. Ventricular rate varies with the degree of block.

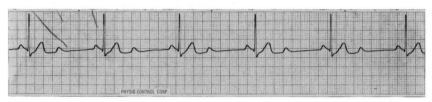

Fig 16–14.—Type II second-degree heart block.

M. Third-degree or complete heart block (Fig 16–15)
   1. P waves are present, similar in configuration to other P waves, but are unrelated to the QRS complexes.
   2. PR interval is completely variable and of no consequence.
   3. QRS complexes are normal in configuration and duration when block occurs at the AV node or bundle of His. QRS complexes are wide and aberrant when block occurs at the bundle branches.
   4. PP and RR intervals are regular but are not equal to each other.
   5. Atrial rate is typically 60–100/minute. Ventricular rate is typically 40–60/minute with block at the AV node and less than 40/minute with infranodal block.

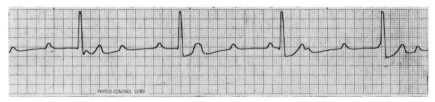

Fig 16–15.—Third-degree or complete heart block.

N. Junctional or nodal rhythm (Fig 16–16)
   1. P waves are typically absent; however, they may be conducted retrogradely and appear anywhere in the cardiac cycle.
   2. PR interval is usually not measurable.
   3. QRS is usually normal in duration and similar in configuration to other QRS complexes.
   4. PP interval usually not measurable. RR interval is regular.
   5. Ventricular rate is typically 40–60/minute.

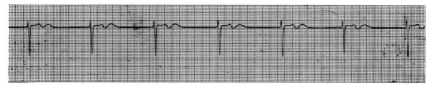

Fig 16–16.—Junctional or nodal rhythm.

O. Supraventricular tachycardia (Fig 16–17)
  1. P waves are usually indiscernible. They may be absent, conducted retrogradely, or buried in the preceding T wave.
  2. PR interval cannot be measured.
  3. QRS complex is normal in duration and similar in configuration to other QRS complexes.
  4. PP interval is not measurable. RR interval is regular and equal to other RR intervals.
  5. Rate is typically greater than 150/minute.

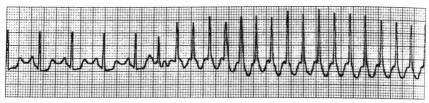

Fig 16–17.—Supraventricular tachycardia.

P. Premature ventricular contraction (PVC) (Fig 16–18)
  1. P waves are typically absent.
  2. PR interval with PVC not measurable.
  3. QRS complex is wide (greater than 0.12 second), bizarre, and unlike normal QRS complexes. It appears earlier in the cardiac cycle than expected and has a T wave on the opposite side of the baseline from the terminal portion of the QRS (PVC) complex.
  4. PP interval with PVC not measurable. RR interval varies with the occurrence of PVC.
  5. PVCs can occur at any rate.

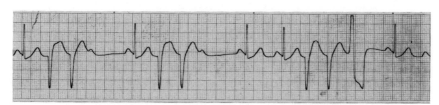

Fig 16–18.—Premature ventricular contraction.

Q. Ventricular tachycardia (Fig 16–19)
1. P waves are generally indiscernible.
2. PR interval is not measurable.
3. QRS complex is wide, bizarre, and generally similar in configuration to other QRS complexes.
4. PP interval is not measurable. RR interval is regular or slightly irregular.
5. Ventricular rate is 100–250/minute.

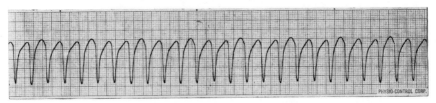

Fig 16–19.—Ventricular tachycardia.

R. Ventricular flutter (Fig 16–20)
1. P waves are absent.
2. PR interval is absent.
3. QRS complex appears as a smooth sinusoidal wave with QRS complex and T waves merged and no clear separation of cardiac cycles.
4. PP interval is absent. RR interval is regular.
5. Ventricular rate is typically 200–300/minute.

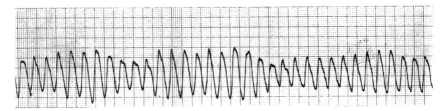

Fig 16–20.—Ventricular flutter.

S. Ventricular fibrillation (Fig 16–21)
1. P waves are absent.
2. PR interval is absent.
3. QRS complexes are absent; however, there is low (fine) or high (coarse) amplitude undulation from the baseline that varies in shape and represents varying degrees of depolarization and repolarization.

4. PP and RR intervals are absent.
5. Rate is absent.

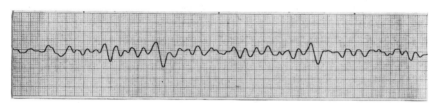

Fig 16–21.—Ventricular fibrillation.

BIBLIOGRAPHY

Conover M.B.: *Exercises in Diagnosing ECG Tracings*, ed. 3. St. Louis, C.V. Mosby Co., 1984.

Dubin D.: *Rapid Interpretation of EKG's*, ed. 3. Tampa, Cover Publishing Co., 1979.

Guyton A.C.: *Textbook of Medical Physiology*, ed. 6. Philadelphia, W.B. Saunders Co., 1981.

Little R.C.: *Physiology of the Heart and Circulation*. Chicago, Year Book Medical Publishers, Inc., 1977.

Marriott H.J.L.: *Practical Electrocardiography*, ed. 6. Baltimore, Williams & Wilkins Co., 1980.

McLaughlin A.J.: *Essentials of Physiology for Advanced Respiratory Therapy*. St. Louis, C.V. Mosby Co., 1977.

Mountcastle V.B.: *Medical Physiology*, ed. 14. St. Louis, C.V. Mosby Co., 1980.

Phillips R.E., Feeney M.K.: *The Cardiac Rhythms*. Philadelphia, W.B. Saunders Co., 1973.

Ross G.: *Essential of Human Physiology*. Chicago, Year Book Medical Publishers, Inc., 1978.

Ruch T.C., Patton H.D.: *Physiology and Biophysics*, ed. 20. Philadelphia, W.B. Saunders Co., 1974.

Rushmer R.F.: *Cardiovascular Dynamics*, ed. 3. Philadelphia, W.B. Saunders Co., 1970.

Schroeder J.S., Daily E.K.: *Techniques in Bedside Hemodynamic Monitoring*, ed. 2. St. Louis, C.V. Mosby Co., 1981.

Shapiro B.A., Harrison R.A., Kacmarek R.M., et al.: *Clinical Applications of Respiratory Care*, ed. 3. Chicago, Year Book Medical Publishers, Inc., 1985.

Spearman C.B., Sheldon R.L., Egan D.F.: *Egan's Fundamentals of Respiratory Therapy*, ed. 4. St. Louis, C.V. Mosby Co., 1982.

17 / Pulmonary Function Studies

I. Lung Volumes and Capacities
  A. The gas in the respiratory system is divided into four basic lung volumes and four lung capacities. All capacities are composed of two or more lung volumes.
    1. Lung volumes
       a. Residual volume (RV): Amount of gas left in the lung after a maximal exhalation.
       b. Expiratory reserve volume (ERV): Amount of gas that can be exhaled after a normal exhalation.
       c. Tidal volume (TV): Amount of gas inspired during a normal inspiration.
       d. Inspiratory reserve volume (IRV): Amount of gas that can be inspired above a normal inspiration.
    2. Lung capacities
       a. Total lung capacity (TLC): Volume of gas contained in the lung at maximum inspiration (RV + ERV + TV + IRV).
       b. Inspiratory capacity (IC): Maximum volume of gas that can be inhaled after a normal exhalation (TV + IRV).
       c. Vital capacity (VC): Maximum volume of gas that can be exhaled after a maximal inspiration (ERV + TV + IRV).
       d. Functional residual capacity (FRC): Volume of gas that remains in the lung after a normal exhalation (RV + ERV).
  B. Normal lung volumes and capacities for a 165-lb, 6 ft tall, 25-year-old man:
    1. TLC = 6,000 cc
    2. VC = 4,800 cc, about 80% of TLC
    3. IC = 3,600 cc, about 60% of TLC
    4. FRC = 2,400 cc, about 40% of TLC
    5. RV = 1,200 cc, about 20% of TLC
    6. ERV = 1,200 cc, about 20% of TLC
    7. TV = 500 cc, about 3 cc per pound of ideal body weight (8%–10% of TLC)
    8. IRV = 3,100 cc, about 50%–55% of TLC
  C. All predicted lung volumes and capacities are based on statistical data from a group of individuals of the stated height, age, and sex.

1. In addition, predicted normal values may vary for different ethnic and racial groups.
2. The acceptable percent deviation from normal in all cases is ±20%. Thus, unless there is greater than 20% variance, the results will be reported as essentially normal.
3. All lung volumes and capacities are expressed at body temperature and pressure saturated (BTPS). Thus, measured values at atmospheric temperature and pressure saturated (ATPS) must be converted to BTPS. Charles' Law (see Chap. 2) is used to make these conversions.
D. Normal values for vital capacities may be taken from various charts or derived from the following formulas:
   1. For males:

$$VC = 27.63 - (0.112 \times age) \times (height\ in\ cm) \qquad (1)$$

   2. For females:

$$VC = 21.78 - (0.101 \times age) \times (height\ in\ cm) \qquad (2)$$

E. All lung volumes and capacities depicted in Figure 17–1 can be measured by direct spirometry except:
   1. RV
   2. FRC
   3. TLC
F. Methods of measuring RV, FRC, and TLC:
   1. Determination of these volumes and capacities is accomplished by using indirect methods of measuring FRC. FRC is measured because it is the most stable of all lung volumes and capacities. Once the FRC is determined, it is used to calculate TLC and RV. In addition, TLC and FRC can be estimated radiologically.
   2. Three basic methods of measuring FRC: nitrogen washout study—open circuit technique; helium dilution study—closed circuit technique; and body plethysmography—total thoracic gas volume determination.
      a. Nitrogen washout study
         (1) The test is always initiated and concluded at the patient's FRC level.
         (2) The patient is connected to a breathing circuit where he inspires 100% oxygen and the total volume of exhaled gas is collected.
         (3) Normally, the test is carried out for 7 minutes or until the percent nitrogen expired is 1%–2.5%.

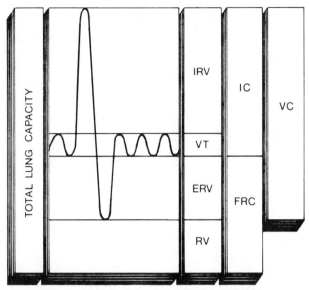

Fig 17–1.—Normal lung volumes and capacities and their relation to each other. Note that with normal spirometry the residual volume *(RV)* cannot be directly determined. Refer to text for further explanation. (From Shapiro B.A.: *Clinical Application of Blood Gases.* ed. 3. Chicago, Year Book Medical Publishers, Inc., 1982. Reproduced by permission.)

(4) Since nitrogen makes up about 80% of FRC when the subject is breathing room air, the volume of nitrogen in the total exhaled gas will equal about 80% of the FRC.

(5) Thus the total gas exhaled is measured for volume and percent nitrogen present.
   Example:

Total volume collected (liters)	50 L
Measured nitrogen concentration	5%
Volume of nitrogen in FRC	2.5 L

(6) The FRC is determined as follows:

$$\frac{2.5 \text{ L}}{0.80 \text{ FRC}} = \frac{x}{1 \text{ FRC}}$$
$$3.125 \text{ L} = x$$

(7) Newer automated spirometers measure % N_2 and exhaled volume breath by breath so that FRC is calculated on an additive basis.

(8) The RV is determined by subtracting ERV from FRC.

(9) The TLC is determined by adding VC to RV.

(10) Problems associated with nitrogen washout study:

   (a) Atelectasis may result from washout of nitrogen from poorly ventilated, partially obstructed areas.

   (b) Elimination of hypoxic drive in carbon dioxide retainers may result in apnea.

   (c) Error in determinations if severe airway obstruction present. The error will be on the low side of actual FRC because of poor distribution of ventilation.

b. Helium dilution study

   (1) Since helium is metabolically inert, a given volume of helium may be distributed throughout the lung bellows system without absorption of a significant volume.

   (2) The test is initiated and concluded at the patient's FRC level.

   (3) The patient is connected to a rebreathing system and a certain volume (%) of helium is placed into a bellows. The patient breathes through the system until a constant helium percentage is read in the lung bellows system.

   (4) Normally the test takes up to 7 minutes to complete.

   (5) A soda lime absorber is placed in the system to remove carbon dioxide. Oxygen is titrated into the system to meet the patient's oxygen demands.

   (6) At the beginning of the test, the concentration of helium in the bellows and the volume of gas in the bellows are measured.

   (7) At the completion of the test, the volume of gas in the bellows and the concentration of helium in the lung bellows system are measured.

   (8) Calculation of FRC

      (a) The amount of helium in the system is constant.

      (b) The volume of helium at the beginning of the test is equal to the volume of helium at the end of the test. Thus:

$$\text{(vol. lung}_B)(\text{conc. lung}_B) + (\text{vol. bellows}_B)(\text{conc. bellows}_B) = \qquad (3)$$
$$\text{(vol. lung}_E)(\text{conc. lung}_E) + (\text{vol. bellows}_E)(\text{conc. bellows}_E)$$

      (c) If the volume of gas in the bellows at the beginning (B) of the test is 2.0 L and the helium concentration is 10%, and at the end (E) of the test the volume in the bellows is 2.0 L and the helium concentration is 3.5%, then the patient's FRC can be calculated using equation 3, the unknown being equal to the FRC.

$$(x) \ (0.0\%) + (2.0 \ \text{L}) \ (0.10) = (x) \ (0.035) + (2.0 \ \text{L}) \ (0.035)$$

$$0.0 + 0.2 \ \text{L} = 0.035x + 0.07 \ \text{L}$$

$$\frac{0.13 \ \text{L}}{0.035} = \frac{0.035x}{0.035}$$

$$3.7 \ \text{L} = x$$

(d) A more commonly used modification of formula 3 is:

$$\text{FRC} = \frac{(\% \ \text{He}_{initial} - \% \ \text{He}_{final})}{\% \ \text{He}_{final}} \times \text{initial vol.} \qquad (4)$$

where $\% \ \text{He}_{initial}$ = initial helium concentration in the system and $\% \ \text{He}_{final}$ = final helium concentration at the conclusion of the test.

$$\text{Initial vol. of system} = \frac{\text{vol. He added}}{\text{initial He conc.}} \qquad (5)$$

(e) Using the same example as above

$$\% \ \text{He}_{initial} = 10\%$$
$$\% \ \text{He}_{final} = 3.5\%$$

$$\text{Initial vol.} = \frac{200 \ \text{ml}}{10\%} = 2{,}000 \ \text{ml or } 2.0 \ \text{L}$$

$$\text{FRC} = \frac{(10\% - 3.5\%)}{3.5\%} \times 2.0 \ \text{L} = 3.7 \ \text{L}$$

(9) Problem associated with the study: Gas distal to severely obstructed airways may not be measured because of poor distribution of ventilation.

c. Body plethysmography
  (1) The patient's total thoracic gas volume is determined. All of the contained gas in the thoracic cavity, even if it is distal to completely obstructed airways, or located in the abdomen or intestines, is measured.
  (2) The overall calculations are based on Boyle's law.
  (3) The total volume of the plethysmograph is known, and

the volume displacement of the patient may be determined by body surface area charts. The volume of gas in the box surrounding the patient is determined by subtracting the volume the patient occupies from the volume of the box.

(4) The patient is sealed in the box and ventilates through a mouthpiece with a pressure transducer attachment and a shutter valve allowing obstruction at the mouthpiece.

(5) During the testing, the patient breathes gas from within the box.

(6) At FRC level, the shutter is closed and the patient inspires against an obstruction. As this occurs, proximal airway pressure and pressure in the plethysmograph are measured simultaneously.

(7) Boyle's law is used to determine the final volume in the plethysmograph itself:

$$P_1V_1 = P_2V_2 \tag{6}$$

where:

P_1 = Original pressure in the plethysmograph is usually equal to atmospheric, or 760 mm Hg

V_1 = Original volume in the plethysmograph minus the volume occupied by patient, e.g., 1,000 L

P_2 = Increased pressure in the plethysmograph as a result of expansion of the thorax, e.g., 760.2 mm Hg

V_2 = Final volume in the plethysmograph

$$(760 \text{ mm Hg})(1,000 \text{ L}) = (760.2 \text{ mm Hg})(x)$$

$$\frac{(760 \text{ mm Hg})(1,000 \text{ L})}{760.2 \text{ mm Hg}} = x$$

$$x = 999.737 \text{ L}$$

(8) The difference (V) between V_1 and V_2 is equal to the decreased volume in the plethysmograph after chest expansion. Since this is a sealed system, the change in volume in the plethysmograph is equal to the change in the volume in the patient's thorax. For the example above:

$$V_1 - V_2 = V \tag{7}$$

$$1,000 \text{ L} - 999.737 \text{ L} = 0.263 \text{ L}$$

(9) As the patient breathes in against an obstruction, the volume in the thorax increases and the pressure in the thorax is decreased. Thus, again applying Boyle's law:

$$Pa_1Va_1 = Pa_2Va_2 \qquad (8)$$

where:

Pa_1 = Proximal airway pressure at resting FRC levels, which would be equivalent to atmospheric (760 mm Hg)

Va_1 = Volume of FRC

Pa_2 = Pressure in airway after inspiring against an obstruction. In this example: 700 mm Hg

Va_2 = Final volume in thorax is equal to original volume Va_1 plus results from equation 7 (V). Thus Boyle's law may be written as:

$$(Pa_1)(Va_1) = (Pa_2)(Va_1 + V)$$

$$(760 \text{ mm Hg})(x) = 700 \text{ mm Hg } (x + 0.263 \text{ L})$$

$$760 \text{ mm Hg } x = 700 \text{ mm Hg } x + 184.1 \text{ mm Hg} \cdot \text{L}$$

$$\frac{60x}{60} = \frac{184.1 \text{ mm Hg} \cdot \text{L}}{60 \text{ mm Hg}}$$

$$x = 3.07 \text{ L} \qquad (9)$$

(10) The thoracic gas volume is equal to 3.07 L.

3. Radiologic estimation of TLC and FRC, from which RV can be calculated.

    a. Estimations are made from standard posteroanterior (PA) and lateral chest x-ray films taken at a standard distance of 72 in. (183 cm).

    b. A transparency is placed over the x-ray film and the lung fields are traced.

    c. Two distinct methods are then available to estimate lung volumes: the ellipsoid method and the planimetry method.

        (1) The ellipsoid method considers the elliptical shape of the lungs and divides them into sections that may be geometrically assessed as cylinders, from which lung volume is determined.

        (2) The planimetry method makes use of regression equations for surface areas of radiologic lung fields that are based on plethysmography measurements.

    d. Patient cooperation and effort must be maximal for proper x-ray representation, regardless of the method employed.

    e. These methods compare well with inert gas and plethysmographic methods.

(1) Usually within 500 ml of the actual TLC

(2) May be more accurate than inert gas methods if severe air trapping exists

G. Closing volume

1. The closing volume is defined as the terminal portion of a slow exhaled VC that indicates the point at which the most gravity-dependent airways start to collapse.

2. Normally during a maximal exhalation, there is a collapsing of peripheral bronchioles. In disease states, the volume of gas present in the lung when peripheral bronchioles begin to collapse increases.

3. A single-breath nitrogen washout study is used to determine the closing volume.

4. If an individual starts at RV level and inspires maximally, the first part of the inspired gas will move from the conducting airways into the apices. At this time, the apices fill only partially. Gas will then start to fill the bases. Toward the end of inspiration, both bases and apices fill. The lung fills in this manner due to transpulmonary pressure differences between apices and bases. An individual in the standing position has a higher transpulmonary pressure in the apices than in the bases. The lower transpulmonary pressure in the bases is essentially a result of lung position and gravity. Thus the alveoli in the apices are considered slow alveoli: they fill first but empty last; the alveoli in the bases are considered fast alveoli: they fill last but empty first. (For further explanation, see Chap. 4.)

5. In the single-breath nitrogen washout study, the patient breathes 100% oxygen from RV level to TLC, then slowly exhales to RV level.

   a. The initial part of the inspiration will go to the apices. This gas will contain a high nitrogen concentration because the volume will be primarily from the conducting airways, which contains 80% nitrogen.

   b. The next volume of gas will move to the bases. This volume will contain nitrogen, but to a lesser extent than the gas that originally moved to the apices.

   c. Finally, the bases and apices will fill to capacity with 100% oxygen.

   d. At maximal inspiration the nitrogen concentration in the apices is much greater than in the bases.

   e. As the patient slowly exhales, gas leaves the area of the lung where compliance is least, i.e., the bases. The bases will empty until the peripheral bronchioles start to collapse. The volume of gas left in the airways at onset of collapsing is referred to as the closing volume.

  f. As the patient continues to exhale, gas starts to leave the apices where the nitrogen concentration is much higher.

6. Graphically plotting the nitrogen concentration against the volume exhaled, a graph similar to that in Figure 17–2 results. This graph depicts the four phases of the single-breath nitrogen washout curve.

  a. Phase 1: The nitrogen concentration is zero, indicating that only gas from the conducting airways is being exhaled.

  b. Phase 2: The steep increase in nitrogen concentration indicates that the gas being exhaled is mixed bronchial and alveolar air.

  c. Phase 3: A very slow increase is evident, indicating that mostly alveolar air is being exhaled.

  d. Phase 4: At closing volume, gas is being exhaled primarily from the apices.

7. Normally the closing volume is expressed as a percentage of the VC.

  a. In young, healthy adults, closing volume is equal to about 10% of VC.

  b. This percentage increases normally with age. An individual aged 60 years or older may have a normal closing volume of 40%.

  c. Increases in closing volume appear to be one of the earliest indications of small airway obstruction.

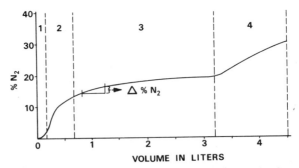

Fig 17–2.—Single-breath nitrogen washout curve shows the four phases associated with the study. Phase 4 is the volume referred to as the closing volume. Δ %N$_2$ is the percent change in nitrogen concentration between the first 750 ml and 1,250 ml of exhaled gas.

8. Closing capacity is a term used to express the percentage of the TLC that the closing volume plus the RV represents. Normally in young, healthy adults this is equal to about 30%.
9. Delta %nitrogen ($\Delta\%N_2$) is an expression used to indicate the change in nitrogen concentration between the first 750 ml and 1,250 ml exhaled.
   a. In normal, healthy adults it is equal to 1.5% or less.
   b. As the $\Delta\%N_2$ increases, it indicates uneven distribution of ventilation.

II. Flow Rate Studies
   A. Forced vital capacity (FVC)
      1. The following flow rate determinations may be calculated from an FVC curve.
         a. The percentage of the vital capacity that is expired in 1 second ($FEV_1\%$) (Fig 17–3)
            (1) The forced expired volume in 1 second (FEV_1) is divided by the FVC:

$$FEV_1\% = \frac{FEV_1}{FVC} \times 100 \qquad (10)$$

            (2) Normally the $FEV_1\%$ is equal to at least 75% of the FVC.
            (3) Decreased values basically indicate obstruction of larger airways.

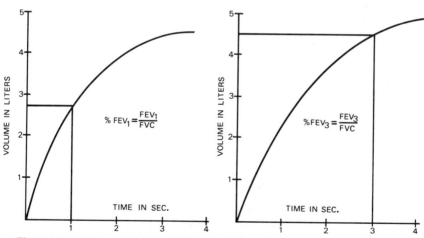

Fig 17–3.—Determination of $FEV_1\%$ and $FEV_3\%$ (see text).

b. The percentage of VC that is expired in 3 seconds ($FEV_3\%$) (see Fig 17–3)

    (1) The forced expired volume in 3 seconds (FEV_3) is divided by the FVC:

$$FEV_3\% = \frac{FEV_3}{FVC} \times 100 \qquad (11)$$

    (2) Normally the $FEV_3\%$ is equal to at least 97% of FVC.

    (3) Decreased values basically indicate obstruction of smaller airways.

c. Forced expiratory flow (FEF) determined between the first 200 ml and 1,200 ml of exhaled volume ($FEF_{200-1,200}$) (Fig 17–4)

    (1) The slope of the line between the first 200 ml and 1,200 ml of exhaled volume is determined and reported as a flow:

$$\text{Slope in L/sec} = \frac{1\text{ L}}{\text{time}} \qquad (12)$$

    (2) The flow in L/sec is then converted to L/min

$$(\text{L/sec})(60\text{ sec/min}) = \text{L/min} \qquad (13)$$

    (3) Since the graph is determined at room temperature (ATPS), the flow must be corrected to body temperature (BTPS).

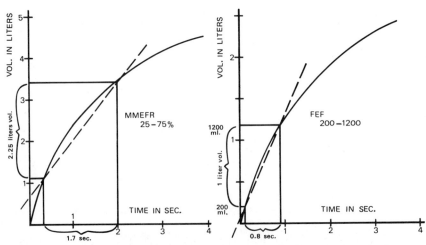

Fig 17–4.—Determination of $MMEFR_{25\%-75\%}$ and $FEF_{200-1,200}$ (see text).

(4) Normally the $FEF_{200-1,200}$ for a young, healthy adult male is about 350–400 L/min.

(5) Decreased values basically indicate obstruction of larger airways.

    d. Maximum midexpiratory flow rate ($MMEFR_{25\%-75\%}$) (see Fig 17–4)

(1) The slope of a line between the first 25% and 75% of exhaled volume is determined and reported as a flow:

$$\text{Slope in L/sec} = \frac{\text{volume}}{\text{time}} \qquad (14)$$

(2) The flow in L/sec is then converted to L/min (see Eq. 13).

(3) Since the graph is determined at ATPS, the flow must be converted to BTPS.

(4) Normally the $MMEFR_{25\%-75\%}$ for a young, healthy adult male is 250–300 L/min.

(5) Decreased values basically indicate obstruction of smaller airways.

B. Maximum voluntary ventilation (MVV) or maximum breathing capacity (MBC)

1. This study is used to determine the maximum volume of gas that a patient can ventilate in a minute.

2. The patient is directed to breathe as rapidly and as deeply as possible for 10–15 seconds.

3. The total volume inspired or expired during the stated period is determined.

4. This volume is converted to the volume per minute. For example, if the patient breathed 30 L in 10 seconds, then:

$$\frac{30 \text{ L}}{10 \text{ seconds}} = \frac{x}{60 \text{ seconds}} \qquad (15)$$

$$x = 180 \text{ L}$$

5. Normal MVV for young healthy adult males is 150–200 L/min.

6. Decreased values basically indicate increased airway resistance or obstruction, decreased lung or thoracic compliance, or weakness of ventilatory muscles.

C. Peak expiratory flow rate

1. Peak expiratory flow normally occurs during the early part of exhalation.

2. Peak flows normally are equal to 400–600 L/min for young, healthy males and 300–500 L/min for young, healthy females.

3. Decreased peak flows indicate larger airway obstruction.
  D. *It is extremely important to remember that all volumes determined must be converted to body temperature and that flow studies are totally patient effort dependent. In order to ensure accuracy, results must be reproducible.*
III. Normal Values
  A. Normal values for all studies discussed are based on the averages of many healthy individuals of a particular sex, age, and height.
  B. Tables are available that give normal values for all tests for both sexes in all age and height categories.
  C. Determined values are considered normal unless they are 20% greater or less than predicted values.
IV. Flow-Volume Loops
  A. A flow-volume loop is the measurement of inspiratory and expiratory flows and volumes.
  B. The test is performed by having the patient maximally inspire, followed by a single forced exhaled vital capacity (FEVC) and forced inspired vital capacity (FIVC loop).
  C. The following data can be determined from a flow-volume loop if a TV loop is superimposed on a VC loop (Fig 17–5).
    1. VC
    2. TV
    3. IRV
    4. ERV
    5. IC
    6. Peak inspiratory and expiratory flows
    7. Inspiratory flows at 25%, 50%, and 75% of VC
    8. Expiratory flows at 25%, 50%, and 75% of VC
  D. The major advantage of flow-volume loops is that they give a quick visual impression of the general disease category (Fig 17–6).
V. Diffusion Studies
  A. Diffusion studies are used to determine how rapidly gases can move across the alveolar-capillary membrane.
  B. Oxygen and carbon monoxide (CO) are used because of their strong affinity for hemoglobin and poor solubility coefficients.
  C. Single-breath method: The patient maximally inhales a mixture of gases containing 0.1%–0.3% CO, helium, and air, followed by breath-holding for 10 seconds.
  D. The pulmonary diffusing capacity for CO (DCO) is equal to:

$$\frac{\text{ml CO transferred/minute}}{\text{mean alveolar CO (mm Hg)} - \text{mean capillary CO (mm Hg)}} \quad (16)$$

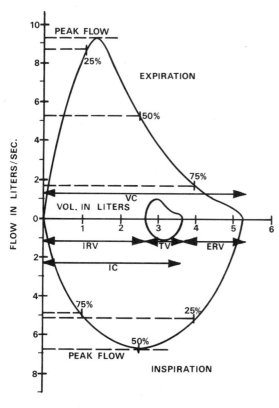

Fig 17–5.—Normal flow-volume loop with superimposed tidal volume (TV) loop. All normal spirometry values plus peak inspiratory and expiratory flows along with flow at 25%, 50%, and 75% of inspiration and expiration may be determined.

    E. Normal resting Dco for the average young adult male is 25 ml/min/mm Hg CO.

    F. The Do_2 may be computed by multiplying the Dco by 1.23:

$$Do_2 = Dco\ (1.23) \qquad (17)$$

VI. Bronchial Provocation Tests

    A. These tests are used to assess the responsiveness of bronchial airways and lung parenchyma to inhaled aerosols and fumes.

    B. Metacholine or histamine inhalation tests

        1. Baseline FEV_1 measurements are made prior to the administration of the drug and following each dose administered.

        2. An aerosol of either drug is inhaled by the patient intermittently or on a continuous basis.

        3. Dosages begin at 0.03 mg/ml of aerosol and increase by doubling to a maximum dose of at least 20 mg/ml.

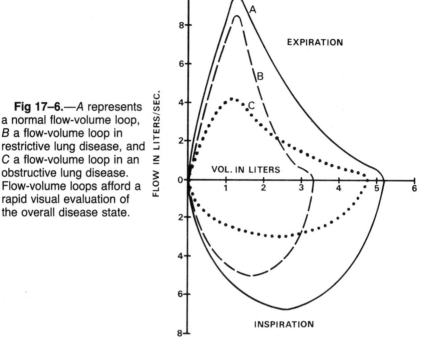

Fig 17–6.—*A* represents a normal flow-volume loop, *B* a flow-volume loop in restrictive lung disease, and *C* a flow-volume loop in an obstructive lung disease. Flow-volume loops afford a rapid visual evaluation of the overall disease state.

4. Increasing dosages are administered and the response is evaluated by FEV_1 determinations until the FEV_1 falls by at least 20% of baseline.

5. The provocation concentration of the drug producing the 20% or greater decrease in FEV_1 is referred to as the PC_{20}.
   a. A PC_{20} value of more than 20 mg/ml is considered asymptomatic for diagnosing asthma.
   b. A PC_{20} between 2 and 20 mg/ml generally corresponds to mild, episodic symptoms of asthma.
   c. Values less than 2 mg/ml are consistent with daily symptomatology and may require bronchodilator therapy.

6. Uses of the test:
   a. To substantiate the diagnosis of asthma in doubtful cases.
   b. To provide an indication of severity and determine treatment requirements.
   c. To document an inducing effect in occupational asthma and subsequent treatment.

7. Normally requires physician supervision.

C. Allergen inhalation tests
  1. Used to determine specific allergic responses.
  2. Methodology similar to metacholine/histamine challenge.
  3. Normally requires physician supervision during testing.
D. Occupational type exposure tests
  1. Used to determine specific occupational sensitivities.
  2. Methodology similar to metacholine/histamine challenge.
  3. Physician supervision required.

BIBLIOGRAPHY

Ayers L.N., Whipp B.J., Ziment I.: *A Guide to the Interpretation of Pulmonary Function Tests.* New York, Roerig, Division of Pfizer Pharmaceuticals, New York Projects in Health, Inc., 1974.

Altose M.D.: The physiological basis of pulmonary function testing. *Clin. Symp.* 3:3–10, 1973.

Altounyan R.E.C.: Variation of drug action on airway obstruction in man. *Thorax* 19:406–415, 1961.

Baldwin E. de F., Cournand A., Richards D.W. Jr.: Pulmonary insufficiency: I. Physiological classification, clinical methods of analysis, standard values in normal subjects. *J. Med.* 27:243–278, 1948.

Barnhard H.J., Pierce J.A., Joyce J.W., et al.: Roentgenographic determination of total lung capacity. *Am. J. Med.* 28:51–60, 1960.

Bates D.V., Macklem P.T., Christie R.V.: *Respiratory Function in Disease.* Philadelphia, W.B. Saunders Co., 1971.

Burrows B., Kasih J.E., Niden A.H., et al.: Clinical usefulness of the single breath pulmonary diffusing capacity test. *Am. Rev. Respir. Dis.* 84:789, 1961.

Cherniack R.N.: *Pulmonary Function Testing.* Philadelphia, W.B. Saunders Co., 1977.

Clausen J.L.: *Pulmonary Function Testing Guidelines and Controversies: Equipment, Methods, and Normal Values.* New York, Academic Press Inc., 1982.

Cockcroft D.W., Killian D.N., Mellon J.J.A., et al.: Bronchial reactivity to inhaled histamine: A method and clinical survey. *Clin. Allergy* 7:235–243, 1977.

Comroe J.H., et al.: *The Lung: Clinical Physiology and Pulmonary Function Tests,* ed. 2. Chicago, Year Book Medical Publishers, Inc., 1962.

Cotes J.E.: *Assessment of Mechanical Attributes in Lung Function; Assessment and Application in Medicine,* ed. 2. Oxford, Blackwell Scientific Publications, 1968.

Dubois A.B., Botehlo S.Y., Bedell G.N., et al.: A rapid plethysmographic method for measuring thoracic gas volume: A comparison with a nitrogen washout method for measuring functional residual capacity in normal subjects. *J. Clin. Invest.* 34:322–326, 1955.

Ferris B.G.: Epidemiology standardization project: Recommended standardized procedure for pulmonary function testing. *Am. Rev. Respir. Dis.* 118:1, 1978.

Forster R.E.: Exchange of gases between alveolar air and pulmonary capillary blood: Pulmonary diffusing capacity. *Physiol. Rev.* 37:391, 1957.

Gardner R.M.: ATS statement: Snowbird workshop on standardization of spirometry. *Am. Rev. Respir. Dis.* 119:831–838, 1979.

Hepper G.G.N., Fowler W.S., Helmholz H.R. Jr.: Relationship of height to lung volume in healthy men. *Dis. Chest* 37:314–320, 1960.

Hyatt R.E., et al.: The flow volume curve. *Am. Rev. Respir. Dis.* 107:191, 1973.

Juniper R.F., Frith P.A., Hargreave F.E.: Airway responsiveness to histamine and metacholine: Relationship to minimum treatment to control symptoms of asthma. *Thorax* 36:575–579, 1981.

Kanner R.E., Morris A.H.: *Clinical Pulmonary Function Testing.* Salt Lake City, Intermountain Thoracic Society, 1975.

Knudson R.J., Slatin R.C., Lebowitz M.D.: The maximal expiratory flow-volume curve: Normal standards, variability, and effects of age. *Am. Rev. Respir. Dis.* 113:587–600, 1976.

Kary R.C., Callahan R., Boren H.G., et al.: The Veterans Administration-Army cooperative study of pulmonary function: I. Clinical spirometry in normal men. *Am. J. Med.* 30:243–258, 1961.

Lapp N.L., Amandus H.E., Hall R.: Lung volumes and flow rates in black and white subjects. *Thorax* 29:185–188, 1974.

McCarthy D.S., Spencer R., Greene R., et al.: Measurement of closing volume as a simple and sensitive test for early detection of small airway disease. *Am. J. Med.* 52:747, 1972.

Needham C.D., Rogar M.D., McDonald J.: Normal standards for lung volumes, intrapulmonary gas mixing, and maximum breathing capacity. *Thorax* 9:313, 1954.

Nicklaus T.M., Watanabe S., Mitchell M.M., et al.: Roentgenographic, physiologic and structural estimations of the total lung capacity in normal and emphysematous subjects. *Am. J. Med.* 42:547–553, 1967.

Ogilvie C.M.: A standardized breath holding technique for the clinical measurement of the diffusing capacity of the lung for carbon monoxide. *J. Clin. Invest.* 36:1, 1957.

Otis A.B.: Mechanical factors in distribution of pulmonary ventilation. *J. Appl. Physiol.* 8:427, 1956.

Pepys J., Hutchcroft B.J.: Bronchial provocation test in etiologic diagnosis and analysis of asthma. *Am. Rev. Respir. Dis.* 112:828–859, 1975.

Ruppel G.: *Manual of Pulmonary Function Testing,* ed. 3. St. Louis, C.V. Mosby Co., 1982.

Ryan G., Dolovich M.B., Roberts R.S.: Standardization of inhalation provocation tests: Two techniques of aerosol generation and inhalation compared. *Am. Rev. Respir. Dis.* 123:195–199, 1981.

Salome C.M., Schoeffel R.E., Waolcock A.J.: Comparison of bronchial reactivity to histamine and metacholine in asthmatics. *Clin. Allergy* 10:541–546, 1980.

Seltzer C., Siegelaub A.B., Freidman G.D.: Differences in pulmonary function related to smoking habits and race. *Am. Rev. Respir. Dis.* 110:598–608, 1974.

Shapiro B.A., Harrison R.A., Walton J.R.: *Clinical Application of Blood Gases,* ed. 2. Chicago, Year Book Medical Publishers, Inc., 1977.

Spearman C.B., Sheldon R.L., Egan D.F.: *Egan's Fundamentals of Respiratory Therapy,* ed. 4. St. Louis, C.V. Mosby Co., 1982.

Suratt P.M., Hooe D.M., Owens D.A., et al.: Effect of maximal versus submaximal effort on spirometric values. *Respiration* 42:233–236, 1981.

Tattersfield A.E.: Measurement of bronchial reactivity: A question of interpretation. *Thorax* 26:561–565, 1981.

Turner J.M., Mead J., Wohl M.E.: Elasticity of human lungs in relation to age. *J. Appl. Physiol.* 25:644–671, 1968.

West J.B.: *Pulmonary Pathophysiology: The Essentials*. Baltimore, Williams & Wilkins Co., 1977.

West J.B.: *Respiratory Physiology: The Essentials*. Baltimore, Williams & Wilkins Co., 1974.

Young J.A., Crocker D.: *Principles and Practice of Respiratory Therapy*, ed. 2. Chicago, Year Book Medical Publishers, Inc., 1976.

18 / Clinical Assessment of the Cardiopulmonary System

I. Physical Assessment of the Chest
   A. Chest assessment includes the following, sequentially performed as listed:
      1. Inspection
      2. Palpatation
      3. Percussion
      4. Auscultation
   B. Inspection is the observation of the patient's chest configuration and pattern of breathing. During inspection the following should be evaluated:
      1. Position
         a. Is the patient sitting comfortably or does he or she require support in order to ventilate?
         b. The position assumed provides information about the patient's use of accessory muscles of ventilation or presence of pain.
      2. Chest configuration
         a. Anteroposterior to lateral diameter is normally in a 1:2 ratio. If the patient is barrel-chested, the ratio approaches 1:1, a common finding in patients with chronic obstructive pulmonary disease.
         b. Bony deformities of the thorax
            (1) Kyphosis—posterior curvature of the thoracic vertebral column.
            (2) Scoliosis—lateral curvature of the spinal column.
            (3) Kyphoscoliosis—combination of kyphosis and scoliosis
            (4) Pectus carinatum—protrusion of the sternum anteriorly
            (5) Pectus excavatum—depression of the sternum
            (6) Any thoracic deformity may result in restriction of ventilation.
      3. Ventilatory pattern
         a. Sequence of lung expansion
            (1) Abdominal protrusion
            (2) Lateral costal expansion

   (3) Upper chest expansion

   (4) Abnormal sequencing may be a result of underlying lung disease or an increase in cardiopulmonary stress.

  b. Uniform bilateral chest expansion

   (1) The chest cage should move equally bilaterally.

   (2) Splinting of an area of the chest may be a result of:

    (a) Pain

    (b) Pneumonia

    (c) Atelectasis

    (d) Pleural effusion

    (e) Pneumothorax

  c. Use of accessory muscles of ventilation

   (1) Normal inspiration requires only contraction of the diaphragm and external intercostals.

   (2) Exhalation is passive.

   (3) Use of accessory muscles is an indication of increased work of breathing (see section II).

  d. Ventilatory rate

   (1) Normal ventilatory rate in the adult is 12–16/min.

   (2) Acute cardiopulmonary stress normally results in an increased ventilatory rate.

   (3) Patients with chronic obstructive lung disease may have a decreased ventilatory rate, while patients with chronic restrictive lung disease may have an increased ventilatory rate.

   (4) Pursed lipped breathing is indicative of chronic airway obstruction.

   (5) Inspiratory to expiratory ratios should be about 1:2.

   (6) Presence of audible wheezes, cackles, or rhonchi is indicative of secretions or bronchospasm.

  e. Cough

   (1) Present without request

   (2) Forceful or weak

   (3) Productive or nonproductive

C. Palpation is the touching of the chest to evaluate movement and underlying lung function:

 1. Symmetric movement of the thoracic cage

 2. Tone of ventilatory muscles

 3. Presence of consolidation, pneumothorax, atelectasis, or pleural effusion. These may cause a shift in the mediastinum. Palpation of the trachea at the suprasternal notch identifies shifting.

4. Fremitus—the vibration produced over the thoracic cage by the conduction of sound waves.
   a. Evaluation of fremitus is performed bilaterally to compare the tactile vibrations between sides of the chest.
   b. Normally fremitus is equal throughout all lung fields. However, it may be increased over the apex of the right lung.
   c. Fremitus is increased if lung density is increased (pneumonia, consolidation).
   d. Fremitus is decreased if atelectasis from obstruction is present or if fluid or air accumulates in the pleural space.
5. Subcutaneous emphysema. If it is present an air leak has allowed gas to enter the tissue.
D. Percussion is the production of audible and tactile vibrations over the chest by tapping the chest wall (Fig 18–1).
   1. If lung tissue is normal, percussion produces a moderately low-pitched sound.
   2. The presence of increased air in the thoracic cavity produces a lower-pitched, more muffled drumlike sound, frequently referred to as hyperresonance.

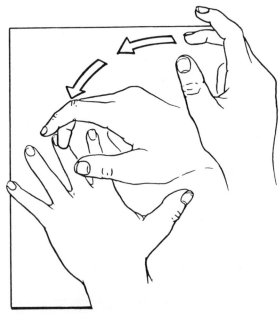

Fig 18–1.—Chest percussion technique. (From DesJardins T.: *Clinical Manifestations of Respiratory Diseases.* Chicago, Year Book Medical Publishers, Inc., 1984. Reproduced by permission.)

      3. Decreased air in the thoracic cavity, consolidation, atelectasis, or a pleural effusion causes the percussion note to be higher pitched but dull or flat.

  E. Auscultation is the evaluation of breath sounds with a stethoscope.

    1. Normal breath sounds

      a. Over the trachea, the sound is loud with a tubular quality, referred to as bronchial or tracheal breath sounds.

      b. Auscultation of the parenchyma reveals a soft muffled sound referred to as vesicular breath sounds. These are usually heard during inspiration but only minimally during exhalation.

      c. The sound heard over the airways is termed bronchovesicular. It is softer than bronchial breath sounds and lower in pitch, being heard during both inspiration and expiration.

    2. Adventitious or abnormal breath sounds

      a. *Crackles* (rales)—a discontinous sound (less than 20 msec) that is perceived as a wet, crackling, bubbling sound associated with gas moving through liquid.

      b. *Rhonchi*—a continuous sound (longer than 25 msec) that is low in pitch and normally indicative of secretions in large airways. In patients who can successfully mobilize their own secretions, rhonchi clear with coughing.

      c. *Wheezes*—a continuous sound (longer than 25 msec) that is high pitched and normally indicative of bronchospasm or mucosal edema in medium to larger airways. Wheezes do not clear with coughing.

II. Work of Breathing

  A. During normal breathing the muscles of ventilation consume 5%–10% of the total oxygen consumed to perform the work of breathing.

  B. The effort required to perform the work of breathing is dependent on the following:

    1. Airway resistance

    2. Compliance

    3. Respiratory rate

    4. Tidal volume

    5. Use of accessory muscles

    6. Ventilatory pattern

  C. Normally the ventilatory pattern a patient assumes is that which requires the least work.

    1. Figure 18–2, A relates the components of the work of breathing to the respiratory rate and tidal volume.

2. Resistance work refers to the amount of work necessary to overcome nonelastic resistance to ventilation. If nonelastic resistance were the only force opposing ventilation, the ideal ventilatory pattern would be a slow rate and a large tidal volume.
3. Elastic work refers to the amount of work necessary to overcome elastic resistance. If elastic resistance were the only force opposing ventilation, a rapid ventilatory rate with a small tidal volume would be ideal.
4. Total work refers to actual work expended with varying ventilatory rates and tidal volumes. Note the ideal rate is about 12–16 per minute with an ideal tidal volume of about 350–550 ml.
5. Figure 18–2, B illustrates the effect an increase in elastic work has on ventilatory pattern.
   a. Since elastic resistance to ventilation has increased, the least amount of work is accomplished at a high ventilatory rate and a small tidal volume.
   b. With most acute pulmonary diseases there is an increase in elastic work; therefore ventilatory rates increase and tidal volumes decrease.
   c. If resistance work were increased the total work curve would shift to the left.

III. Ventilatory Reserve
   A. The ability of the organism to respond to increased levels of cardiopulmonary stress.
   B. During normal breathing, the efficiency of the ventilatory muscles is poor. About 90% of the oxygen consumed to perform the work of breathing is lost as heat.
   C. The efficiency of the ventilatory muscles is further reduced with chronic pulmonary disease and with an increased minute ventilation.
   D. Figure 18–3, A depicts the relationship between minute volume and percentage of oxygen consumed for breathing in patients without chronic pulmonary disease *(solid line)* and patients with chronic pulmonary disease *(dotted line)*.
      1. The percentage of oxygen consumed for breathing markedly increases as minute volume increases.

Fig 18–2.—A is a graphic representation of total work of breathing when minute ventilation is unchanged but ventilatory pattern (tidal volume and frequency) is varied. Note that for any minute ventilation there is a ventilatory pattern that

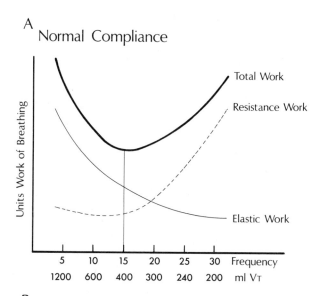

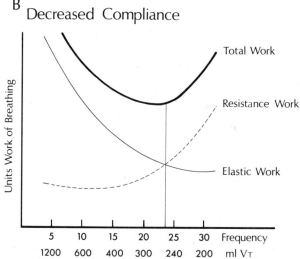

requires minimal work. Of course, total work is the summation of resistance work (nonelastic resistance) and elastic work (elastic resistance). If elastic work is increased, as in **B,** the pattern of ventilation at which the minute volume can be achieved with minimal work is dramatically altered. This is a schematic representation of the principle that work of breathing is a major factor determining ventilatory pattern (see text). (From Shapiro B.A., Harrison R.A., Kacmarek R.M., et al.: *Clinical Application of Respiratory Care,* ed. 3. Chicago, Year Book Medical Publishers, Inc., 1985. Reproduced by permission.)

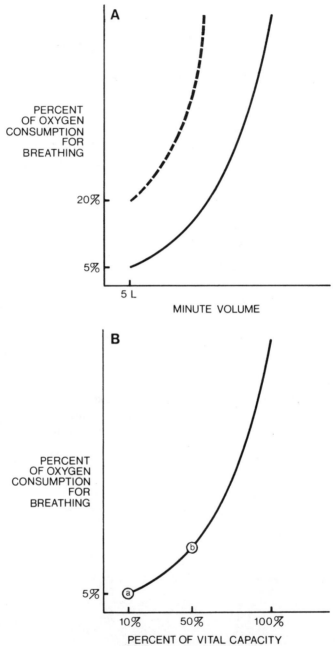

Fig 18–3.—See legend on facing page.

2. In patients with chronic pulmonary disease the percentage of oxygen consumed for breathing at basal level is already increased (20%). With increased minute volume there is a tremendous increase in oxygen consumption. These patients have lower reserves than patients without chronic pulmonary disease.

E. Figure 18–3, B illustrates the relationship between percentage of oxygen consumed for breathing and the percentage of the vital capacity that is the tidal volume.

1. As the tidal volume becomes a greater percentage of the vital capacity, the amount of oxygen consumed for breathing increases.

2. When the tidal volume is 50% of the vital capacity, limited ventilatory reserves exist and the likelihood of sustained spontaneous ventilation is questionable.

IV. Vital Capacity/Negative Inspiratory Force

A. A normal vital capacity is about 70–90 ml/kg.

B. Vital capacities are frequently used as an estimate of the patient's ventilatory reserve.

C. If the vital capacity is above 15 ml/kg of ideal body weight, it is assumed that the individual has the capability to respond to increased levels of cardiopulmonary stress.

D. However, if the vital capacity is less than 10 ml/kg, prolonged sustained spontaneous ventilation is questionable. This individual has virtually no reserves.

E. At vital capacities between 10 and 15 ml/kg, reserves are marginal and appropriate monitoring should be instituted.

F. Negative inspiratory force (NIF) is also a parameter used to assess ventilatory reserves.

G. If the NIF is more negative than -20 to -25 cm H_2O in a 20-second period the individual has adequate ventilatory reserves and sustained spontaneous ventilation is highly probable.

H. However, if the NIF is more positive than -20 cm H_2O in a 20-second period, sustained spontaneous ventilation is questionable.

I. An NIF of -20 to -25 cm H_2O correlates well with a vital capacity of 15 ml/kg of ideal body weight.

←**Fig 18–3.—A,** the work of breathing in relation to vital capacity (see text). In **B,** point *a* represents a VT of 500 ml with a VC of 5 L; point *b* represents a VT of 500 ml with a VC of 1 L. (From Shapiro B.A., Harrison R.A., Walton J.R.: *Clinical Application of Blood Gases,* ed. 3. Chicago, Year Book Medical Publishers, 1982. Reproduced by permission.)

J. The use of vital capacity or NIF as an estimate of ventilatory reserves is least accurate in patients with chronic pulmonary disease.
V. Assessment of Peripheral Perfusion
  A. Adequacy of peripheral perfusion can be estimated by:
    1. Sensorium
    2. Urinary output
    3. Capillary refill
    4. Skin turgor
    5. Cyanosis
    6. Peripheral pulses
    7. Skin temperature
  B. Sensorium
    1. Confusion, agitation, and disorientation are all signs of cerebral hypoxia that can be caused by decreased oxygen carriage or decreased cerebral perfusion.
    2. Somnolence and drowsiness are signs of increased arterial P_{CO_2} levels.
  C. Urinary output
    1. Normal urinary output is about 40–60 ml/hour.
    2. Decreased urinary output is frequently a sign of decreased peripheral perfusion.
  D. Capillary refill decreases as peripheral perfusion decreases.
  E. Skin turgor also decreases as peripheral perfusion decreases.
  F. Cyanosis
    1. Cyanosis is a blueish discoloration of nail beds, lips, mucous membranes and skin.
    2. Cyanosis is present if 5 gm % of hemoglobin is reduced.
    3. Decreased peripheral perfusion may cause sufficient pooling of blood also allowing cyanosis to be noticed.
    4. However, cyanosis is normally noted when oxygen content is decreased in arterial blood.
    5. Anemic patients are least likely to demonstrate cyanosis, while polycythemic patients are most likely.
  G. Thready, faint, or distant peripheral pulses are noted as peripheral perfusion decreases.

BIBLIOGRAPHY

Cherniack R.M., Cherniack L.: *Respiration in Health and Disease*, ed. 3. Philadelphia, W.B. Saunders Co., 1983.
George R.B., Light R.W., Matthay R.A.: *Chest Medicine*. New York, Churchill Livingstone, 1983.
Pare J.A.P., Fraser R.G.: *Synopsis of Diseases of the Chest*. Philadelphia, W.B. Saunders Co., 1983.

Parot S., Miara B., Milic-Emili J., et al.: Hypoxemia, hypercarbia, and breathing pattern in patients with chronic obstructive pulmonary disease. *Am. Rev. Respir. Dis.* 126:882–886, 1982.

Petty T.L.: *Intensive and Rehabilitative Respiratory Care,* ed. 3. Philadelphia, Lea & Febiger, 1982.

Rarey K.P., Youtsey J.W.: *Respiratory Patient Care.* Englewood Cliffs, N.J., Prentice-Hall, Inc., 1981.

Shapiro B.A., Harrison R.A., Kacmarek R.M., et al.: *Clinical Application of Respiratory Care,* ed. 3. Chicago, Year Book Medical Publishers, Inc., 1985.

Tisi G.M.: *Pulmonary Physiology in Clinical Medicine,* ed. 2. Baltimore, Williams & Wilkins Co., 1983.

Whitcomb M.E.: *The Lung: Normal and Diseased.* St. Louis, C.V. Mosby Co., 1982.

19 / Obstructive Pulmonary Diseases

I. General Comments
  A. The acronym COPD is applied to patients with long-term chronic obstructive pulmonary disease, who show persistent airway obstruction normally manifested by decreased expiratory flow rates.
  B. Prevalence
    1. From 1960 to 1970, the increase in deaths from emphysema was about 150%.
    2. In 1981, 60,000 deaths were attributed to emphysema.
    3. There are about 7.5 million Americans with chronic bronchitis, 2.1 million with emphysema, and 6.4 million with asthma.
    4. There seems to be a much greater incidence of COPD in men than in women.
    5. On autopsy some degree of emphysema appears in a large percentage of the population.
    6. Emphysema is the second leading cause of disability, arteriosclerotic heart disease being first.
  C. General causes of COPD
    1. Smoking
      a. Inhibits ciliary function.
      b. Causes bronchospasm.
      c. Affects macrophage activity.
      d. Affects alveolar septal wall and capillary endothelium.
    2. Air pollutants, both particulate and gaseous.
    3. Occupational exposure to dusts and fumes.
    4. Infection, which may cause decreased pulmonary clearance, resulting in an increased incidence of recurrent infection.
    5. Heredity
      a. $Alpha_1$ antitrypsin deficiency, which results in emphysematous changes measurable in the third and fourth decades (see section III).
      b. Cystic fibrosis (see Chap. 22).
      c. Asthma (see section VII).
    6. Allergies (e.g., chronic asthma), which can lead to permanent pulmonary changes.

300

7. Aging, which causes natural degenerative changes in the respiratory tract resembling emphysematous changes.

D. Physical appearance of patient
  1. *Barrel-chested* as a result of increased air trapping (anteroposterior diameter increased).
     a. Increase in anteroposterior diameter
     b. Increase proportional to increase in FRC
  2. Clubbing (pulmonary hypertrophic osteopathy), bulbous enlargement of terminal portion of the digits altering the angle of the nailbed, is frequently exhibited.
  3. Cyanosis, a result of hypoxemia coupled with secondary polycythemia.
  4. Decreased and adventitious breath sounds.
  5. Often a hyperresonant chest.
  6. Ventilatory pattern
     a. Increased use of accessory muscles
     b. Paradoxical movement of the abdomen frequently observed
     c. Prolonged expiratory time
     d. Active exhalation
     e. Pursed-lip breathing
  7. Malnourished, secondary to loss of appetite (anorexia)
  8. Anxious
  9. General muscle atrophy
  10. May be edematous with jugular vein distention if congestive heart failure present

E. General pulmonary function changes (Table 19–1)
  1. Frequently an increase in pulmonary compliance.
  2. Increased airway resistance as a result of mucosal edema and bronchiolar wall weakening.

TABLE 19–1.—COMPARISON OF
PULMONARY FUNCTION STUDY RESULTS IN
PATIENTS WITH OBSTRUCTIVE AND
RESTRICTIVE PULMONARY DISEASES

PFT STUDY	OBSTRUCTIVE	RESTRICTIVE
TLC	↔ or ↑	↓
VC	↔ or ↓	↓
FRC	↑	↔ or ↓
RV	↑	↔ or ↓
RV/TLC	↑	↔
FEV$_1$%	↓	↔
MMEFR$_{25-75}$	↓	↔ or ↓

3. Prolonged expiratory times when #1 and #2 are present.
4. Increased FRC.
5. Increased RV.
6. Increased RV/TLC ratio.
7. Increased or normal TLC.
8. Decreased or normal VC.
9. Decreased or normal IC and IRV.
10. Increased ERV.
11. Decreased expiratory flow studies: $FEV_1\%$, $FEV_3\%$, $MMEFR_{25\%-75\%}$, $FEF_{200-1,200}$, and MVV may all be reduced.

F. General x-ray findings
1. Increased anteroposterior diameter
2. Flattened hemidiaphragms
3. Hyperinflation
4. Pulmonary vascular engorgement with increased vascular markings
5. Increased retrosternal airspace
6. Normal or increased heart shadow
7. Normal or thin elongated mediastinum
8. Hypertranslucency
9. Possible peripheral bullae or blebs
10. In severe cases or end-stage disease, right ventricular hypertrophy also may be seen.

G. Dyspnea
1. In all patients dyspnea on exertion is one of the first noticeable symptoms.
2. As the disease process progresses, dyspnea becomes apparent even at rest.
3. Dyspnea normally increases as the work of breathing progressively increases.
4. The percentage of the oxygen consumed to ventilate is increased, severely limiting the patient's level of physical exertion.

H. Arterial blood gases of COPD patients with CO_2 retention
1. Patients may experience a regular, predictable pattern of blood gas changes as the disease progresses.
2. Because of the pathophysiology of COPD, ventilation/perfusion inequalities develop.
3. Mismatching of ventilation and blood flow results in hypoxemia. It should be noted that hypoxemia normally is the first measured blood gas abnormality (see Chap. 12).

4. Hypoxemia becomes increasingly worse as the disease process progresses, resulting in stimulation of peripheral chemoreceptors.

5. Stimulation of peripheral chemoreceptors results in hyperventilation—the body's attempt to correct hypoxemia.

6. Hyperventilation persists and the kidneys compensate for the acid-base imbalance. Blood gas analysis reveals compensated respiratory alkalosis (chronic alveolar hyperventilation) with hypoxemia.

7. Hyperventilation continues until oxygen consumption by the patient's respiratory musculature exceeds the benefits received by hyperventilation.

8. The percentage of total oxygen consumption being used for ventilation becomes greatly increased because the efficiency of the respiratory system is greatly reduced by disease and increased accessory muscle use.

9. The body can no longer maintain the level of alveolar ventilation necessary to maintain adequate oxygen tensions without severely compromising oxygen delivery to other organs.

10. An inbred instinct in the survival of any organism in conservation of energy. Thus the body's instinctive response is to hypoventilate in an attempt to conserve energy.

11. This results in further progression of the hypoxemia.

12. The total oxygen reservoir may be decreased even further. This is counterbalanced to a degree by a reduction in oxygen consumption by the respiratory muscles, a decrease in the patient's overall level of activity, and secondary polycythemia.

13. Alveolar ventilation continues to decrease. This is evidenced by increasing CO_2 levels and further development of hypoxemia.

14. With time, the patient begins to retain CO_2. Blood gases at this time would reveal compensated respiratory acidosis (chronic ventilatory failure) with moderate to severe hypoxemia.

15. It is at the point where CO_2 starts to be retained that the patient's primary stimulus to breathe becomes oxygen. This abnormal primary stimulus to ventilation is known as the hypoxic drive.

16. If oxygen were administered in sufficient amounts, the hypoxic stimulus to breathe would be reduced, potentially to the point of apnea.

17. The disease continues to progress with increasing levels of CO_2 retention and more severe hypoxemia.
18. The disease process becomes end-stage and terminal. The patient's level of physical activity is severely limited and he is reduced to a pulmonary cripple.

I. Cor Pulmonale

1. Cor pulmonale denotes right ventricular hypertrophy secondary to abnormalities of lung structure and function. Congestive heart failure may or may not be present.
2. A frequent sequel to chronic bronchitis and cystic fibrosis.
3. Pathogenesis
   a. Developing pulmonary disease results in increasing hypoxemia, which causes constriction of the pulmonary capillary system.
   b. Constriction causes pulmonary hypertension. The decreased capillary bed seen with advancing pulmonary disease also contributes to development of pulmonary hypertension.
   c. Pulmonary hypertension causes the right side of the heart to work harder. With time, right ventricular hypertrophy develops.
   d. Pulmonary hypertension, if not controlled, precipitates the development of right ventricular failure in addition to cor pulmonale.
   e. This results in peripheral edema due to increased resistance to venous return and decreased right ventricular function.
   f. Failure of the right side of the heart is more frequently seen in association with pulmonary disease than is left-sided heart failure.

II. Management of COPD

A. The process is treatable to a certain extent but is not reversible.
B. Management revolves mainly around symptomatic treatment of the presenting problem.
   1. Relief of airway obstruction
      a. Mucosal edema: Sympathomimetics (alpha drugs), steroids and aerosol.
      b. Bronchospasm: Sympathomimetics (beta drugs).
      c. Secretions: Mobilization by aerosol therapy and chest physiotherapy.
   2. Prevention and treatment of bronchopulmonary infection by use of antibiotics and proper patient education.

3. Improvement of patient's exercise tolerance by general graded body toning and stamina-developing exercises.
4. Treatment of severe hypoxemia with oxygen therapy.
5. Maintenance of cardiovascular status by treatment of congestive heart failure.
6. Avoidance of exposure to all types of airway irritants.
7. Proper education and psychological and sociologic support.

III. Emphysema
   A. Characterized by enlargement of air spaces distal to terminal bronchioles, with loss of elastic fibers and destruction of alveolar septal wall.
   B. Etiology
      1. Smoking (high correlation with emphysema).
      2. High correlation with environmental conditions (e.g., air pollution).
      3. Occupational hazards, dust, fumes, and similar factors.
      4. Heredity
         a. Alpha$_1$ antitrypsin deficiency, a lack of the enzyme that metabolizes trypsin, a digestive enzyme.
         b. If the trypsin is not metabolized, it will cause destruction of normal pulmonary tissue.
   C. Types of emphysema
      1. Centrilobular
         a. Destructive changes primarily in the respiratory bronchioles.
         b. Much higher incidence in men.
         c. Primary lesions appear in upper lobes.
         d. A very high correlation with centrilobular emphysema and smoking; frequently a sequel to chronic bronchitis.
         e. Rare occurrence in nonsmokers.
      2. Panlobular
         a. Changes at alveolar level where destruction of septa predominates.
         b. Effects seemingly generalized in distribution.
         c. Seen with alpha$_1$ antitrypsin deficiency and the natural aging process.
      3. Bullous
         a. Destructive changes at the alveolar and respiratory bronchiolar level
         b. Prominent bleb and bullae formation
   D. Clinical manifestations
      1. Shortness of breath, developing very gradually

 2. Nonproductive cough
 3. Frequent respiratory infections
 4. Cyanosis
 5. Barrel-chested appearance
 6. Hyperresonant chest
 7. Polycythemia
 8. Use of accessory muscles
 9. Clubbing
 10. Anorexia
 11. Muscle atrophy
 12. Suprasternal retractions
E. Chest x-ray findings
 1. Flattened hemidiaphragms
 2. Hypertranslucency
 3. Increased retrosternal air space
 4. Attenuated peripheral pulmonary vasculature
 5. Small heart
 6. Elongated cardiac silhouette
F. Pulmonary function studies: As outlined in section I.
G. Management: As outlined in section II.
IV. Bronchitis
A. Acute bronchitis
 1. Acute inflammation of tracheobronchial tree with production of excessive mucus.
 2. Clinical manifestations
  a. Mucosal edema
  b. Increased sputum production
  c. Hacking paroxysms of cough
  d. Raw, burning substernal pain
 3. Causes
  a. Infectious: viral, bacterial, or fungal
  b. Allergic
  c. Chemical, smoke, irritant gases, and similar factors
 4. Treatment: Usually by administration of antibiotics, expectorants, aerosol therapy, and occasionally antitussives.
 5. Normally a self-limiting process without serious complications or residual effects.
B. Chronic bronchitis
 1. Chronic cough with excessive sputum production of unknown specific etiology for 3 months per year for 2 or more successive years.

2. Cause basically is frequent acute episodes of bronchitis, which may result from:
   a. Smoking (by far the leading cause)
   b. Air pollution
   c. Chronic infections
3. Clinical manifestations
   a. Onset normally insidious with patient rarely aware of its development.
   b. Steps in development
      (1) Smoker's cough, followed by a
      (2) Morning cough, leading to
      (3) Continual cough, especially during cold weather and exacerbations.
   c. Sputum
      (1) Normally a slow increase until there is continual abnormal production.
      (2) Sputum usually thick, gray, and mucoid until chronic infections develop, then turning mucopurulent.
4. Pathophysiology
   a. Mucosal glands
      (1) Size increases in relation to wall thickness; normally gland size is about one third of height of bronchial walls.
      (2) In chronic bronchitis, gland size is about two thirds of height of bronchial walls.
      (3) Increase in number of mucus-secreting glands.
   b. Submucosal gland hypertrophy.
   c. Increased population of goblet cells replacing ciliated columnar cells (epithelial metaplasia).
   d. Submucosal infiltration.
   e. Mucosal edema.
   f. Smooth muscle hypertrophy.
   g. All the above collectively result in:
      (1) Diminished airway lumen
      (2) Secretion accumulation
      (3) Submucosal infiltration
      (4) General increase in sputum production
      (5) Loss of ciliated cells
      (6) Sputum production in nonciliated airways
      (7) Impaired clearance mechanism
5. Chest x-ray findings

a. Early in the disease, x-ray changes are not significant, especially if the disease is associated only with larger airways.
b. If the disease has moved to the periphery, hyperinflation with a flattened hemidiaphragm may be noticed.
c. May show prominent peripheral pulmonary vasculature.
d. Enlarged cardiac shadow.
e. Pulmonary vascular engorgement.
f. X-ray usually is of little use in establishing diagnosis.
g. A positive patient history usually is the best diagnostic tool.

6. Pulmonary function studies
   a. In early stages, all pulmonary function studies may be normal, except for slight decreases in expiratory flow rates.
   b. As the disease process progresses, pulmonary function results are consistent with those presented in section I.

7. Treatment
   a. Most important: Removal of patient from irritants.
   b. Aerosol and bronchodilator therapy.
   c. Antibiotics if indicated.
   d. Treatment regimen fairly consistent with that outlined in section II.

V. Bronchiectasis
   A. Permanent abnormal dilation and distortion of bronchi and/or bronchioles.
   B. Classification
      1. Cylindrical (tubular)
         a. Bronchial walls are dilated, with regular outlines.
         b. Least severe type, as bronchiectatic areas drain fairly well.
      2. Fusiform (cystic)
         a. Bronchial walls have large, irregularly shaped distortions with bulbous ends.
         b. Evidence of bronchitis or bronchiolitis often is present.
      3. Saccular
         a. Complete destruction of bronchial walls.
         b. Replacement of normal bronchial tissue by fibrous tissue.
         c. Most severe type and has worst prognosis.
   C. Etiology
      1. Despite controversy, probable contributing factors are as follows:
         a. Recurrent infection, gram-negative infections being prominent.

   b. Complete airway obstruction.

   c. Atelectasis.

   d. Congenital abnormalities.

D. Pathophysiology

  1. Loss of cilia

  2. Inflammatory infiltration

  3. Sloughing of mucosa with ulceration and possible abscess formation.

  4. Adjacent and distal lung tissue generally has reduced volume with patchy scarring and consolidation, all believed to be secondary to the obstruction of the bronchi.

E. Diagnosis

  1. The bronchogram is the only absolute diagnostic tool.

  2. Bronchoscopy may afford direct visualization of bronchiectatic lesions.

  3. Chest x-ray findings (see below).

  4. Sputum examination (see below).

F. Clinical manifestations

  1. Chronic loose cough, often exacerbated by change of position.

  2. Clubbing of fingers.

  3. Recurrent infections.

  4. Increased sputum production of a characteristic three-layer nature upon standing

   a. Top layer: Thin, frothy.

   b. Middle layer: Turbid, mucopurulent.

   c. Bottom layer: Opaque, mucopurulent to purulent with mucous plugs (Dittrich's plugs), sometimes foul-smelling.

  5. Hemoptysis (common).

  6. Severe ventilation/perfusion abnormalities.

  7. Hallitosis.

G. Chest x-ray findings

  1. Usually normal unless disease is advanced.

  2. May show multiple cysts with associated fluid level.

  3. May show cor pulmonale.

H. Pulmonary function studies

  1. Cylindric type may show no changes or decreases in expiratory flow rates.

  2. The saccular or cystic type shows decreased flow rates, especially if associated with bronchitis, emphysema, or cystic fibrosis.

I. Management

  1. Aggressive bronchial hygiene with aerosol and chest physiotherapy.

2. Appropriate antibiotic therapy.

3. Possible lung resection if lesions are localized.

VI. Asthma

A. Asthma, according to the American Thoracic Society, is "characterized by an increased responsiveness of the trachea and bronchi to various stimuli and is manifested by widespread narrowing of the airways that changes in severity either spontaneously or as the result of treatment."

B. Categories of asthma

1. *Allergic* or *extrinsic:* Implies that asthma is a result of an antigen-antibody reaction on mast cells of the respiratory tract. This reaction causes release of histamine, bradykinins, ECF-A (eosinophilic chemotactic factor of anaphylaxis) and SRS-A (slow-reacting substance of anaphylaxis). These substances then elicit the clinical responses associated with an asthmatic attack and cause high serum IgE levels along with sputum and serum eosinophilia.

2. *Idiopathic* or *intrinsic:* Implies that asthma is a result of imbalance of the autonomic nervous system, i.e., response of beta- and alpha-adrenergic sites, as well as cholinergic sites of the autonomic nervous system are not properly coordinated.

3. *Nonspecific:* Implies that the origin of asthmatic reactions is unknown. The asthmatic attack may follow viral infection, emotional changes, or exercise.

C. Etiology

1. In general, the complete causes are unknown, but heredity plays a significant role. Allergies and environmental factors also are frequently implicated.

2. If the disease develops between ages 5 through 15, it usually has an allergic basis.

3. If onset is after age 30, the disease normally is considered nonspecific.

4. Incidence

a. About 5%–15% of the population under age 15 is asthmatic.

b. About 1% of the adult population is asthmatic.

c. Normally at the onset of adolescence, the disease begins to disappear.

D. Diagnosis

1. Depends on skin testing for antibodies and on patient's and family history.

2. In allergic asthma, antibody IgE serum levels are about six times that of normal.

3. In idiopathic asthma, patients show an abnormal response to drug therapy: decreased beta sympathetic response and increased alpha sympathetic response.
4. In nonspecific asthma, frequent presenting symptoms are nasal polyps and aspirin intolerance.
5. Eosinophilia of sputum and blood are common.

E. Pathophysiology
   1. Thickening of subepithelial membranes.
   2. Hypertrophy of mucous glands.
   3. Eosinophilic infiltrates common in both sputum and serum.
   4. Decrease in number of pulmonary mast cells.
   5. Mucosal edema and bronchoconstriction.
   6. Increased production of thick viscid secretions.

F. Clinical manifestations
   1. Severe respiratory distress.
   2. Rapid, shallow respiratory pattern.
   3. Wheezing that is often audible without a stethoscope.
   4. Weak cough.
   5. Tachycardia and hypertension.
   6. Sometimes diaphoresis.
   7. Cyanosis may be present.
   8. Barrel-chested appearance with hyperresonance.
   9. Anxious.
   10. Intercostal, substernal, subcostal retractions.
   11. Paradoxical chest movement.
   12. Accessory muscle usage.
   13. Shortness of breath.
   14. Prolonged expiratory time.

G. Chest x-ray findings
   1. During an attack a classic hyperinflation pattern is seen.
   2. Between attacks the chest x-ray may be normal.

H. Pulmonary function studies
   1. During an attack expiratory flow rates and vital capacity are decreased. Bronchodilator therapy during pulmonary function testing often results in a significant improvement in test results.
   2. Between attacks pulmonary function studies may be normal or show decreased expiratory flow rates.

I. Status asthmaticus
   1. Sustained asthmatic attack that does not respond to conventional therapy.
   2. Severe hypoxemia is normally present.

3. Possible results:
   a. Lactic acidosis
   b. Respiratory failure
   c. Mechanical ventilation
   d. Death
J. Management
   1. Primarily drug oriented
      a. Sympathomimetics
         (1) Aerosolized by metered mist or mechanical aerosol generator.
         (2) Subcutaneous epinephrine, 1 ml of 1:1,000 solution × 3 every 20–30 minutes.
         (3) IV Isuprel has been successfully employed in the treatment of pediatric patients with status asthmaticus.
      b. Cromolyn sodium
      c. Steroids
      d. Xanthines
   2. Systemic fluid administration
   3. Arterial blood gas monitoring
   4. Ventilatory and cardiovascular monitoring
   5. Use of IPPB and aerosol therapy is controversial and depends on patient tolerance
   6. Oxygen therapy if hypoxemia is present
   7. If status asthmaticus results in ventilatory failure, mechanical ventilation is indicated
      a. Management is difficult and may require significant sedation and/or paralysis with muscle relaxants.
      b. Pneumothorax frequently develops.

BIBLIOGRAPHY

Abraham A.S.: The management of patient with chronic bronchitis and cor pulmonale. *Heart Lung* 6:104, 1977.
Bates D.V., Macklem P.T., Christie R.V.: *Respiratory Function in Disease*. Philadelphia, W.B. Saunders Co., 1971.
Bracchi G., Barbaccio P., Vezzoli F., et al.: Peripheral pulmonary wedge sengiography in chronic obstructive pulmonary disease. *Chest* 71:718–724, 1977.
Cherniack R.M., Cherniack L.: *Respiration in Health and Disease,* ed. 3. Philadelphia, W.B. Saunders Co., 1983.
Committee of the Oregon Thoracic Society, Chronic Obstructive Pulmonary Disease: *C.O.P.D. Manual.* New York, American Lung Association, 1977.
Crofton J., Douglas A.: *Respiratory Diseases,* ed. 2. London, Blackwell Scientific Publications, 1975.
Farzan S.: *A Concise Handbook of Respiratory Diseases.* Reston, Virginia, Reston Publishing Co., 1978.

Gates A.J.: Bronchiolitis or asthma: Differential diagnosis and treatment. *Respir. Care* 20:1153, 1975.

George R.B., Light R.W., Matthay R.A.: *Chest Medicine.* New York, Churchill Livingstone, 1983.

Goldsmith J.R.: *Health Effects of Air Pollution.* New York, American Thoracic Society. *Basics of Respiratory Diseases,* vol. 4, 1975.

Hedley-Whyte J., Burgess G.E., Feeley T.W., et al.: *Applied Physiology of Respiratory Care.* Boston, Little, Brown & Co., 1976.

Higgins M.W., Keller J.B., Metzner H.L.: Smoking, socioeconomic status and chronic respiratory disease. *Am. Rev. Respir. Dis.* 116:403–409, 1977.

Joint Committee of the Allergy Foundation of America and the American Thoracic Society: *Asthma: A Practical Guide for Physicians.* New York, National Tuberculosis and Respiratory Disease Association, 1973.

Martin T.R., Lewis S.W., Albert R.K.: The prognosis of patients with chronic obstructive pulmonary disease after hospitalization for acute respiratory failure. *Chest* 82:310–314, 1982.

Pare J.A.P., Fraser R.G.: *Synopsis of Diseases of the Chest.* Philadelphia, W.B. Saunders Co., 1983.

Parot S., Miara B., Milic-Emili J., et al.: Hypoxemia, hypercarbia, and breathing pattern in patients with chronic obstructive pulmonary disease. *Am. Rev. Respir. Dis.* 126:882–886, 1982.

Petty T.L.: *Intensive and Rehabilitative Respiratory Care,* ed. 3. Philadelphia, Lea & Febiger, 1982.

Pontoppidan H., Geffin B., Lowenstein E.: *Acute Respiratory Failure in the Adult.* Boston, Little, Brown & Co., 1973.

Rarey K.P., Youtsey J.W.: *Respiratory Patient Care.* Englewood Cliffs, N.J., Prentice-Hall, Inc., 1981.

Shapiro B.A., Harrison R.A., Kacmarek R.M., et al.: *Clinical Application of Respiratory Care,* ed. 3. Chicago, Year Book Medical Publishers, Inc., 1985.

Said S.I.: *The Lung in Relationship to Hormones.* New York, American Thoracic Society, *Basics of Respiratory Diseases,* vol. 1, No. 3, 1973.

Tisi G.M.: *Pulmonary Physiology in Clinical Medicine,* ed. 2. Baltimore, Williams & Wilkins Co., 1983.

Thurlbeck W.M.: *Chronic Bronchitis and Emphysema.* New York, American Thoracic Society, *Basics of Respiratory Diseases,* vol. 3, No. 1, 1974.

Ward J.: Cromolyn sodium: A new approach to treatment of asthma. *Heart Lung* 4:415, 1975.

West J.B.: *Pulmonary Pathophysiology: The Essentials.* Baltimore, Williams & Wilkins Co., 1977.

Whitcomb M.E.: *The Lung: Normal and Diseased.* St. Louis, C.V. Mosby Co., 1982.

Wintrobe M.M., Thorn G.W., Adams R.D., et al.: *Harrison's Principles of Internal Medicine,* ed. 7. New York, McGraw-Hill Book Co., 1974.

Witek T.J., Schachter E.N.: Air pollution and respiratory health. *Respir. Care* 28:442–446, 1983.

20 / Restrictive Lung Diseases

I. General Comments
   A. A restrictive lung disease is any disease in which the ability to inhale is affected. Generally the characteristic feature is an inability to expand the lung fully.
   B. Restrictive diseases of pulmonary origin are frequently associated with an increase in pulmonary fibrous tissue. The result is an overall increase in pulmonary elastance and a decrease in pulmonary compliance.
   C. Characteristic pulmonary function findings (Table 20–1)
      1. Decreased or normal TV (tidal volume).
      2. Decreased or normal RV (residual volume).
      3. Decreased or normal ERV (expiratory reserve volume).
      4. Decreased or normal IRV (inspiratory reserve volume).
      5. Decreased TLC (total lung capacity).
      6. Decreased VC (vital capacity).
      7. Decreased IC (inspiratory capacity).
      8. Decreased or normal FRC (functional residual capacity).
      9. In pure restrictive lung diseases flow rate studies usually are normal; however, flow rates may be decreased when an obstructive component is also present.
      10. Pulmonary and/or thoracic and total compliance is usually severely decreased.
      11. There is a progressive increase in the work of breathing as the severity of the disease increases.
         a. Initially alveolar minute ventilation is normal or increased but, as the disease progresses, alveolar minute ventilation progressively decreases.
         b. Arterial blood gases may follow the same pattern as that seen in obstructive lung disease. The initial presenting symptom may be chronic respiratory alkalosis with hypoxemia but, as the disease progresses, chronic respiratory acidosis with hypoxemia may develop.
   D. Categories of restrictive diseases
      1. Pulmonary
      2. Thoracoskeletal

314

TABLE 20–1.—COMPARISON OF
PULMONARY FUNCTION STUDY RESULTS IN
OBSTRUCTIVE AND RESTRICTIVE
PULMONARY DISEASES

PFT STUDY	OBSTRUCTIVE	RESTRICTIVE
TLC	↔ or ↑	↓
VC	↔ or ↓	↓
FRC	↑	↔ or ↓
RV	↑	↔ or ↓
RV/TLC	↑	↔
$FEV_1\%$	↓	↔
$MMEFR_{25-75}$	↓	↔ or ↓

   3. Neurologic-neuromuscular

   4. Abdominal

II. Pulmonary Restrictive Lung Diseases

  A. Pulmonary fibrosis: A disease characterized by the excessive formation of connective tissue in the process of repairing chronic or acute tissue injury.

    1. Etiology: Any permanent injury to the lung, inflammation, allergy, etc.

    2. Type: Localized or diffuse

      a. Causes of localized fibrosis

        (1) Tuberculosis

        (2) Unresolved pneumonias

        (3) Fungal infections

        (4) Abscess formation

      b. Causes of diffuse fibrosis

        (1) Chronic exposure to various inhalants. Specific pneumoconioses are listed in Table 20–2.

TABLE 20–2.—SPECIFIC PNEUMOCONIOSES

DISEASE	CAUSATIVE AGENT
Silicosis	Silica dust
Farmer's lung	Moldy hay
Stannosis	Tin dust
Silo-fillers' disease	Nitrogen dioxide
Coal workers' pneumoconiosis	Coal dust
Asbestosis	Asbestos
Berylliosis	Beryllium
Siderosis	Iron dust
Talcosis	Talc
Barritosis	Barium
Aluminosis	Aluminum

(2) Acute exposure to toxic inhalants may also cause diffuse fibrosis (i.e., chlorine gas, ammonia, polyvinyl chloride, smoke inhalation, radiation therapy).

(3) Diseases of unknown etiology that often show diffuse fibrosis:

   (a) Hamman-Rich syndrome
   (b) Eosinophilic granuloma
   (c) Sarcoidosis
   (d) Familial fibrocystic dysphagia
   (e) Chronic interstitial pneumonia
   (f) Collagen diseases

3. Pathophysiology

   a. Inflammatory reaction in response to organic or inorganic foreign agents.

   b. Inflammation is followed by cellular infiltration and acute vasculitis with local hemorrhage and thrombus formation, resulting in scar tissue.

4. Clinical presentation

   a. Primary symptom: Progressive dyspnea on exertion and ultimately at rest.

   b. Nonproductive cough.

   c. As disease continues, progressive respiratory impairment and often cor pulmonale.

   d. Physical examination findings:

      (1) Clubbing
      (2) Cyanosis
      (3) Restricted chest wall and diaphragmatic movement
      (4) Diffuse, dry, crackling rales
      (5) Increased work of breathing
      (6) Use of accessory muscles of ventilation
      (7) Tachypnea with shallow tidal volumes

   e. Chest x-ray

      (1) Small lung with large heart and elevated diaphragm.
      (2) Fine reticular or nodular pattern involving entire lung but predominantly the lower lobes.

   f. Arterial blood gases and pulmonary function studies as outlined in section I.

4. Treatment

   a. Removal of patient from environment causing the fibrotic changes.

   b. Therapy for underlying disease entity.

       c. Symptomatic management of pulmonary problems, emphasizing:
- (1) Bronchial hygiene
- (2) Overall nutrition
- (3) Graded exercise programs
- (4) Oxygen therapy
- (5) Corticosteroids in early stages

B. Pleural effusion: Accumulation of fluid in pleural space.
1. Normally the fluid lining of the pleura is produced by the capillary network of the visceral pleural surface, and any excess is removed by the lymphatic system.
2. Any disturbance in production of this fluid or in its removal can lead to development of pleural effusion.
3. Primary causes: Inflammation and circulatory disorders.
   a. Malignancy
   b. Congestive heart failure
   c. Infection
   d. Pulmonary infarction
   e. Trauma
4. The effusion compresses the lung on the affected side.
5. The effusion is gravity dependent and may shift with positional change.
6. Types of effusions:
   a. Hydrothorax—a thin clear transudate caused by congestive heart failure, chronic nephritis, or pulmonary neoplasm.
   b. Empyema (pyrothorax)—an effusion consisting entirely of pus caused by a bacterial infection.
   c. Hemothorax—frank blood caused by a malignancy, pulmonary infarction, or ruptured blood vessel.
   d. Chylothorax—accumulation of chyle resulting from the obstruction or trauma of the thoracic duct.
   e. Fibrothorax—an accumulation of fibrous tissue normally secondary to a prolonged effusion.
7. Treatment:
   a. Primary: Removal of fluid from pleural space
      - (1) Thoracentesis or insertion of chest tubes
      - (2) Fluid allowed to resorb into pulmonary lymphatic system.
   b. Secondary: Treatment of underlying disease.

C. Pneumothorax: Accumulation of air within the pleural space.

1. If air enters the pleural space, the pressure within the space changes from subatmospheric to atmospheric or supra-atmospheric pressure.
   a. The increased pressure will compress lung tissue and result in atelectasis.
   b. Ventilation of the lung on the affected side is decreased as a result of elimination of the subatmospheric intrapleural pressure.
2. Types: Open and under tension
   a. In an open pneumothorax, there is no buildup of pressure because the gas is allowed to move freely in and out of the pleural space.
   b. A tension pneumothorax results from the presence of a one-way valve, which allows gas only to enter the pleural space—not to leave it. This results in significant increases in pressure within the pleural space.
      (1) Clinical signs:
         (a) Increased difficulty in ventilating. If patient is on a ventilator, airway pressure will increase with each breath.
         (b) Patient's vital signs will begin to deteriorate as mean intrathoracic pressure increases.
         (c) Breath sounds will be absent on affected side.
         (d) Affected side will be hyperresonant to percussion.
         (e) Trachea and mediastinum may be shifted toward unaffected side as extent of tension pneumothorax increases.
         (f) Possible pleuritic pain.
         (g) Dry hacking cough.
         (h) These clinical signs are more predominant if patient is on a mechanical ventilator than if he is ventilating spontaneously. This is due to the greater pressure gradients developed, forcing more gas into the pleural space.
      (2) Treatment: Decompression of the thorax by chest tube insertion.
D. Cardiogenic pulmonary edema: Active movement of fluid across alveolar capillary membrane into alveoli as a result of increased capillary hydrostatic pressures.
   1. Normally a fine balance exists among capillary colloid osmotic (oncotic) pressure, capillary hydrostatic pressure, interstitial

hydrostatic pressure, and interstitial colloid osmotic (oncotic) pressure across the pulmonary capillary bed (see Chap. 15).

2. Usually a very small net pressure forces fluid into the interstitial space. This interstitial fluid is drained by the lymphatics.
3. If capillary hydrostatic pressure increases significantly, the net pressure forcing fluid into the interstitial space increases and eventually fluid will move directly into the alveoli.
4. Primary cause: Acute left ventricular failure (congestive heart failure).
   a. The hydrostatic pressure of the pulmonary vascular bed is increased because of the inability of the left side of the heart to accept the blood presented to it.
   b. This increased pressure offsets the normal pressure dynamics at the alveolar capillary membrane.
5. Secondary cause: Increased vascular volume causing an increase in pulmonary capillary hydrostatic pressure.
6. Treatment
   a. Primary: Pharmacologic
      (1) Furosemide (Lasix)
      (2) Morphine
      (3) Digitalis
   b. Pulmonary management
      (1) Oxygen at a high F_{IO_2}
      (2) IPPB with ethyl alcohol
      (3) PEEP and mechanical ventilation in severe cases
7. Acute right ventricular failure (congestive heart failure)
   a. Systemic edema develops as a result of right ventricular failure.
   b. The inability of the right heart to accept the blood presented to it results in blood pooling in the periphery.
   c. Dependent edema (pedal edema), neck vein distention, and hepatomegaly are common clinical findings.
   d. It is not unlikely for patients with right-sided failure to eventually develop left-sided failure and those with left-sided failure to develop right-sided failure.
E. Noncardiogenic pulmonary edema
   1. The development of interstitial or true pulmonary edema from noncardiogenic origins.
   2. Pathophysiologic etiologies
      a. Altered permeability of capillary endothelial cells allowing an increased quantity of fluid into the interstitial space.

  b. Decreased capillary colloid osmotic pressure, which increases the pressure gradient, allowing more fluid to enter the interstitial space.

  c. Altered lymphatic function, preventing normal drainage of the pulmonary interstitium, thereby allowing fluid to accumulate.

  d. Alveolar epithelial damage, allowing fluid to enter the alveoli.

3. Clinical etiologies

  a. Neurogenic origin

   (1) Primarily a result of an acute insult to the CNS.

   (2) Causing an increased sympathetic discharge leading to a sudden intravascular fluid shift into the pulmonary circulation.

   (3) The imbalance in hydrostatic and osmotic pressures created causes fluid to enter the interstitial space.

  b. Drug overdose

   (1) Exact mechanism poorly defined.

   (2) It is presumed that drugs, especially narcotics and sedatives, have a direct effect on increasing pulmonary capillary membrane permeability.

  c. High-altitude pulmonary edema

   (1) Mechanism poorly understood.

   (2) Thought to be the result of severe hypoxemia and vasoconstriction of the microcirculation.

   (3) As blood flows under high pressure through the patent portion of the microvasculature, edema develops.

  d. Reexpansion edema

   (1) Develops after the sudden reexpansion of a lung that had been collapsed for several hours.

   (2) The sudden reexpansion causes a negative pressure in the interstitium, creating a large pressure gradient across the capillary membrane and an increased transudation of fluid.

   (3) The rapid removal of pleural effusion fluid (greater than 1,000 ml) may produce edema.

  e. Pulmonary edema associated with renal disease

   (1) Mechanism poorly defined.

   (2) May occur in patients with acute glomerulonephritis or nephrotic syndrome.

   (3) Also seen in chronically uremic patients and in patients on long-term hemodialysis.

    f. Other clinical conditions known to lead to noncardiogenic pulmonary edema:
- (1) Sepsis
- (2) Shock
- (3) Pancreatitis
- (4) Toxic gas or smoke inhalation
- (5) Aspiration
- (6) Pulmonary infections

4. Clinical presentation
   - a. Responsive hypoxemia
   - b. Decreased compliance
   - c. Diffuse atelectasis
   - d. Minimal decrease in FRC
5. Treatment
   - a. Oxygen therapy
   - b. Fluid therapy
   - c. Diuretics
   - d. Low levels of PEEP therapy
6. Many consider noncardiogenic pulmonary edema to be the early form of adult respiratory distress syndrome.

F. Adult respiratory distress syndrome (ARDS)
1. Terms representing the same clinical syndrome
   - a. Oxygen toxicity
   - b. Oxygen pneumonitis
   - c. Wet lung
   - d. Congestive atelectasis
   - e. Stiff lung syndrome
   - f. Respiratory lung syndrome
   - g. Postpump lung
   - h. Posttraumatic pulmonary insufficiency
   - i. Shock lung
2. Clinical features of the syndrome's pathophysiologic processes
   - a. Refractory hypoxemia (hypoxemia that does not respond to an increasing F_{IO_2})
   - b. Decrease in pulmonary compliance
   - c. Decrease in FRC
   - d. Chest x-ray: Diffuse alveolar infiltrates throughout entire lung field (honeycomb effect)
   - e. Complete reversal of disease process except for any residual fibrotic changes
3. Postmortem pulmonary findings
   - a. Beefy lung, which does not collapse on removal from thoracic cavity

    b. Hyaline membrane formation on pulmonary parenchyma

    c. Interstitial edema and fibrosis

    d. Pneumocyte hyperplasia

4. Cause

    a. Probably a reaction of the respiratory tract to high levels of physiologic stress for prolonged periods. This stress may be associated with any of the organ systems.

    b. Clinical problems associated with the development of ARDS:

       (1) Oxygen toxicity

       (2) Chest trauma

       (3) Aspiration

       (4) Chemical irritation of respiratory tract

       (5) Blood transfusion

       (6) Emboli formation

       (7) Sepsis

       (8) Shock

       (9) Radiation injury

       (10) Near drowning

       (11) Pancreatitis

5. Pathophysiology of ARDS resulting from oxygen toxicity

    a. F_{IO_2} maintained above 0.50–0.60 for prolonged periods may cause acute pulmonary changes (see Chap. 24).

       (1) Interference with pulmonary enzyme systems, which disrupts pulmonary metabolism.

       (2) Type II alveolar cell dysfunction, which results in altered surfactant production.

       (3) Inhibition of mucociliary activity.

       (4) Increased permeability of capillary endothelium.

       (5) Nitrogen washout and atelectasis (absorption atelectasis).

    b. Primary symptoms noted by patient

       (1) Substernal distress

       (2) Cough

       (3) Nausea and vomiting

       (4) Paresthesia

       (5) Shortness of breath

       (6) Tachypnea

       (7) Tachycardia

    c. Functional changes

       (1) Decrease in compliance secondary to

         (a) Altered surfactant levels

(b) Dilution of surfactant by transudate

(c) Atelectasis

(2) Decrease in FRC secondary to

(a) Altered surfactant levels

(b) Nitrogen washout atelectasis

(3) Increased work of breathing

(4) Refractory hypoxemia

d. Pathophysiology of ARDS resulting from clinical problems presented in #4 follows the general pattern seen with oxygen toxicity. The actual mechanism by which these changes develop is unclear.

6. Treatment

a. Maintain adequate oxygenation state (see Chap. 33).

(1) Administer PEEP therapy.

(2) Titrate PEEP in an attempt to reduce F_{IO_2} below 0.50.

(3) Maintain P_{O_2} at a minimum of approximately 60 mm Hg.

(4) Maintain adequate tissue perfusion.

b. Mechanical ventilation is indicated if the work of breathing becomes excessive and an adequate ventilatory state cannot be maintained.

c. Fluid therapy.

d. Diuretic therapy.

e. Steroid therapy: In early stages of management, steroids, especially methylprednisolone sodium succinate (Solu-Medrol), may help stabilize endothelial cells and type II pneumocytes if they are administered in large doses for short periods.

G. Pneumonia: Pneumonitis caused by a microorganism.

1. Pneumonias are a leading cause of death in the United States and account for 10% of admissions to general medical floors.

2. Pathophysiology of pneumonia

a. Microorganisms cause inflammation of pulmonary mucosa, resulting in edema and phagocytic infiltration.

b. Results in exudation and consolidation.

c. Consolidation is typically localized, as in lobar pneumonias.

3. Bacterial pneumonia (Table 20–3)

a. Common clinical signs and symptoms

(1) Onset normally is abrupt.

(2) Very high fevers, with chills, sometimes lasting longer than 20 minutes.

TABLE 20–3.—COMPARISON OF CLINICAL AND
LABORATORY MANIFESTATIONS OF BACTERIAL
AND VIRAL PNEUMONIAS

SYMPTOM	BACTERIAL	VIRAL
Onset	Abrupt	Gradual
Fever	High	Low-grade
Chills	Common	Uncommon
Sputum	Purulent, thick	Thin, mucoid
Tachycardia	Frequent	Rare
Hypoxemia	Common	Uncommon
Chest x-ray	Consolidation	Consolidation uncommon
WBC	>10,000/cu mm	<10,000/cu mm
Pleuritic pain	Occasional	Uncommon

      (3) Large volumes of thick, purulent sputum.

      (4) Frequently tachypnea and tachycardia, sometimes a pleuritic type pain.

      (5) X-ray: Consolidation.

      (6) White blood cell count: Frequently greater than 10,000/cu mm.

      (7) Hypoxemia secondary to shunting.

  3. Nonbacterial (viral or fungal) pneumonia (see Table 20–3)

    a. Clinical signs and symptoms (occasionally mild and frequently undiagnosed)

      (1) Onset normally is very gradual.

      (2) Fevers normally are low grade, chills are uncommon.

      (3) Sputum production is minimal, usually thin and mucoid.

      (4) Tachypnea and tachycardia are rare; pleuritic pain is uncommon.

      (5) X-ray: Consolidation uncommon.

      (6) White blood cell count: Commonly less than 10,000/ cu mm.

  4. Treatment

    a. Appropriate antibiotic therapy (bacterial and fungal)

    b. Oxygen therapy

    c. Fluid therapy

    d. IPPB, aerosol, and chest physiotherapy, if indicated

H. Pulmonary embolism

  1. The occlusion of the pulmonary artery or one of its branches by a substance carried in the blood, normally a blood clot.

  2. A blood clot that is attached to its site of origin is referred to as a thrombus. Once detached it is referred to as an embolus.

3. The actual substance may be fat, blood, air, amniotic fluid, or a tissue fragment.
4. Etiology and pathogenesis
   a. The most common sites of thrombus formation are the deep veins of the lower extremities and pelvis and within the right side of the heart.
   b. Thrombus development is most prevalent in patients who are immobilized due to pain or who are debilitated, paralyzed, or require prolonged bed rest.
   c. Factors facilitating thrombus formation
      (1) Abnormal vessel wall
      (2) Stagnation of blood
      (3) Increased coagulability
   d. Dependent lung regions are most commonly involved with pulmonary emboli.
   e. Pulmonary infarction occurs in about 10% of patients with pulmonary emboli, especially if there is a history of cardiac disease.
5. Pathophysiology
   a. Deadspace ventilation is significantly increased.
   b. Total ventilation markedly increases in an effort to maintain normal P_{CO_2}.
   c. A minute volume – P_{CO_2} disparity develops (see Chap. 12).
   d. With large emboli, pulmonary artery pressures increase, especially if there is underlying cardiac disease.
6. Clinical presentation
   a. Dyspnea and chest pain.
   b. Hemoptysis may develop.
   c. Frequently cough, faintness, and anxiety accompany pulmonary embolus.
   d. Thrombophlebitis is often noted (frequently at the site of embolus formation).
   e. If a massive embolus is present:
      (1) Tachypnea
      (2) Tachycardia
      (3) Cyanosis
      (4) Decreased breath sounds
      (5) Wheezing and rales
      (6) Pleural friction rub
   f. Less common findings:
      (1) Fever
      (2) Cardiac arrhythmias

        (3) Shock

  7. Chest x-rays

    a. In some cases decreased lung volume, atelectasis, pleural effusion, and signs of pulmonary infarction may be present.

    b. In rare cases there is a local reduction in vascular markings and an enlarged pulmonary artery.

  8. Laboratory findings

    a. Decreased lung volumes and capacities.

    b. Flow studies usually normal.

    c. Arterial blood gases usually reveal hypoxemia with a normal acid base balance or a respiratory alkalosis.

    d. ECG may reveal arrhythmias.

  9. Radioisotope lung scanning

    a. Ventilation/perfusion scans may help differentiate pulmonary embolism from other perfusion abnormalities.

    b. Findings must be correlated with patient's clinical findings and history.

  10. Pulmonary angiography is considered definitive in the diagnosis of pulmonary embolism.

  11. Treatment

    a. Intravenous streptokinase or urokinase.

    b. Anticoagulation therapy with heparin.

    c. Oxygen therapy.

    d. Intubation and ventilation in severe cases.

    e. Occasionally embolectomy is performed; however, this procedure is controversial.

I. Pulmonary alveolar proteinosis

  1. A disease characterized by alveoli filled with a liquid high in protein and lipid.

  2. Alveolar walls are normal but only scattered macrophages are noted.

  3. Pathogenesis

    a. Origin unknown, but it is theorized that type II alveolar epithelial cells produce an excess of surfactant, lipid, and protein.

    b. This substance is poorly cleared by defective macrophages.

  4. Prevalence

    a. Most commonly develops in age groups 20–50 years, with 2:1 male-female ratio.

    b. Some cases described in infants.

  5. Clinical manifestations

    a. One third of all patients are asymptomatic.

    b. Common clinical findings:
      (1) Shortness of breath on exertion
      (2) Cough
      (3) Fatigue
      (4) Weight loss
      (5) Pleuritic pain
      (6) Possible low-grade fever
      (7) Clubbing of digits
6. Chest x-ray reveals infiltrates in perihilar regions and bases of the lung.
7. Pulmonary function studies may be normal but diffusing capacity is decreased.
8. Diagnosis is made primarily by open lung biopsy, bronchoalveolar lavage, or the measurement of lactic dehydrogenase levels.
9. Prognosis
    a. Clinical course is variable.
    b. Disease may spontaneously resolve but reappear at a later date.
    c. One third of patients die, primarily due to predisposition to infection.
10. Treatment
    a. No specific therapy defined.
    b. Corticosteroids used but controversial.
    c. Lung lavage helpful in some patients.

III. Thoracoskeletal Restrictive Lung Diseases
  A. Deformities of thoracic cage that result in limited movement of the chest demonstrate pulmonary function patterns consistent with restrictive lung disease.
  B. If the deformity is severe enough, a significant increase in the work of breathing results.
  C. Increased work of breathing eventually leads to hypoxemia, hypercapnia, and possible heart failure.
  D. Most commonly encountered thoracic abnormalities leading to restrictive lung disease are:
    1. Scoliosis: Gradual curvature of vertebral column in lateral plane of body.
      a. One of the most common thoracic deformities.
      b. May occur at various levels of the vertebral column.
      c. May develop with age as a result of poor posture.
    2. Kyphosis: Posterior curvature of thoracic vertebral column, resulting in a bony hump.

   a. Frequently develops in older individuals with degenerative osteoarthritis.
   b. May develop in individuals with chronic obstructive pulmonary disease.
   3. Kyphoscoliosis: Combination of thoracic scoliosis and kyphosis.
      a. In severe cases of kyphoscoliosis, one lung becomes severely compressed, the other overdistended.
      b. Cardiopulmonary disability may be very pronounced in severe kyphoscoliosis.
IV. Neurologic-Neuromuscular Restrictive Lung Diseases
   A. Weakness or paralysis of the muscles of ventilation results in a pulmonary function pattern consistent with restrictive lung disease.
   B. Myasthenia gravis: A disease of the myoneural junction in which transmission of impulses across the motor end-plate is inhibited.
      1. Etiology: Unknown. Functionally it appears that acetylcholine is improperly released, synthesized, or prematurely hydrolyzed before crossing the neuromuscular junction (see Chap. 8).
      2. The disease is most common in women in their 20s to 40s, but it affects individuals of both sexes and of all ages, with about 10% of patients having a tumor of the thymus gland.
      3. The disease is manifested by generalized muscle weakness and most commonly demonstrates a descending paralysis.
      4. The primary symptoms normally are ocular, progressing to facial muscle weakness or paralysis followed by pharyngeal and laryngeal weakness and finally respiratory muscle weakness.
      5. Patients frequently present with a chief complaint of easy fatigability.
      6. Diagnosis
         a. Primarily based on history and symptomatology.
         b. The administration of a parasympathomimetic of the cholinesterase inhibitor type confirms the diagnosis. Increased muscle strength is normally noted shortly after the administration of the drug.
      7. Treatment
         a. Maintenance with cholinesterase inhibitors.
            (1) Prostigmine (neostigmine) drug of choice, but also:
            (2) Pyridostigmine (mestinon)
            (3) Ambenonium (mytelase)
         b. Treatment with atropine to reverse the side effects of the cholinesterase inhibitor.

c. Thymectomy in severe cases: in some patients complete remission has been reported.
d. A 10-day course of adrenocorticotropic hormone (ACTH). Symptoms deteriorate during administration; however, remission is frequent after a 10-day course.
e. In severe cases intubation and mechanical ventilation as supportive measures until drug therapy is titrated.
8. Myasthenic vs. cholinergic crisis
a. An acute exacerbation of the disease process producing weakness is termed a myasthenic crisis.
b. An acute decrease in muscle strength as a result of the excessive use of cholinesterase inhibitors is termed a cholinergic crisis.
c. The Tensilon (generic name edrophonium chloride) test is used to differentiate between a myasthenic and cholinergic crisis. Tensilon is a short acting (5 minutes) cholinesterase inhibitor.
   (1) If the patient is suffering from a myasthenic crisis, the administration of Tensilon will improve muscle strength.
   (2) If a cholinergic crisis is present, Tensilon will increase muscle weakness and exacerbate symptomatology.
   (3) Muscle strength can be evaluated by serial vital capacity or NIF measurements.
9. Monitoring of cardiopulmonary status
a. Patients in acute exacerbation require very close cardiopulmonary monitoring.
b. Evaluation of the patient's ventilatory reserve (see Chap. 18) is used to determine changes in ventilatory muscle strength.
c. Vital capacity is monitored as frequently as every hour in acute situations.
d. Deterioration of the vital capacity may signal the need for further medical intervention.
C. Guillain-Barré syndrome: Polyneuritis primarily affecting the peripheral motor and sensory neurons.
1. Etiology: Unclear. The disease may be viral or traumatic in nature. An increase in the number of cases has been reported following vaccination against poliomyelitis and swine flu.
2. The syndrome affects all ages but is more prevalent in adults.
3. The signs and symptoms show a symmetric ascending pattern of sensory abnormalities that may progress to actual paralysis.

4. The disease is normally self-limiting and is reversible with time. The amount of residual effects is dependent on the extent of demyelination occurring during the active disease state.
5. Diagnosis is made by the presentation of the disease, a high protein content in the cerebral spinal fluid, and the reversible nature of the disease.
6. Treatment is purely symptomatic, the patient frequently requiring ventilatory support.
7. As with myasthenia gravis, careful monitoring of the patient's ventilatory reserves is indicated.

D. Other neuromuscular or neurologic diseases that may show a restrictive lung disease pattern
  1. Spinal cord diseases
    a. Paraplegia or quadriplegia
    b. Poliomyelitis
  2. Tetanus
  3. Muscular dystrophy
  4. Tick bite paralysis
  5. Congenital myotonia

V. Abdominal Restrictive Lung Diseases
A. Increased size of abdominal contents results in limited movement and elevation of the diaphragm.
B. The limited diaphragmatic movement will demonstrate pulmonary function findings consistent with those of restrictive lung disease.
C. Conditions that may show a restrictive pattern
  1. Abdominal tumors
  2. Obesity
  3. Third-trimester pregnancy
  4. Diaphragmatic hernias
  5. Ascites
D. Pickwickian syndrome
  1. Also referred to as obesity-hypoventilation syndrome.
  2. The syndrome is characterized by:
    a. Severe obesity
    b. Alveolar hypoventilation (more pronounced with sleep), with episodes of sleep apnea
    c. Somnolence
    d. Severe hypoxemia (more pronounced with sleep)
    e. Polycythemia
    f. Pulmonary hypertension (not related to hypoxemia)
    g. Cor pulmonale

3. Etiology is unclear.
   a. Weight loss may reverse the syndrome.
   b. A high percentage of patients experience upper airway obstruction during sleep, especially in the supine position. The obstruction is believed to be soft tissue obstruction.
4. Frequently the hypoxemia and hypoventilation develop only during sleep.
   a. A significant decrease in total compliance is present at all times and is increased further when the subject assumes the supine position.
   b. This results in an increased work of breathing, followed by decreased tidal volumes. This, coupled with possible soft tissue upper airway obstruction, leads to hypoventilation and hypoxemia.
   c. The sleep of these patients is commonly broken and restless, leading to generalized somnolence.
5. Treatment
   a. Primary treatment is weight loss.
   b. Respiratory stimulants have been used but with questionable success.
   c. Tracheostomy may be done when obstruction is identified by sleep studies.
   d. Continuous positive airway pressure by nasal mask.
VI. Smoke Inhalation and Carbon Monoxide Poisoning
   A. Smoke inhalation
      1. Etiology: The inhalation of byproducts of a fire—smoke and other noxious gases.
         a. Aldehydes
         b. Oxides of nitrogen and sulfur
         c. Ammonia
      2. Pathophysiology
         a. Edema, congestion, sloughing of mucosal membranes of the oral and nasal pharynx, larynx, trachea, and bronchi.
         b. Obliterative bronchiolitis and alveolar edema.
         c. Development of pulmonary edema.
         d. Atelectasis caused by airway obstruction with fibrin, edema, fluid, carbon particles, white cells, and epithelial debris.
      3. Clinical presentation (it may take 24–48 hours for symptoms to develop fully)
         a. Coughing and dyspnea
         b. Hypoxemia

       c. Tachypnea and tachycardia

       d. Facial burns, singed nasal hairs, stridor, and grunting are all indicative of upper airway burns.

       e. X-ray studies are negative for first 24–48 hours; however, signs of pulmonary edema, atelectasis, and infiltrates subsequently develop.

    4. Treatment

       a. Establish an artificial airway. This is imperative if upper airway burns accompany the smoke inhalation. If an airway is not established early, subsequent edema may prevent cannulation of the airway.

       b. Oxygen therapy (100% if CO poisoning is also present).

       c. Fluid and electrolyte therapy.

       d. Bronchodilator therapy.

       e. Steroid therapy.

       f. Antibiotic therapy.

B. CO Poisoning

    1. A result of inspiring byproducts of the incomplete combustion of carbon or carbon-containing material.

    2. Pathophysiology

       a. CO combines strongly with hemoglobin to form carboxyhemoglobin (hemoglobin's affinity for CO is 210 times that of O_2).

       b. The total capability of the organism to carry oxygen to the tissues is reduced (anemia hypoxia).

       c. In addition, the oxyhemoglobin dissociation curve is shifted to the left, further limiting the amount of O_2 available at the tissue level.

       d. The likelihood of tissue hypoxia increases as COHb %sat. increases.

    3. Clinical manifestations (symptomatology based on carboxyhemoglobin levels)

       a. Less than 20%: normally asymptomatic.

       b. 20%–60%: headache, exertional dyspnea, impaired judgment, nausea and vomiting.

       c. 60%–80%: loss of consciousness, convulsions, deep coma.

    4. X-ray findings: Chest x-ray may show abnormalities consistent with pulmonary edema, usually interstitial in location.

    5. Diagnosis

       a. Analysis of arterial blood for carboxyhemoglobin levels.

       b. History.

c. Frequently a metabolic acidosis caused by lactic acid accumulation is noted.
6. Treatment
   a. Oxygen therapy: 100% O_2 is indicated until COHb levels reach 10%–15% or less. Increasing the arterial Po_2 decreases the half-life of COHb. On inhalation of room air, the half-life of COHb is about 5–6 hours, while the inhalation of 100% O_2 decreases the half-life to about 90 minutes. Hyperbaric conditions (3 atm) can decrease the half-life of COHb to 23 minutes.
   b. With high COHb levels (>40%–50%), intubation and mechanical ventilation may be necessary.

BIBLIOGRAPHY

Albert R.K.: Factors affecting transvascular fluid and protein movement in pulmonary edema and ARDS. *Semin. Respir. Med.* 2:109–113, 1981.

Amandus H.E., et al.: The pneumoconioses: Methods of measuring progression. *Chest* 63:736, 1973.

Bates D.V., Macklem P.T., Christie R.V.: *Respiratory Function in Disease*, ed. 2. Philadelphia, W.B. Saunders, 1971.

Bendixen H.H., et al.: *Respiratory Care*. St. Louis, C. V. Mosby Co., 1965.

Brigham K.L.: Primary (high permeability) pulmonary edema. *Semin. Respir. Med.* 4:285–288, 1983.

Brigham K.L.: Therapy of pulmonary edema. *Semin. Respir. Med.* 4:313–316, 1983.

Cherniack R.M., Cherniack L.: *Respiration in Health and Disease*, ed. 3. Philadelphia, W.B. Saunders Co., 1983.

Crofton J., Douglas A.: *Respiratory Diseases*, ed. 2. London, Blackwell Scientific Publications, 1975.

Cushing R.: Pulmonary infections. *Heart Lung* 5:611, 1976

Farzan S.: *A Concise Handbook of Respiratory Diseases*. Reston, Virginia, Reston Publishing Co., 1978.

Fink J.N., et al.: Clinical survey of pigeon breeders. *Chest* 62:277, 1972.

George R.B., Light R.W., Matthay R.A.: *Chest Medicine*. New York, Churchill Livingstone, 1983.

Gracey D.R.: Adult respiratory distress syndrome. *Heart Lung* 4:280, 1975.

Griswold K., Guanci M.M., Ropper A.H.: An approach to the care of patients with Guillain-Barré syndrome. *Heart Lung* 13:66–72, 1984.

Hudson L.D.: Ventilatory management of patients with adult respiratory distress syndrome. *Semin. Respir. Med.* 2:128–139, 1981.

Hyers T.M.: Pathogenesis of adult respiratory distress syndrome: Current concepts. *Semin. Respir. Med.* 2:104–108, 1981.

Kealy S.L.: Respiratory care in Guillaine-Barré syndrome. *Am. J. Nurs.* 22:58, 1977.

Lakshminarayan S., Stanford R.E., Petty T.L.: Prognosis after recovery from adult respiratory distress syndrome. *Am. Rev. Respir. Dis.* 113:7, 1976.

Mathewson H.S.: Oxygen: The specific antidote to carbon monoxide. *Respir. Care.* 27:986–987, 1982.

Pore J.A., Fraser R.G.: *Synopsis of Diseases of the Chest.* Philadelphia, W.B. Saunders Co., 1983.

Petterson J.E., Stewart R.D.: Absorption and elimination of carbon monoxide by inactive young men. *Arch. Environ. Health* 21:165–171, 1970.

Petty T.L.: Adult respiratory distress syndrome: Historical perspective and definition. *Semin. Respir. Med.* 2:99–103, 1981.

Petty T.L.: *Intensive and Rehabilitative Care,* ed. 3. Philadelphia, Lea & Febiger, 1982.

Safar P. (ed.): *Respiratory Therapy.* Philadelphia, F.A. Davis Co., 1965.

Selecky P.A., Ziment I.: Prolonged respirator support for the treatment of intractable myasthenia gravis. *Chest* 65:207, 1974.

Shapiro B.A., Cane R.D.: Metabolic malfunction of lung: Noncardiogenic edema and adult respiratory distress syndrome. *Surg. Annu.* 22:271–298, 1981.

Shapiro B.A., et al.: Case study: Myasthenia gravis. *Respir. Care* 19:460, 1974.

Shapiro B.A., Harrison R.A., Kacmarek R.M., et al.: *Clinical Application of Respiratory Care,* ed. 3. Chicago, Year Book Medical Publishers, Inc., 1985.

Shulman J.A.: Errors and hazards in the diagnosis and treatment of bacterial pneumonias. *Ann. Intern. Med.* 62:41, 1965.

Snider G.L.: *Clinical Pulmonary Medicine.* Boston, Little, Brown & Co., 1981.

Solliday N.H., Shapiro B.A., Gracey D.R.: Adult respiratory distress syndrome. *Chest* 69:207, 1976.

Tisi G.M.: *Pulmonary Physiology in Clinical Medicine,* ed. 2. Baltimore, Williams & Wilkins, 1983.

Urbanitle J.S.: Carbon monoxide poisoning. *Prog. Clin. Biol. Res.* 51:355–385, 1981.

Whitcomb M.E.: *The Lung: Normal and Diseased.* St. Louis, C.V. Mosby Co., 1982.

Wintrobe M.M., Thorn G.W., Adams R.D., et al.: *Harrison's Principles of Internal Medicine,* ed. 7. New York, McGraw-Hill Book Co., 1974.

Ziskind M.M.: *The Acute Bacterial Pneumonia in the Adult.* New York, American Lung Association, 1974.

21 / Neonatal Anomalies and Diseases

I. Infant Respiratory Distress Syndrome (IRDS); (Idiopathic Respiratory Distress Syndrome or Hyaline Membrane Disease)
   A. Factors increasing the incidence of IRDS
      1. Premature birth at less than 35 weeks
      2. Low birth weight
         a. Neonates of less than 1,000 gm very frequently develop IRDS.
         b. At birth weights of 1,000–1,500 gm, IRDS is common.
         c. At birth weights of 1,500–2,000 gm, some infants develop IRDS.
         d. In general, the lower the birth weight and/or gestational age, the higher the incidence of IRDS.
   B. Early signs and symptoms
      1. Expiratory grunting
      2. Sternal and intercostal retractions
      3. Nasal flaring
      4. Cyanosis
      5. Rapid respiratory rates
      6. Edematous extremities
      7. X-ray: Ground glass appearance with an air bronchogram
   C. Physiologic changes
      1. Decreased surfactant production
      2. Increased capillary endothelial cell permeability
      3. Atelectasis
      4. Decreased pulmonary compliance
      5. Increased intrapulmonary shunting
      6. Severe hypoxemia
      7. Decreased functional residual capacity
      8. Hyaline membrane formation
   D. Etiology: Primarily decreased surfactant production as a result of decreased L/S ratio associated with premature birth.
   E. Course
      1. Normally a self-limiting process, the first 48-hour period being critical.

2. Process is totally reversible.
F. Management
   1. Supportive in nature.
   2. Oxygenation with least $F_{I_{O_2}}$ necessary to attain an acceptable P_{O_2}.
      a. Maintenance of P_{O_2} between 50 and 70 mm Hg.
      b. Application of PEEP via CPAP in early phases or in moderate cases.
      c. Possible ventilatory support in severe cases or if the infant tires and blood gases indicate acute or impending ventilatory failure.
   3. Reduction of stress on neonate and decrease of overall level of activity to reduce oxygen consumption to a minimum.
   4. Maintenance of adequate cardiovascular function.
   5. Forty-eight hours prior to delivery of known premature infant, administration of betamethasone (steroid) to mother may increase lung maturity.
II. Bronchopulmonary Dysplasia (BPD)
   A. BPD is a disease process associated with ventilator therapy, a high $F_{I_{O_2}}$, high peak inspiratory pressures and prolonged inspiratory times that causes chronic pulmonary changes.
   B. Frequently BPD develops during the course of therapy for IRDS.
   C. BPD is divided into four stages.
      1. Period of acute RDS: Diagnosed retrospectively. This stage lasts 2–3 days and cannot be distinguished from IRDS.
      2. Period of regeneration: Chest x-ray is almost completely opaque. This stage lasts 4–10 days.
      3. Period of transition to chronic disease: Chest x-ray shows atelectasis with small rounded areas of radiolucency throughout the lungs. This stage lasts 10–20 days.
      4. Period of chronic disease: Chest x-ray shows an increase in the size of the radiolucencies. This stage lasts at least 1 month. Pulmonary hypertension and right heart failure are frequent sequelae.
   D. Pathophysiologic pulmonary changes
      1. Damage to alveolar and bronchiolar epithelium
      2. Bronchiolar metaplasia
      3. Peribronchial and interstitial fibrosis
   E. Chronic pulmonary changes show a slow clearing during infancy, and most individuals are clinically and radiologically normal by age 6 months to 2 years.

F. Treatment
1. Stage 1: Same as for IRDS.
2. Stage 2:
   a. O_2 therapy
   b. Chest physiotherapy
   c. Symptomatic support

III. Meconium Aspiration
A. Meconium: Normal contents of the intestinal tract of the fetus. Usually it is not passed from fetal gastrointestinal tract until after birth.
1. Composition
   a. Dark brownish green semisolid material, tarry in texture.
   b. Bile, intestinal secretions, and other pancreatic secretions.
2. Presence in amniotic fluid
   a. In full-term and postmature neonates, meconium may be free in the amniotic fluid, making its aspiration likely.
   b. Whenever meconium is found in the amniotic fluid, its aspiration should be suspected.
   c. It has been *hypothesized* that meconium is passed in utero following an anoxic episode of the fetus.

B. Aspiration
1. At birth, all attempts to suction the oral and nasal pharynx should be made before ventilating an infant suspected of meconium aspiration.
2. Results of irritation to respiratory tract from meconium
   a. Obstruction (check valve type) associated with pneumothorax.
   b. Chemical pneumonitis.
   c. Bacterial infection.
3. Management: Symptomatic
   a. In severe cases, possible CPAP and CPPV.
   b. Oxygen therapy.
   c. Aggressive chest physiotherapy and suctioning (unless persistent fetal circulation (PFC) and birth asphyxia are present).
   d. Mechanical hyperventilation if PFC is present.

IV. Persistent Fetal Circulation
A. Normally seen in full-term infants.
B. Characterized by:
1. A patent ductus arteriosus (PDA) and/or
2. A patent foramen ovale
3. Persistent cyanosis (right-to-left shunt)

    C. Pulmonary hypertension in which pressures often exceed systemic pressures.

    D. Right-to-left shunting through PDA diagnosed by comparing PO_2 values obtained simultaneously from right radial, brachial, or temporal arteries (preductal sample) and umbilical arteries (postductal sample). PDA will cause the preductal arterial blood sample to have a significantly higher PO_2 than the postductal sample.

    E. Treatment

        1. Mechanical hyperventilation (PCO_2, 25–30 mm Hg, with pH of 7.50–7.55) and hyperoxemia (PO_2, 90–110) to dilate pulmonary vasculature.

        2. Tolazoline HCl (Priscoline): An alpha-adrenergic blocker administered to promote pulmonary vasodilation.

  V. Transient Tachypnea of the Newborn (TTN)

    A. Occurs during the first hours of life.

    B. Thought to be caused by delayed absorption of fetal lung fluid.

    C. Occurs in normal term infants.

    D. Characterized by:

        1. Tachypnea (RR 80–140 breaths/min).

        2. Slight cardiomegaly (ECG normal) on chest x-ray.

        3. Breath sounds are normal without rales and rhonchi.

    E. Treatment

        1. Usually symptomatic.

        2. Condition is normally self-limiting, lasting about 3–5 days.

        3. Cardiopulmonary monitoring, including arterial blood gases.

        4. Low levels of oxygen therapy are required to maintain an adequate PO_2.

 VI. Pulmonary Dysmaturity (Mikity-Wilson Syndrome)

    A. Characterized by late onset (1–5 weeks after birth) of respiratory distress with tachypnea not connected to IRDS or BPD.

    B. Etiology unclear. May be due to abnormal distribution of ventilation with air trapping.

    C. Chest x-ray is normal at birth but then reveals a pattern of infiltrates interspersed with cystic foci.

    D. Occurs in premature infants usually weighing less than 1,500 gm.

    E. Treatment

        1. Supportive, including:

           a. Oxygen therapy.

           b. PEEP therapy.

           c. Ventilation (rarely required).

        2. The disease tends to resolve in those who survive, and the chest x-ray returns to normal in 1–6 months.

VII. Rh Incompatibilities
   A. Occurs when an Rh-negative mother gives birth to an Rh-positive infant.
   B. The mother produces antibodies to the fetal antigens because the mother lacks the Rh-positive antigens.
   C. These antibodies cross the placenta, attach to the fetal antigens, and cause hemolysis of the fetal blood and anemia.
   D. Rh incompatibilities include:
      1. Erythroblastosis fetalis: caused by maternal immunization against antigens of fetal blood.
      2. Hydrops fetalis: a more serious form of Rh incompatibility which results in massive edema, pleural effusions, and ascites with severe anemia.
   E. Treatment
      1. Amniocentesis is performed late in pregnancy to diagnose incompatibility if Rh factor problems are suspected from the maternal history.
      2. Intrauterine transfusion may be performed to support infant until birth.
      3. Exchange transfusion is performed after birth.
VIII. Neonatal Pneumonia
   A. Acquired in utero, during delivery, or after birth.
   B. May be bacterial, fungal, viral, or chemical in origin.
   C. Chest x-ray normally shows unilateral infiltrates.
   D. Treatment
      1. Culture and sensitivity study to identify cause.
      2. Antibiotic therapy.
      3. Oxygen therapy.
      4. Mechanical ventilation (if necessary).
IX. Cardiac Anomalies
   A. Patent Ductus Arteriosus (PDA) (Fig 21–1)
      1. Acyanotic anomaly (left-to-right shunt).
      2. Develops because of a failure of the ductus arteriosus to close at birth.
      3. Because of the difference between pulmonary artery and aortic pressures, left ventricular output flows into the pulmonary artery via the patent ductus arteriosus.
      4. Right ventricular work greatly increases, resulting in congestive heart failure (CHF).
      5. Entity is most common among preterm infants with IRDS.
      6. Treatment:
         a. Indomethacin (Indocin), a prostaglandin inhibitor that causes constriction of the ductus arteriosus.

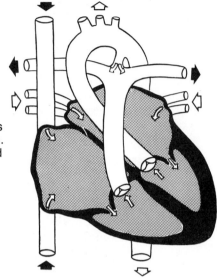

Fig 21–1.—Patient ductus arteriosus. (From Ross Laboratories Clinical Education Aid No. 7 (G163). Columbus, Ohio, 1978. Reproduced by permission.)

      b. Surgical correction may be necessary.
   B. Atrial Septal Defects (ASD) (Fig 21–2).
      1. Acyanotic anomaly (left-to-right shunt).
      2. Reflects failure of the foramen ovale to close or failure of the atrial septum to form correctly.

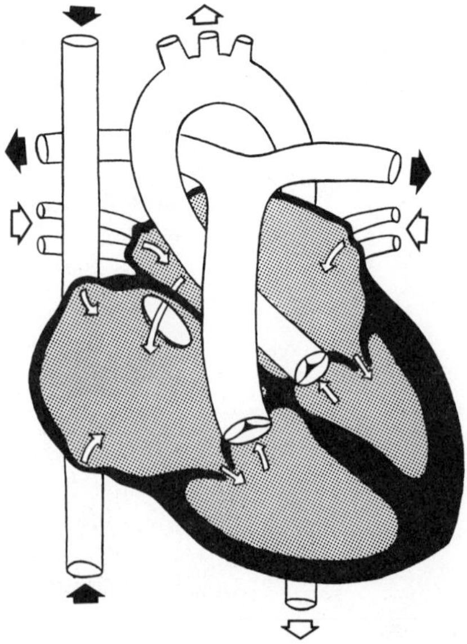

Fig 21–2.—Atrial septal defect. (From Ross Laboratories Clinical Education Aid No. 7 (G163). Columbus, Ohio, 1978. Reproduced by permission.)

3. Basic types of defects
   a. Ostium primum: Occurs low in the atrial wall and usually involves the mitral and tricuspid valves.
   b. Ostium secundum: Isolated defect occurring high in the atrial wall.
4. Because of the pressure difference between the left and right atria, blood moves from the left atrium to the right atrium via the ASD.
5. Right heart work frequently increases, resulting in CHF.
6. Treatment: Surgical correction, either by direct closure or using a plastic prosthesis via open heart surgery.

C. Ventricular Septal Defects (VSD) (Fig 21–3)
   1. Acyanotic anomaly (left-to-right shunt).
   2. Vary considerably in size and may develop in either the membranous or muscular portion of the septal wall.
   3. Small defects may cause minor left-to-right shunting and normally close spontaneously.
   4. With large defects, significant left-to-right shunting occurs.
      a. Left and right ventricular pressures equilibrate.
      b. Since pulmonary vascular resistance is only about one fifth systemic vascular resistance, the majority of cardiac output is forced through the lung.
      c. As a result, CHF develops.
   5. Treatment:
      a. Small defects—spontaneous closure.

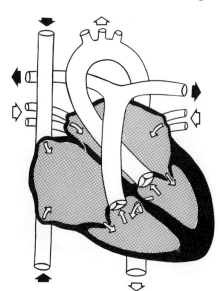

Fig 21–3.—Ventricular septal defect. (From Ross Laboratories Clinical Education Aid No. 7 (G163). Columbus, Ohio, 1978. Reproduced by permission.)

        b. Large defects—surgical correction necessary.

D. Aortic Stenosis (subaortic stenosis) (Fig 21–4)

    1. Acyanotic anomaly.

    2. Obstructive outflow lesion of the left ventricle.

    3. Develops as a result of a fibrous lesion at the aortic semilunar valve.

    4. Left ventricular hypertrophy develops as a result of the increased resistance to cardiac output.

    5. Treatment: Surgical correction may be necessary, achieved by performing an aortic valvulotomy or by a division of the fibrous obstruction below the aortic semilunar valve.

E. Coarctation of the Aorta (Fig 21–5)

    1. Acyanotic or cyanotic anomaly.

    2. Characterized by a narrowed aortic lumen.

    3. Majority of cardiac output moves to the head and upper extremities.

    4. Hypertension frequently develops in the upper extremities and hypotension in the lower extremities.

    5. Types of coarctation

        a. Preductal coarctation: Stenosis of the aorta proximal to the entrance of the ductus arteriosus. This will cause cyanosis (right-to-left shunting).

        b. Postductal coarctation: Stenosis of the aorta distal to the ductus arteriosus. This will not cause cyanosis (left-to-right shunting).

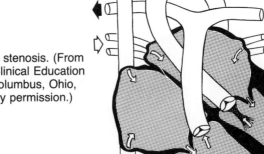

Fig 21–4.—Aortic stenosis. (From Ross Laboratories Clinical Education Aid No. 7 (G163). Columbus, Ohio, 1978. Reproduced by permission.)

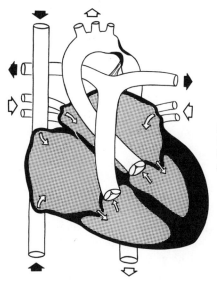

Fig 21–5.—Coarctation of the aorta. (From Ross Laboratories Clinical Education Aid No. 7 (G163). Columbus, Ohio, 1978. Reproduced by permission.)

6. Treatment:
   a. Medical treatment with digitalis for heart failure.
   b. Surgical correction is usually necessary, by resection of the coarctation.
F. Tricuspid Atresia (Fig 21–6)
   1. Cyanotic anomaly (right-to-left shunting).

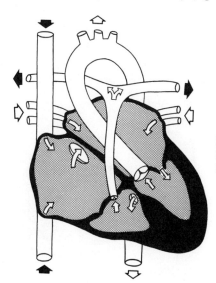

Fig 21–6.—Tricuspid atresia. (From Ross Laboratories Clinical Education Aid No. 7 (G163). Columbus, Ohio, 1978. Reproduced by permission.)

2. Obstructive lesion—the normal pathway of blood from the right atrium to the right ventricle through the tricuspid valve is partially blocked.
3. Characterized by the following:
   a. Small right ventricle.
   b. Large left ventricle.
   c. Diminished pulmonary circulation.
4. Blood from the right atrium passes through an ASD into the left atrium, where it mixes with oxygenated blood from pulmonary veins.
5. Then blood flows into the left ventricle and can go into the aorta or through a VSD to the right ventricle and into the pulmonary circulation.
6. Treatment: Surgical correction is necessary and entails anastomosis of the aorta to the pulmonary artery and/or anastomosis of the superior vena cava to the right pulmonary artery to increase pulmonary blood flow.

G. Tetralogy of Fallot (Fig 21–7)
   1. Cyanotic anomaly (right-to-left shunt).
   2. Characterized by the following:
      a. VSD
      b. Stenosis of the pulmonic valve
      c. Dextroposition of the aorta
      d. Hypertrophy of the right ventricle

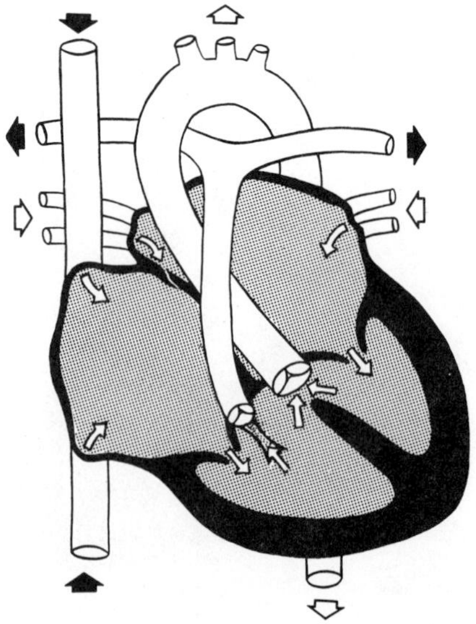

Fig 21–7.—Tetralogy of Fallot. (From Ross Laboratories Clinical Education Aid No. 7 (G163). Columbus, Ohio, 1978. Reproduced by permission.)

3. Obstruction to right ventricular outflow because of pulmonary stenosis causes right ventricular hypertrophy. Blood will then be shunted through the VSD into the dextropositional aorta. This will cause blood from the right side of the heart to pass directly into the systemic system unoxygenated. Right ventricular pressure will be equal to left ventricular pressure.
4. Treatment: Medical management, including adequate hydration. Surgery may be necessary to create an anastomosis between systemic and pulmonary circulations to increase pulmonary blood flow.

H. Truncus Arteriosus (Fig 21–8)
1. Cyanotic anomaly (right-to-left shunt)
2. Characterized by:
   a. VSD associated with a common blood vessel leaving both ventricles.
   b. Branching of pulmonary arteries from the common vessel (truncus), which continues as the aorta.
   c. Variable pulmonary blood flow, dependent on level of the stenosis distal to branching of the pulmonary arteries.
   d. Variable pulmonary symptoms, depending on amount of pulmonary circulation.
   e. Both right and left ventricular hypertrophy is common.
3. An admixture of venous and arterial blood from the right and left ventricle empties into a common vessel (bulbar trunk) at

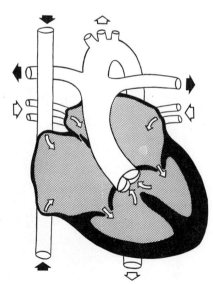

Fig 21–8.—Truncus arteriosus. (From Ross Laboratories Clinical Education Aid No. 7 (G163). Columbus, Ohio, 1978. Reproduced by permission.)

systemic pressure. Blood will either continue out the trunk to the systemic circulation or enter the pulmonary arteries. Pulmonary hypertension is often present.

4. Treatment: No surgical correction is available at this time. Medical management is used to reduce pulmonary hypertension and infections.

I. Complete Transposition of the Great Vessels (Fig 21–9)
1. Cyanotic anomaly (right-to-left shunt).
2. Characterized by:
   a. Reversed position of aorta and pulmonary arteries (i.e., the aorta comes off the right ventricle and the pulmonary artery comes off the left ventricle).
   b. Frequently a PDA and ASO are present.
3. Two separate circulations occur with the aorta emanating from the right ventricle and returning through systemic veins into the right atrium and the pulmonary artery emanating from the left ventricle and returning to the left atrium via the pulmonary veins. Venous and arterial blood may mix through an ASD, VSD, or PDA (Table 21–1).
4. Treatment: Surgical correction may be necessary.

J. Anomalous venous return of the pulmonary veins (Fig 21–10)
1. Cyanotic anomaly (right-to-left shunt).
2. Characterized by oxygenated blood returning from the lungs to the right atrium by one or more pulmonary veins.

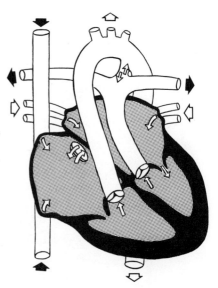

Fig 21–9.—Complete transposition of the great vessels. (From Ross Laboratories Clinical Education Aid No. 7 (G163). Columbus, Ohio, 1978. Reproduced by permission.)

TABLE 21–1.—CARDIAC ANOMALIES

DEFECT	CHARACTERISTIC FEATURES	DIRECTION OF SHUNT	PRESENCE OF CYANOSIS	TREATMENT
Patent Ductus Arteriosus (PDA)	Failure of DA to close at birth	Left to right	Acyanotic	Indomethacin (Indocin); surgical correction
Atrial Septal Defect (ASD)	Failure of foramen ovale to close or septum to form correctly	Left to right	Acyanotic	Surgical correction
Ventricular Septal Defect (VSD)	Failure of the septal wall to form properly	Left to right	Acyanotic	Surgical correction if large
Aortic Stenosis	Fibrous lesion at the aortic semilunar valve causing ventricular hypertrophy	No shunt present	Acyanotic	Surgical correction if severe
Coarctation of Aorta:				
Preductal	Stenosis of aorta proximal to entrance of ductus arteriosus	Right to left	Cyanotic	Standard therapy for heart failure
Postductal	Stenosis of aorta distal to entrance of ductus arteriosus	Left to right	Acyanotic	Surgical resection
Tricuspid Atresia	Blockage of the tricuspid valve: Small rt. ventricle Large lf. ventricle ASD	Right to left	Cyanotic	Surgical correction
Tetralogy of Fallot	VSD Stenosis of pulmonic valve Dextroposition of aorta Hypertrophic rt. ventricle	Right to left	Cyanotic	Surgical correction may be necessary
Truncus Arteriosus	VSD with common vessel leaving both ventricles; pulmonary arteries branch from common vessel, which continues as aorta RT. and lf. ventricular hypertrophy	Right to left	Cyanotic	No surgical correction available Treat hypertension
Complete Transposition of Great Vessels	Reversed position of aorta and pulmonary arteries Frequently PDA or ASD	Right to left	Cyanosis	Surgical correction usually necessary
Anomalous Venous Return	Pulmonary veins (one or more) returning to right atrium	Right to left	Cyanosis	Surgical correction usually necessary

3. Types of anomalous return:
   a. Complete: All pulmonary and systemic veins enter the right atrium. Interatrial communication is needed for oxygenated blood to reach the systemic circulation.
   b. Partial: Some pulmonary veins enter the left atrium.

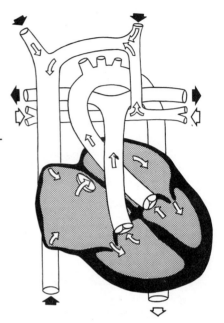

Fig 21–10.—Anomalous venous return of the pulmonary veins. (From Ross Laboratories Clinical Education Aid No. 7 (G163). Columbus, Ohio, 1978. Reproduced by permission.)

4. Treatment:
   a. Complete anomalous return requires transplanting anomalous pulmonary veins from the right atrium to the left atrium and closing the ASD.
   b. With partial anomalous return, surgical correction may not be necessary.
X. Pulmonary Anomalies
   A. Choanal atresia: Blockage of the opening into the nasopharynx by a membranous tissue, usually with bony implants.
      1. If bilateral, the condition is a respiratory emergency because it inhibits nasal ventilation.
      2. If a nasal suction catheter cannot be passed, choanal atresia should be suspected in a neonate with severe respiratory distress.
      3. Treatment: Surgical correction is necessary.
   B. Esophageal atresia: Malformation of esophagus, with tracheoesophageal fistulas a common complication.
      1. Types
         a. Atresia of upper esophagus, with lower esophagus connected to trachea or mainstem bronchi.
         b. An intact trachea, but unattached stomach and esophagus.
         c. H-type fistula: A normal trachea and esophagus connected by a small tubelike fistula.

2. Clinical signs
   a. Accumulation of oral secretions
   b. Continuous or sporadic respiratory distress
   c. Abdominal distention as a result of air entry
   d. Treatment: Surgical correction is necessary.
C. Diaphragmatic hernia: Result of incomplete development of diaphragm, allowing abdominal organs to enter the thoracic cavity.
   1. Respiratory and cardiovascular stress is pronounced.
   2. Most hernias occur on the left side, frequently causing a shift of the mediastinum and atelectasis.
   3. Treatment: Immediate surgical correction is necessary.
D. Congenital laryngeal stridor or partial airway obstruction: Result of incomplete development of larynx
   1. May cause mild respiratory distress.
   2. Usually improves with maturing of laryngeal and tracheal cartilage.
E. Lung hypoplasia and aplasia
   1. A partial (hypoplasia) or complete (aplasia) lack of development of the parenchyma of a lung.
   2. Results from in utero failure to develop an adequate circulation to the affected lung, lobe, or segment, causing a reduction in lung parenchyma.
   3. If only a small portion of the lung is involved, physiologic effects are minimal.
   4. If lungs are aplastic, the reduction in lung parenchyma means a reduction in pulmonary vasculature. This causes pulmonary hypertension and right heart failure.
   5. Lung aplasia or hypoplasia can be seen with other anomalies.
   6. Treatment: Symptomatic; no specific intervention is specified.

BIBLIOGRAPHY
Alfery D.D., Ward C.F., Plumer M.H., et al.: Management of tracheal atresia with tracheoesophageal fistula. *Anesthesiology* 53:242–246, 1980.
Avery G.B. (ed.): *Neonatology, Pathophysiology and Management of the Newborn,* ed. 2. Philadelphia, J.B. Lippincott Co., 1981.
Avery M.E.: *The Lung and Its Disorders in the Newborn Infant,* ed. 2. Philadelphia, W.B. Saunders Co., 1981.
Avery M.E., Gatewood D.B., Brumley G.: Transient tachypnea of the newborn. *Am. J. Dis. Child.* 111:380–385, 1966.
Ballard R.A., Ballard P.L., Granberg J.P., et al.: Prenatal administration of betamethasone for prevention of respiratory distress syndrome. *J. Pediatr.* 94:97–101, 1979.
Bearman R.E. (ed.): *Neonatology and Diseases of the Fetus and Infant.* St. Louis, C.V. Mosby Co., 1973.

Berg T.J., Pagtakhan R.D., Reed M.H., et al.: Bronchopulmonary dysplasia and lung rupture in hyaline membrane disease: Influence of continuous distending pressure. *Pediatrics* 55:51–54, 1975.

Burgess W.R., Chernick V.: *Respiratory Therapy in Newborn Infants and Children.* New York, Thieme & Stratton, Inc., 1982.

Coates A.L., Bergsteinsson H., Desmond K., et al.: Long-term pulmonary sequelae of premature birth with and without idiopathic respiratory distress syndrome. *J. Pediatr.* 90:611–616, 1977.

Farrell P.M., Avery M.E.: Hyaline membrane disease. *Am. Rev. Respir. Dis.* 111:657–688, 1975.

Fox W.W., Dvara S.: Persistent pulmonary hypertension in the neonate: Diagnosis and management. *J. Pediatr.* 103:505–514, 1983.

Goldsmith J.P., Karotkin E.M. (eds.): *Assisted Ventilation of the Neonate.* Philadelphia, W.B. Saunders Co., 1981.

Goodwin J.W.: *Perinatal Medicine—The Basic Science Underlying Clinical Practice.* Baltimore, Williams & Wilkins Co., 1976.

Gregory G.A., Kitterman J.A., Phibbs R.H., et al.: Treatment of the idiopathic respiratory distress syndrome with continuous positive airway pressure. *N. Engl. J. Med.* 284:1333–1340, 1971.

Helms M.B., Stocks J.: Lung function in infants with congenital pulmonary hypoplasia. *J. Pediatr.* 101:918–922, 1982.

Kelly D.H., Shannon D.C.: Treatment of apnea in excessive periodic breathing in the full term infant. *Pediatrics* 68:183–186, 1981.

Klaus M.H., Fanaroff A.A.: *Care of the High-Risk Neonate,* ed. 2. Philadelphia, W.B. Saunders Co., 1979.

Korones S.B.: *High-Risk Newborn Infants,* ed. 3. St. Louis, C.V. Mosby Co., 1981.

Lough M.D., Williams T.J., Rawson J.E.: *Newborn Respiratory Care.* Chicago, Year Book Medical Publishers, Inc., 1979.

Murphy J.D., Rabinovitch M., Goldstein J.D., et al.: The structural basis of persistent pulmonary hypertension of the newborn infant. *J. Pediatr.* 98:962–967, 1981.

Naeye R.L.: Neonatal apnea: Underlying disorders. *Pediatrics* 63:8–12, 1979.

Northway W.H., Rosan R.C., Porter D.V.: Pulmonary disease following respirator therapy of hyaline-membrane disease–bronchopulmonary displasia. *N. Engl. J. Med.* 276:357–368, 1967.

Philip A.G.S.: Oxygen plus pressure plus time: The etiology of bronchopulmonary dysplasia. *Pediatrics* 55:44–50, 1975.

Ross Laboratories Clinical Education Aids No. 1–18. Ross Laboratories, Columbus, Ohio, 1976.

Scarpelli E.M.: *Pulmonary Physiology of the Fetus, Newborn and Child.* Philadelphia, Lea & Febiger, 1975.

Storer J.S.: Respiratory problems unique to the newborn. *Respir. Care* 20:1146–1152, 1975.

Strang L.B.: *Neonatal Respiration: Physiologic and Clinical Studies.* Philadelphia, J.B. Lippincott Co., 1974.

Thibeault D.W., Gregory G.A.: *Neonatal Pulmonary Care.* Philadelphia, Addison-Wesley Publishing Co., 1979.

Wesenberg R.L.: *The Newborn Chest.* Hagerstown, Md., Harper & Row, Publishers, 1973.

William J.W.: *Handbook of Neonatal Respiratory Care.* Riverside, Calif., Bourns, Inc., 1977.

Wilson M.G., Mikity V.G.: A new form of respiratory disease in premature infants. *Am. J. Dis. Child.* 99:489–499, 1960.

Yanagi R.M., Wilson A., Newfield E.A., et al.: Indomethacin treatment for symptomatic patent ductus arteriosus: A double-blind controlled study. *Pediatrics* 67:647–652, 1981.

22 / Pediatric Pulmonary Diseases

I. Cystic Fibrosis (Mucoviscidosis)
   A. A generalized genetic abnormality of the exocrine glands resulting primarily in malfunction of pancreas, sweat glands, salivary glands, and respiratory mucosal glands.
   B. Etiology and incidence
      1. A non-sex-linked autosomal recessive trait primarily affecting Northern European Caucasians.
      2. About one of every 2,000 Caucasians is born with the disease.
   C. Prognosis
      1. Extremely poor: Patients usually die before age 25.
      2. A mortality of 90%, associated with respiratory complications.
   D. Clinical manifestations
      1. Chronic pulmonary disease.
      2. Pancreatic insufficiency.
      3. Increased electrolyte concentration in sweat.
   E. Clinical symptoms
      1. Gastrointestinal
         a. Pancreatic enzyme deficiency resulting from obstruction of the pancreatic duct in 80%–85% of patients.
         b. Very large appetite with little or no weight gain.
         c. Incomplete digestion of food (especially fats and proteins).
         d. Large, bulky, loose stools, pale and foul smelling.
         e. Protruding abdomen.
         f. Intestinal obstruction in 5%–10% of patients at birth (meconium ileus).
         g. Some 95% of cystic males are sterile.
      2. Pulmonary
         a. Initially a dry, hacking cough
         b. With time, development of a loose and more productive cough
         c. Eventually paroxysmal coughing
         d. Fatigability
         e. Shortness of breath
         f. Fever

      g. Barrel-chested appearance

      h. Clubbing of fingers

      i. Cyanosis

      j. Frequent infections

  F. Diagnosis

     1. Positive diagnosis normally is dependent on a "sweat test" or iontophoresis, which measures the chloride content of the sweat. Normally 18 mEq/L of chloride is contained in the sweat. If more than 60 mEq/L of chloride is found, diagnosis is positive.

     2. Increased amount of fat in stool.

     3. Decreased amount of trypsin in stool.

     4. Decreased blood chloride and sodium levels.

  G. X-ray

     1. If pulmonary problems are not significant, the chest x-ray may be normal.

     2. As the disease progresses, pulmonary manifestations show a hyperinflation pattern on x-ray studies.

     3. If end-stage cardiac decompensation is present, vascular engorgement and myocardial hypertrophy may be seen.

  H. Management

     1. Gastrointestinal problems

       a. Pancreatic enzyme substitutes.

       b. Diet: Low fat, high protein, and high caloric intake.

     2. Respiratory problems

       a. Aggressive bronchial hygiene with aerosol and chest physiotherapy on a daily basis.

       b. Mucolytics to improve clearance of secretions.

       c. IPPB therapy generally not indicated because of presence of bullous lung disease and potential for pneumothorax.

       d. Appropriate antibiotic administration, when indicated by infection.

       e. Oxygen therapy if necessary in acute exacerbation and in end-stage disease.

II. Bronchiolitis

  A. Inflammation of the bronchioles primarily associated with children, aged 6 months to 3 years, but also may occur in adults, especially those with chronic bronchitis or emphysema.

  B. Etiology: Respiratory syncytial virus (RSV), in children primarily.

  C. Clinical manifestations in children

     1. Fever

    2. Cough

    3. Audible expiratory wheezing

    4. Increased anteroposterior chest diameter with hyperresonance

    5. Subcostal, intercostal, and suprasternal retractions commonly noted

    6. Inspiratory and expiratory wheezes as well as rhonchi frequently noted

  D. X-ray: Hyperinflation.

  E. Treatment: Symptomatic; artificial airways and mechanical ventilation sometimes required.

III. Croup

  A. Inflammation of larynx and trachea, confined to subglottic area; also referred to as laryngotracheobronchitis.

  B. Etiology: Almost exclusively *viral infection*.

    1. Most common causative viruses:

      a. Parainfluenza virus

      b. Respiratory syncytial virus (RSV)

      c. Influenza virus

      d. Adenovirus

  C. Diagnosis: Based on lateral x-ray of neck on which the epiglottis is seen as normal, whereas the area of the larynx and trachea is hazy indicating inflammation.

  D. Clinical manifestations

    1. Normally occurs between ages 6 months and 3 years.

    2. Primarily a dry, barking cough.

    3. Inspiratory stridor and noisy, labored breathing.

    4. Onset of symptoms progress over a period of 1–2 days before cough reaches maximum severity.

  E. Laboratory analysis: Normal WBC count compatible with a viral infection.

  F. Treatment

    1. Cool aerosol mist

    2. Racemic epinephrine

    3. Systemic hydration

    4. Oxygen therapy

    5. Cough suppressant

IV. Epiglottitis

  A. Acute inflammation of supraglottic area, having the potential of causing complete upper airway obstruction.

  B. Etiology: *Bacterial, Haemophilus influenzae* being the most frequent agent in children.

  C. Diagnosis

1. Lateral x-ray of neck, in which the epiglottis appears as a large, round, dense tissue mass covering the opening of the trachea. Subglottic area appears normal.
2. Visualization of epiglottis by direct laryngoscopy should be performed with extreme caution because of increased potential of spasm of epiglottis and complete obstruction.

D. Clinical manifestations
   1. Epiglottitis normally occurs in older children (between ages 2 and 8 years).
   2. Primary feature: Rapid onset. Symptoms may progress to the point of partial or complete airway obstruction in about 8 hours.
   3. Patient complains of a sore throat and has noisy, labored breathing, inspiratory stridor, hoarseness, and fever.
   4. Speech and cough are muffled due to dampening effect of the swollen epiglottis.
   5. Patient is unable to swallow; drooling is common.
   6. Patient assumes a sitting position with lower jaw thrust forward.

E. Laboratory analysis: Elevated WBC count compatible with bacterial infection.

F. Treatment
   1. Artificial airway
   2. Appropriate antibiotic therapy
   3. Symptomatic treatment of fever (Table 22–1)

V. Sudden Infant Death Syndrome (SIDS)
   A. Defined as the sudden death of an infant or young child, unexpected by history, in which a thorough postmortem examination fails to reveal an adequate cause of death.
   B. Common etiologic factors
      1. Infant's age usually between 1 month and 1 year with greatest incidence in infants aged 2–4 months.
      2. Nonwhites affected most, with American Indians, Alaskan natives, and socioeconomically disadvantaged blacks having the highest risk.
      3. Typically the mother is less than 20 years old, unmarried, poor, had little or no prenatal care, and has smoked cigarettes and/or abused drugs (especially narcotics).
   C. Probable causes
      1. Apnea caused by immature neurologic control of ventilation.
      2. Upper respiratory tract infection present on autopsy in 50% of all SIDS victims.

TABLE 22–1.—COMPARISON OF CROUP AND EPIGLOTTITIS

FACTOR	CROUP	EPIGLOTTITIS
Etiology	Virus: *Parainfluenza*	Bacteria: *Haemophilus influenzae*
WBC	Normal	Elevated
Onset	Gradual	Sudden
Cough	Dry, barking	Muffled
Lateral neck x-ray	Subglottic inflammation	Supraglottic inflammation
Treatment	Symptomatic	Artificial airway

     3. Airway obstruction during sleep.
     4. Triggering of mammalian diving reflex.
  D. Treatment
     1. Cardiopulmonary resuscitation
     2. Pneumograms
     3. Apnea monitors

BIBLIOGRAPHY

Burgess W.R., Cherniack V.: *Respiratory Therapy in Newborn Infants and Children.* New York, Thieme & Stratton, 1982.

Coates A.L., Bergsteinssen H., Desmond K., et al.: Long-term pulmonary sequelae of premature birth with and without idiopathic respiratory distress syndrome. *J. Pediatr.* 90:611–616, 1977.

Desmond K.J., Schsunk W.F., Thomas E., et al.: Immediate and long-term effects of chest physiotherapy in patients with cystic fibrosis. *J. Pediatr.* 103:538–542, 1983.

Eigen H.: Croup or epiglottis: Differential diagnosis and treatment. *Respir. Care* 20:1158–1164, 1975.

Fogel J.M., Berg J., Gerber M.A., et al.: Racemic epinephrine in the treatment of croup: Nebulization alone versus nebulization with intermittent positive pressure breathing. *J. Pediatr.* 101:1028–1031, 1982.

Goodwin J.W., et al.: *Perinatal Medicine—The Basic Science Underlying Clinical Practice.* Baltimore, Williams & Wilkins Co., 1976.

Kelly D.T., Shannon D.C., O'Connell K.: Care of infants with near miss sudden infant death syndrome. *Pediatrics* 61:511–514, 1978.

Keuskamp D.H.C.: *Neonatal and Pediatric Ventilation.* Boston, Little, Brown & Co., 1974.

Lough M.D., Doershuk C.F., Stern R.C.: *Pediatric Respiratory Therapy,* ed. 2. Chicago, Year Book Medical Publishers, Inc., 1979.

Moss A.J.: The cardiovascular system in cystic fibrosis. *Pediatrics* 70:728–741, 1982.

Myer C.M., Cotton R.T.: Nasal obstruction in the pediatric patient. *Pediatrics* 72:766–777, 1983.

Nash G., Blennerhassett J.B., Pontoppidan H.: Pulmonary lesions associated with oxygen therapy and artificial ventilation. *N. Engl. J. Med.* 276:368–374, 1967.

Neonatal Screening for Cystic Fibrosis: Position Paper of the Cystic Fibrosis Foundation. *Pediatrics* 72:741–745, 1983.

Nowakowski L.: *Pediatrics: Specific Anatomic Variables, Newborn Respiratory Tract.* Washington, D.C., Robert J. Brady Co., 1974.

Ross Laboratories Clinical Education Aids No. 1–18. Ross Laboratories, Columbus, Ohio, 1976.

Scarpelli E.M.: *Pulmonary Physiology of the Fetus, Newborn and Child.* Philadelphia, Lea & Febiger, 1975.

Scarpelli E.M.: *Pulmonary Diseases of the Fetus, Newborn and Child.* Philadelphia, Lea & Febiger, 1978.

Schenker M.B., Samet J.M., Speizer F.E.: Risk factors for childhood respiratory diseases. *Am. Rev. Respir. Dis.* 128:1038–1043, 1983.

Selbst S.M.: Epiglottitis. *Am. J. Emerg. Med.* 3:342–350, 1983.

Shannon D.C., Kelly D.A.: SIDS and near SIDS. *N. Engl. J. Med.* 306:959–965, 1022–1028, 1982.

Slonim N.B.: *Pediatric Respiratory Therapy: An Introductory Text.* Sarasota, Glenn Educational Medical Services, Inc., 1974.

Southall D.P.: Home monitoring and its role in the sudden infant death syndrome. *Pediatrics* 72:133–138, 1983.

Valdes-Dapens M.A.: Sudden infant death syndrome: A review of the medical literature. *Pediatrics* 66:597–614, 1980.

Welliver R.C., Wong D.T., Middleton E., et al.: Role of parainfluenza virus-specific IgE in pathogenesis of croup and wheezing subsequent to infection. *J. Pediatr.* 101:889–896, 1982.

23 / Gas Therapy

I. Medical, Laboratory, and Therapeutic Gases and Mixtures
   A. Ethylene (C_2H_4)
   B. Nitrous oxide (N_2O)
   C. Cyclopropane [$(CH_2)_3$]
   D. Oxygen (O_2)
   E. Nitrogen (N_2)
   F. Carbon dioxide (CO_2)
   G. Helium (He)
   H. Oxygen/nitrogen (21% O_2/79% N_2)
   I. Oxygen/carbon dioxide (90%–98% O_2/2%–10% CO_2)
   J. Helium/oxygen (40%–80% He/20%–60% O_2)
II. Flammable Gases
   A. Ethylene
   B. Cyclopropane
III. Nonflammable Gases
   A. Nitrogen
   B. Carbon dioxide
   C. Helium
IV. Gases That Support Combustion
   A. Oxygen
   B. Helium/oxygen
   C. Oxygen/carbon dioxide
   D. Oxygen/nitrogen
   E. Nitrous oxide
V. Gas Cylinders
   A. Cylinder types and composition
      1. Type 3AA: Seamless, high-quality, heat-treated steel, spun chrome molybdenum
      2. Type 3A: Seamless, low carbon, heat-treated steel (no longer produced)
   B. Cylinder markings: Markings are located at the neck of the cylinder in two groupings (Fig 23–1)
      1. Front
         a. Line 1: ICC or DOT, 3A or 3AA, 2015
            (1) ICC or DOT: The organization governing the transport of cylinder

358

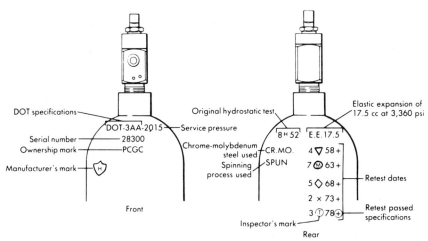

DOT specifications

Serial number
Ownership mark

Manufacturer's mark

DOT-3AA-2015 — Service pressure
28300
PCGC

Front

Original hydrostatic test

Chrome-molybdenum
steel used
Spinning
process used

Inspector's mark

Rear

8 H 52   E.E. 17.5

CR.MO.   4 ▽ 58 +
SPUN   7 Ⓝ 63 +

5 ◇ 68 +

2 × 73 +

3 ① 78 ⊕

Elastic expansion of
17.5 cc at 3,360 psi

Retest dates

Retest passed
specifications

Fig 23–1.—Typical markings for cylinders containing medical gases, front and back views. (From Spearman C.B., Sheldon R.L., Egan D.F.: *Egan's Fundamentals of Respiratory Therapy,* ed. 4. St. Louis, C.V. Mosby Co., 1982. Reproduced by permission.)

(a) ICC: Interstate Commerce Commission. The agency that regulated construction, transport, and testing of compressed gas cylinders from 1948 to 1970.

(b) DOT: Department of Transportation. The federal agency responsible for construction, transport, and testing of compressed gas cylinders since 1970.

(2) 3A or 3AA: Cylinder type

(3) 2,015: Maximum working pressure in pounds per square inch (psi), which normally can be exceeded by 10% (2,200 psi).

b. Line 2: 28300, Serial number

c. Line 3: PCGC

(1) PCGC: Initial of owner

d. Line 4: Manufacturer's mark

2. Rear: Refer to Figure 23–1

C. Cylinder size

1. Large cylinders using hexagonal nut connections

a. H or K: 9 in. diameter, 55 in. height

b. G: 8½ in. diameter, 55 in. height

c. M: 7⅛ in. diameter, 46 in. height

d. F: 5½ in. diameter, 55 in. height

2. Small cylinders using yoke connections

    a. E: 4¼ in. diameter, 30 in. height
    b. D: 4¼ in. diameter, 20 in. height
    c. B: 3½ in. diameter, 16 in. height
    d. A: 3 in. diameter, 10 in. height

D. Cylinder capacities for oxygen
  1. D: 12.7 cu ft
  2. E: 22 cu ft
  3. G: 187 cu ft
  4. H or K: 244 cu ft

E. Maximum filling pressure of 3AA oxygen cylinders: 2,015 psi plus 10% (2,200 psi).

F. Calculation of duration of flow from oxygen and compressed air cylinders.
  1. One cubic foot of gas = 28.3 L.
  2. The volume of gas in liters in a full cylinder = cubic foot volume × 28.3 L/cu ft.
  3. Dividing the above determined value by the maximum filling pressure of 2,200 psi results in the calculation of a factor indicating the number of liters per pound per square inch:

$$\text{Factor for duration of flow} = \frac{(\text{cu ft vol})(28.3 \text{ L/cu ft})}{2,200 \text{ psi}} \tag{1}$$

  4. For a D size cylinder:

$$\frac{(12.7 \text{ cu ft})(28.3 \text{ L/cu ft})}{2,200 \text{ psi}} = 0.16 \text{ L/psi}$$

  5. Liters per psi factors for oxygen cylinders
    a. D: 0.16 L/psi
    b. E: 0.28 L/psi
    c. G: 2.41 L/psi
    d. H or K: 3.14 L/psi
  6. Calculation of duration of flow in minutes
    a. Gauge pressure multiplied by duration of flow factor (L/psi) equals the number of liters in the cylinder.
    b. Dividing the result of 6a by the flow in liters per minute results in the time in minutes that the cylinder will last:

$$\text{Time in minutes cylinder will last} = \frac{(\text{Gauge pressure})(\text{Duration of flow factor})}{(\text{Flow in L/min})} \tag{2}$$

c. Example for E cylinder:

Gauge pressure	1,500 psi
Duration of flow factor	0.28 L/psi
Flow in L/min	10 L/min

$$42 \text{ min} = \frac{(1{,}500 \text{ psi})(0.28 \text{ L/psi})}{10 \text{ L/min}}$$

The cylinder will deliver 10 L/min for 42 minutes before it is completely empty.

d. Clinically, it is advisable to subtract 500 psi from the gauge pressure to provide a safety margin before calculating duration of flow.

G. Color code for E cylinders (color coding is mandatory for E size cylinders only; other size cylinders are not required to follow any coding system).

1. Oxygen: Green (universal code: white)
2. Helium: Brown
3. Ethylene: Red
4. Cyclopropane: Orange
5. Nitrous oxide: Light blue
6. Carbon dioxide: Gray
7. Oxygen and carbon dioxide: Green and gray
8. Oxygen and helium: Green and brown

H. Hydrostatic testing of cylinders

1. Periodic high-pressure testing of gas cylinder integrity.
2. Cylinder expansion is determined by measuring water displacement of an empty cylinder compared to that cylinder when filled to ⅗ of its maximum pressure.
3. All cylinders must be retested every 5–10 years, depending on elastic expansion of the original testing.

I. Cylinder stem pop-off valves

1. Large cylinders use a frangible disk designed to rupture at a pressure within 5% of cylinder-bursting pressure.
2. Small cylinders use a fusable plug designed to melt at a temperature of 150°–170° F.

VI. Regulation of Gas Flow

A. High-pressure gas regulators

1. Regulators limit flow in a system by reducing maximum working pressure.
2. Regulators reduce cylinder pressures to a usable working pressure of 50 psi or less.

3. Single-stage regulators
   a. Cylinder pressure is reduced to a working pressure of up to 50 psi in one step or stage.
   b. One high-pressure pop-off valve is incorporated in the regulator and set at about 200 psi.
4. Multistage regulators
   a. Cylinder pressure is reduced to a working pressure of up to 50 psi in a series of steps or stages.
   b. A high-pressure pop-off valve is incorporated into each stage of the regulator, with the final stage pop-off set at about 200 psi.
5. Preset regulators (Fig 23–2)

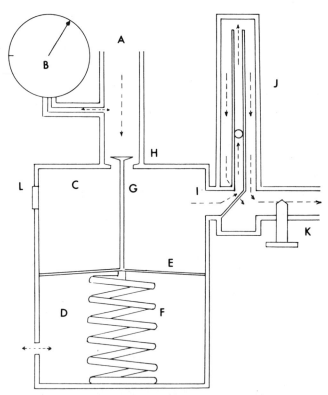

Fig 23–2.—Diagram of preset, high-pressure gas regulator. *A*, Attachment to cylinder; *B*, pressure gauge; *C*, pressure chamber; *D*, ambient pressure chamber; *E*, Flexible diaphragm; *F*, spring; *G*, valve stem; *H*, gas entry valve; *I*, outflow port; *J*, Thorpe tube flowmeter; *K*, needle valve; *L*, pop-off valve. (From Spearman C.B., Sheldon R.L., Egan D.F.: *Egan's Fundamentals of Respiratory Therapy*, ed. 4. St. Louis, C.V. Mosby Co., 1982. Reproduced by permission.)

a. Pressure is reduced in one or more stages to a fixed working pressure of 50 psi.
b. Normally a low-pressure gas-regulating device (e.g., Thorpe tube) is incorporated to reduce flows to working levels.
c. Preset regulators are used without a Thorpe tube when connected to a system utilizing a 50 psi pressure source (e.g., ventilators).

6. Adjustable regulators (Fig 23–3)

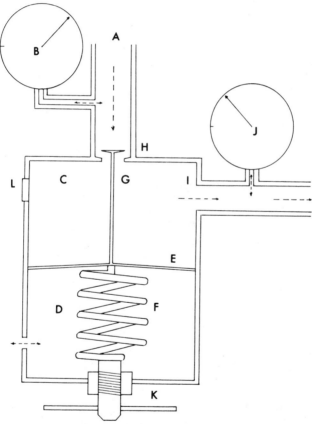

Fig 23–3.—Diagram of an adjustable, high-pressure gas regulator. *A,* attachment to cylinder; *B,* pressure gauge; *C,* pressure chamber; *D,* ambient pressure chamber; *E,* flexible diaphragm; *F,* spring; *G,* valve stem; *H,* gas entry valve; *I,* outflow port; *J,* Bourdon flow gauge; *K,* threaded gas flow control; *L,* pop-off valve. (From Spearman C.B., Sheldon R.L., Egan D.F.: *Egan's Fundamentals of Respiratory Therapy,* ed. 4. St. Louis, C.V. Mosby Co., 1982. Reproduced by permission.)

a. Pressure is reduced in one or more stages to a final working pressure adjustable to between 0 and 50 psi.

b. Normally a Bourdon pressure gauge calibrated in liters per minute indicates flow leaving the final stage of the adjustable regulator.

B. Low-pressure gas regulators (flowmeters)

  1. Bourdon gauge (Fig 23–4)

    a. A pressure-sensitive gauge that uses an expandable copper coil to indicate pressure readings.

    b. Bourdon gauges can be calibrated to indicate flow and are used as flow-measuring devices.

    c. If back pressure is applied distal to the gauge, it will indicate a flow higher than actual flow.

  2. Thorpe tube flowmeters (Fig 23–5): Gas flow is measured by the vertical displacement of a float in an increasing diameter tube. Flow is regulated by a needle valve placed proximal or distal to the float.

    a. Compensated Thorpe tubes are designed to function accurately at a working pressure of 50 psi at 70° F.

      (1) The needle valve is always located distal to the float.

      (2) If backpressure is applied distal to the needle valve, the float will indicate the actual flow delivered.

    b. Uncompensated Thorpe tubes are designed to function at variable working pressures.

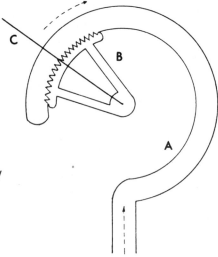

Fig 23–4.—Internal function of a Bourdon gauge. *A,* curved, flexible, closed tube; *B,* gear mechanism; *C,* indicator needle, reflecting flow or pressure on face of valve. (From Spearman C.B., Sheldon R.L., Egan D.F.: *Egan's Fundamentals of Respiratory Therapy,* ed. 4. St. Louis, C.V. Mosby Co., 1982. Reproduced by permission.)

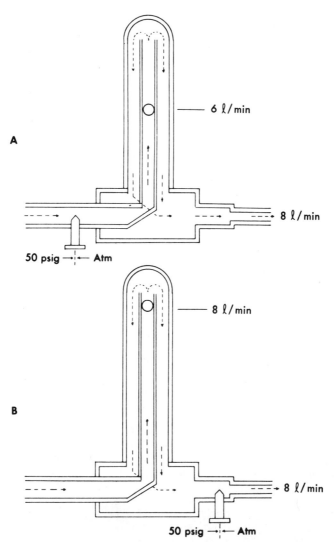

Fig 23–5.—Comparison of pressure-uncompensated **(A)** and pressure-compensated **(B)** flowmeters. In the former, the flow-control valve is proximal to the meter, and the gauge records less than the actual output. In the latter, location of the valve distal to the meter correlates the gauge reading with the output. (From Spearman C.B., Sheldon R.L., Egan D.F.: *Egan's Fundamentals of Respiratory Therapy,* ed. 4. St. Louis, C.V. Mosby Co., 1982. Reproduced by permission.)

(1) The needle valve is always located proximal to the float.

(2) If backpressure is applied distal to the float, the float will always indicate a flow lower than the actual flow delivered.

VII. Safety Systems Incorporated in Gas Flow Systems and Cylinders

  A. Pin Index Safety System (PISS) (Fig 23–6)

    1. This system is only used on *E size cylinders or smaller.*

    2. It is used on connections where the maximum working pressure is greater than 200 psig (pounds per square inch gauge).

    3. It incorporates a yoke type of connection where two pins on the regulator connection (yoke) are matched to holes on the cylinder stem.

    4. Ten possible combinations are available, nine currently in use.

    5. Pin positions 2–5 are used for oxygen.

  B. American Standard Compressed Gas Cylinder Valve Outlet and Inlet Connections Safety System (Fig 23–7)

    1. This system is only used on cylinders *larger than* E size.

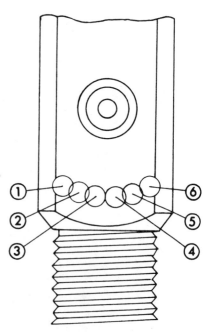

Fig 23–6.—Location of the Pin-Index Safety System holes in the cylinder valve face, various pairs of which constitute indices for different gases. See text for complete pairings. (From Spearman C.B., Sheldon R.L., Egan D.F.: *Egan's Fundamentals of Respiratory Therapy*, ed. 4. St. Louis, C.V. Mosby Co., 1982. Reproduced by permission.)

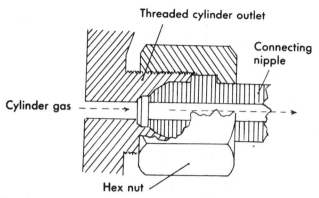

Fig 23–7.—Structure of a typical American Standard connection, such as might be used to attach a reducing valve to a large high-pressure cylinder. The hexagonal nut is held onto the nipple of the reducing valve by a circular collar, seen as a cross-sectional projection on the nipple. As the hexagonal nut is tightened on the threaded cylinder outlet, the end of the nipple is snugly seated into the conical outlet. (From Spearman C.B., Sheldon R.L., Egan D.F.: *Egan's Fundamentals of Respiratory Therapy,* ed. 4. St. Louis, C.V. Mosby Co., 1982. Reproduced by permission.)

    2. It is used on connections where the maximum working pressure is greater than 200 psig.

    3. It incorporates a hexagonal nut and specific nipple on the regulator fitted to an externally threaded cylinder connection.

    4. For oxygen the connection is CGA-540, 0.903-14 NGO, RH-Ext. A Compressed Gas Association connection No. 540 is used with a 0.903-in. threaded outlet diameter and 14 threads per inch of the National Gas Outlet type. The threads are external and right-handed.

  C. Diameter-Index Safety System (DISS) (Fig 23–8)

    1. Used on all connections distal to the regulator where maximum working pressures are less than 200 psig.

    2. Used for connections of flowmeters to regulators or other connections where frequent equipment changes are made.

    3. It incorporates a hexagonal nut and a nipple designed with two shoulders fitted into a body and externally threaded with two concentric borings.

    4. DISS connection for oxygen is No. 1240 with a 0.5625-in. diameter and 18 threads per inch.

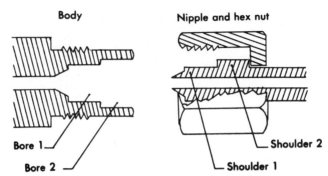

Fig 23–8.—Components of a representative DISS connection. The two shoulders of the nipple allow the nipple to unite only with a body having corresponding borings. If the match is incorrect, the hexagonal nut will not engage the body threads. (From Spearman C.B., Sheldon R.L., Egan D.F.: *Egan's Fundamentals of Respiratory Therapy,* ed. 4. St. Louis, C.V. Mosby Co., 1982. Reproduced by permission.)

VIII. Agencies Regulating Medical Gases
   A. Food and Drug Administration (FDA): Determines purity standards and labeling for all medical gases listed in the United States Pharmacopeia (USP).
   B. Compressed Gas Association (CGA): Sets standards and makes recommendations to manufacturers and municipal authorities on manufacture of gases and on safety standards for cylinders.
   C. National Fire Prevention Agency (NFPA): Sets standards and makes recommendations to manufacturers and municipal authorities on storage and handling of cylinders.
   D. Department of Transportation (DOT): The federal agency responsible for construction, transport, and testing of compressed gas cylinders since 1970.
IX. Fractional Distillation of Air
   A. The gas is filtered to remove all dust and impurities.
   B. The gas is dried to remove all water vapor.
   C. The gas is compressed to 200 atm pressure.
   D. The heat of compression is removed by heat exchangers until the temperature returns to ambient.
   E. The gas is then rapidly and repeatedly decompressed by dropping the pressure 5 atm. The reduction in pressure allows tremendous cooling by expansion to occur, bringing the temperature below the boiling point and liquifying all gases in the air.
   F. The temperature of the liquid is then increased and the various gases evaporated and collected at their respective boiling points.

BIBLIOGRAPHY

Burton G.G., Gee G.N., Hodgkin J.E.: *Respiratory Care: A Guide to Clinical Practice*. Philadelphia, J.B. Lippincott Co., 1977.

Compressed Gas Association: *Handbook of Compressed Gases*. New York.

Compressed Gas Association: Pamphlet V-1: *American Standard Compressed Gas Cylinder Valve Outlet and Inlet Connections*. 500 Fifth Ave., New York, NY 10036.

Compressed Gas Association: Pamphlet V-5: *Diameter Index Safety System*. 500 Fifth Ave., New York, NY 10036.

McPherson S.P.: *Respiratory Therapy Equipment*, ed. 2. St. Louis, C.V. Mosby Co., 1981.

Rarey K.P., Youtsey J.W.: *Respiratory Patient Care*. Englewood Cliffs, N.J., Prentice-Hall, Inc., 1981.

Rau J.L., Rau M.Y.: *Fundamental Respiratory Therapy Equipment: Principles and Use of Operation*. Sarasota, Fla., Glenn Educational Medical Services, Inc., 1977.

Spearman C.B., Sheldon R.L., Egan D.F.: *Egan's Fundamentals of Respiratory Therapy*, ed. 4. St. Louis, C.V. Mosby Co., 1982.

Young J.A., Crocker D.: *Principles and Practice of Respiratory Therapy*, ed. 2. Chicago, Year Book Medical Publishers, Inc., 1976.

24 / Oxygen Therapy

I. General Characteristics of Oxygen
   A. Colorless
   B. Odorless
   C. Tasteless
   D. Molecular weight: 32 gm
   E. Density at STP: 1.43 gm/L
   F. Boiling point at 1 atm: $-297.4°$ F $(-183°$ C)
   G. Melting point at 1 atm: $-361.1°$ F $(-216.6°$ C)
   H. Critical temperature: $-181.1°$ F $(-118.4°$ C)
   I. Critical pressure: 736.9 psia (pounds per square inch absolute)
   J. Triple point: $-361.89°$ F $(-218.7°$ C) at 0.2321 psia
   K. Forms oxides with all elements except inert gases
   L. Constitutes about 20.95% of atmosphere
   M. Used at cellular level as the final electron acceptor in electron transport chain located in mitochondria of cell
II. Hypoxia: Inadequate Quantities of Oxygen at the Tissue Level
   A. Anemic hypoxia: Decreased carrying capacity of blood for oxygen
      1. Anemia
      2. Carbon monoxide poisoning
      3. Methemoglobinemia
      4. Shift of the oxyhemoglobin dissociation curve to the right
      5. Hypoxemia may or may not be present
   B. Stagnant hypoxia: Decreased cardiac output, resulting in increased systemic transit time
      1. Shock
      2. Cardiovascular instability
      3. Regional vasoconstriction
   C. Histotoxic hypoxia: Inability of tissue to utilize available oxygen
      1. Cyanide poisoning
      2. Rarely accompanied by hypoxemia
   D. Hypoxemic hypoxia: Decrease in diffusion of oxygen across alveolar capillary membrane
      1. Low inspired F_{IO_2}
      2. Ventilation/perfusion inequalities
      3. Increased true shunt

4. Cardiac anomalies
5. Diffusion defects

III. Hypoxemia: Inadequate Quantities of Oxygen in the Blood
    A. Evaluation of hypoxemia
        1. Pa_{O_2} 80–100 mm Hg—normal
        2. Pa_{O_2} 60–79 mm Hg—mild hypoxemia
        3. Pa_{O_2} 40–59 mm Hg—moderate hypoxemia
        4. Pa_{O_2} <40 mm Hg—severe hypoxemia
        5. For individuals over 60 years of age, the lower level of acceptable Pa_{O_2} decreases because the normal aging process of the lung effects oxygenation capabilities.
           a. The lower limit of normal Pa_{O_2} is decreased 1 mm Hg for each year over 60. *Example:* For a 70-year-old patient, a Pa_{O_2} down to 70 mm Hg is acceptable.
              (1) Pa_{O_2} less than 60–65 mm Hg is always considered hypoxemia.
           b. More precisely acceptable lower limits for Pa_{O_2} can be determined by the following (at sea level):
              (1) For patients in the supine position:
$$Pa_{O_2} = 103.5 - (.42 \times age) \pm 4 \text{ mm Hg}$$
              (2) For patients in the sitting position:
$$Pa_{O_2} = 104.2 - (.27 \times age) \text{ mm Hg}$$
    B. Causes of hypoxemia (see Chaps. 12 and 13)
        1. True shunting
        2. Ventilation/perfusion inequalities
        3. A decreased mixed venous P_{O_2} may intensify the hypoxemic effect of 1 and 2 above.
    C. Responsive versus refractory hypoxemia
        1. Refractory hypoxemia is hypoxemia demonstrating a negligible increase in the Pa_{O_2} with the application of oxygen.
           a. If the $F_{I_{O_2}}$ is greater than or equal to 0.50 while the Pa_{O_2} is less than 60 mm Hg, the hypoxemia is refractory.
           b. If a 0.20 increase in the $F_{I_{O_2}}$ results in less than a 10 mm Hg increase in the Pa_{O_2}, the hypoxemia is refractory.
           c. Refractory hypoxemia is a result of true shunting.
        2. Responsive hypoxemia is hypoxemia that demonstrates a significant response to an increase in the $F_{I_{O_2}}$.
           a. A 0.20 increase in the $F_{I_{O_2}}$ results in a greater than 10 mm Hg increase in the Pa_{O_2}.
           b. Responsive hypoxemia is a result of ventilation/perfusion inequalities.
    D. Clinical manifestations of hypoxemia

1. Tachycardia and hypertension.
   a. If cardiovascular status is poor, bradycardia and hypotension may result.
2. Tachypnea and hyperpnea.
3. Pulmonary hypertension (constriction of pulmonary vascular bed).
4. Vasoconstriction of vascular beds supplying skin, muscles, and abdominal viscera (with moderate to severe hypoxemia).
5. Vasodilatation of vascular beds supplying heart and brain, resulting in increased blood flow.
6. Development of cyanosis (if hypoxemia is severe and hemoglobin content is increased or normal).
7. Lactic acidosis if coupled with poor perfusion.
8. Confusion and/or disorientation.
9. Secondary polycythemia (with chronic hypoxemia).

IV. Indications for Oxygen Therapy
   A. Hypoxemia
      1. Oxygen therapy increases alveolar P_{O_2}, thus increasing the pressure gradient for oxygen diffusion into the bloodstream.
      2. Increasing the pressure gradient may cause an increase in Pa_{O_2}.
   B. Excessive work of breathing
      1. Hypoxemia stimulates peripheral chemoreceptors, causing an increase in the rate and depth of ventilation and increasing the work of breathing.
      2. Oxygen therapy, by increasing alveolar P_{O_2}, may increase arterial P_{O_2}. This will reduce stimulation of peripheral chemoreceptors and reduce the work of breathing.
   C. Excessive myocardial work
      1. The primary compensatory response to hypoxemia is an increase in force and rate of contraction of the heart.
      2. Oxygen therapy may correct hypoxemia and decrease the stimulus to increase cardiac output.

V. Hazards of Oxygen Therapy.
   A. Retrolental fibroplasia (RLF)
      1. The presence of opaque fibrotic tissue behind the lens of the eye, resulting in retinal detachment and blindness.
      2. Pa_{O_2} greater than 100 mm Hg may result in RLF in the premature infant.
      3. Pathophysiology of RLF
         a. Phase 1: Hyperoxia causes vasoconstriction of the retinal blood vessels. This is followed by vascular obliteration if the hyperoxia persists (≥ 3 days).

      b. Phase 2: Vasoproliferation with elimination of the hyperoxic state; additional capillaries develop in the immature retina to the point that light penetration is impaired and blindness results.

    4. Normally only seen in neonates.

    5. Maintaining Pa_{O_2} values below 80 mm Hg greatly reduces the risk of RLF.

B. Oxygen toxicity

    1. A series of reversible pathophysiologic inflammatory changes of lung tissue.

    2. Free radical theory of oxygen toxicity

       a. The following free radicals of oxygen can be produced at the cellular level:

         (1) Hydrogen peroxide H_2O_2

         (2) Superoxide radical O_2^-

         (3) Hydroxyl radical $OH\cdot$

         (4) Singlet excited oxygen $^1O_2$

       b. The following enzymes are important cellular defenses against oxygen free radicals:

         (1) Superoxide dismutase (SOD), which converts O_2^- to O_2.

         (2) Catalase (CAT), which converts H_2O_2 to H_2O and O_2.

         (3) Additional intracellular defenses against oxygen free radicals include:

           (a) Glutathione peroxide

           (b) Glutathione

           (c) Cysteine

           (d) Cysteamine

           (e) Vitamin E in lipid membrane

           (f) Vitamin C (intracellular)

       c. The quantity of oxygen free radicals is dependent on PA_{O_2}. The greater the PA_{O_2}, the greater the quantity of free radicals.

       d. Effects of oxygen free radicals

         (1) Inhibition of glycolysis

         (2) Interference with surfactant transport and production

         (3) Nucleic acid (DNA) damage

         (4) Cross-linkage of DNA molecules

         (5) Cell and organelle membrane disruption

         (6) Enzyme inhibition

    3. Pathophysiology of oxygen toxicity

       a. Cellular susceptibility to hyperoxia (100% O_2)

         (1) Pulmonary capillary endothelium (most susceptible)

     (2) Alveolar Type I epithelial cells
     (3) Alveolar Type II epithelial cells
     (4) Alveolar Type III epithelial cells (least susceptible)
  b. With continued exposure to 100% O_2 Type I alveolar cells are destroyed and replaced by Type II cells.
  c. Early or acute exudative phase is characterized by perivascular, interstitial, and intra-alveolar edema with destruction and necrosis of endothelial cells. Alveolar congestion and fibrinous exudation (hyaline membrane) develop.
  d. Late or chronic proliferative phase is characterized by a progressive reabsorption of the exudate and a thickening of the alveolar septa.
  e. Clinical manifestations
     (1) Tracheobronchitis
     (2) Cough
     (3) Substernal pain
     (4) Nausea and vomiting
     (5) Anorexia
     (6) Paresthesia
     (7) Refractory hypoxemia
     (8) Diffuse patchy bilateral infiltrates
     (9) Alveolar atelectasis
     (10) Decreased compliance
4. Susceptibility and risk factors associated with the development of oxygen toxicity:
  a. Exposure to F_{IO_2} values greater than 0.40 for lengthy periods of time.
  b. Previous development of severe acute pulmonary disease decreases the risk of toxicity. The acute disease is believed to induce the production of SOD and glutathione, thus reducing the oxygen free radical levels.
5. Prevention: Judicious use of oxygen therapy.
6. Treatment: Appropriate use of PEEP therapy, diuretics, and fluids while reducing the F_{IO_2} to "safe" levels.
C. Oxygen-induced hypoventilation
1. This is observed in patients with chronic CO_2 retention or CNS depression (see Chap. 19).
2. The increased Pa_{O_2} decreases or eliminates the hypoxic drive, inducing greater levels of hypoventilation.
3. Intermittent use of oxygen therapy may cause arterial PO_2 to fall below pretreatment levels.
D. Absorption atelectasis (Fig 24–1)

1. Nitrogen is metabolically inactive and constitutes 80% of alveolar gas. Nitrogen is essential in maintaining alveolar stability.
2. Administration of high F_{IO_2} (>0.70) washes out nitrogen.
3. In poorly ventilated alveoli more oxygen is removed per unit time by the perfused blood than can be replaced by normal ventilation.
4. This results in a decrease in alveolar size.
5. As alveoli reach their critical volume, collapse and atelectasis occur.
6. This commonly occurs in patients with small tidal volumes and/or poor distribution of ventilation due to partial airway obstruction.

VI. Oxygen Delivery Systems
  A. In general, delivery systems are divided into two categories: high-flow and low-flow.
  B. High-flow systems
    1. The patient's entire inspired atmosphere is consistently and predictably delivered by the system.
    2. To maintain a consistent F_{IO_2} the apparatus flow must exceed the peak inspiratory flow of the patient.
    3. Peak inspiratory flows are difficult to measure, but may be approximated by delivering a total flow at least *four times* the patient's measured minute volume.
      a. Normal peak inspiratory flows are about four times the patient's measured minute volume.
      b. This flow usually will provide adequate volume in the face of a changing ventilatory pattern.
    4. Typical high-flow systems
      a. Air entrainment masks: Deliver a specific F_{IO_2} up to 0.50 (Table 24–1).
        (1) Care should be taken to ensure the air entrainment mask provides sufficient flow to meet a patient's need. This is especially true with masks delivering higher F_{IO_2} levels.
      b. Mechanical aerosol systems: Set up singly or in tandem to deliver high humidity along with a specific F_{IO_2} (see Table 24–1).
        (1) Again, care should be taken to ensure sufficient flow.
      c. Cascade-type humidifier systems
        (1) Volume and concentration of gas determined by titration of compressed air and oxygen or use of oxygen blender.

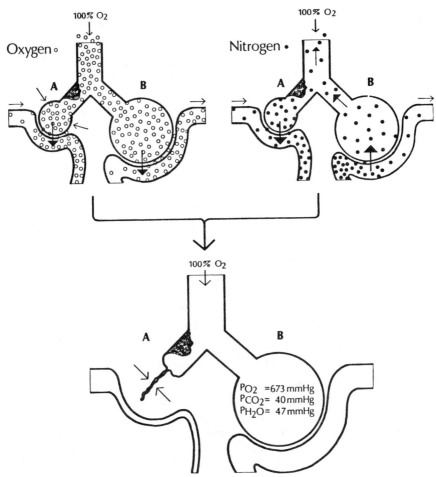

Fig 24–1.—Schematic representation of primary mechanisms causing denitrogenation absorption atelectasis. *Top drawings* represent the alveolar-capillary units shortly after administration of 100% inspired oxygen. *White circles* represent oxygen molecules which have increased in concentration in both units *A* and *B*. The ablation of alveolar hypoxia in unit *A* results in loss of vasoconstriction with considerably increased blood flow. The increased blood flow to this still poorly ventilated alveolus results in significantly increased oxygen extraction, which results in diminished gas volume. *Black circles* represent nitrogen, which is rapidly depleted from all units secondary to the fact that inspired nitrogen concentration is now zero. Initially, more nitrogen leaves the blood and the body via unit *B* because it is better ventilated. However, as the blood P_{N_2} level progressively decreases, nitrogen will start to leave alveolus *A* via the blood. This results in further loss of gas volume from alveolus *A* since it remains poorly ventilated but well perfused. Thus, nitrogen is depleted from all units within 5–15 minutes.

TABLE 24–1.—ENTRAINMENT RATIOS AND OUTPUTS OF SPECIFIC
AIR ENTRAINMENT SYSTEMS*

SYSTEM	$F_{I_{O_2}}$	ENTRAINMENT RATIO	FLOW AT WHICH OPERATED	TOTAL FLOW (L/MIN)
Ventimasks	0.24	1–25	4	104
	0.28	1–10	4	44
	0.31	1–7	6	48
	0.35	1–5	8	48
	0.40	1–3	8	32
	0.50	1–1.7	12	32
Mechanical	0.60	1–1	12	24
Aerosol	0.70	1–0.6	12	19

*Clinical trials indicate some variation in $F_{I_{O_2}}$ levels provided by air entrainment masks.

    (2) Virtually any $F_{I_{O_2}}$ level is available.
    (3) Virtually any flow is available.
    (4) Systems are extremely versatile and may be applied to a patient via an aerosol mask or standard artificial airway attachment.
  d. Determination of $F_{I_{O_2}}$ with any system combining gas flows:

$$F_{I_{O_2}} = \frac{(F_{I_{O_2}} \text{ of A})(\text{flow of A}) + (F_{I_{O_2}} \text{ of B})(\text{flow of B}) + \text{etc.}}{\text{total flow of combined systems}} \quad (1)$$

C. Low-flow systems
  1. The total minute volume is not delivered by the apparatus.
  2. The $F_{I_{O_2}}$ delivered to the patient depends on
    a. Flow of gas from equipment
    b. Patient anatomical reservoir (oral and nasal cavity)
      (1) Normal anatomical reservoir in adults is about 50 ml.
      (2) Normal end-expiratory pause may allow for filling of anatomical reservoir with 100% oxygen.
    c. Reservoir of equipment
    d. Patient respiratory rate, tidal volume, and minute volume
  3. *The $F_{I_{O_2}}$ delivered with any low-flow system is extremely variable and unpredictable.*

The *bottom* drawing represents the final steady state in which increased oxygen and nitrogen extraction has caused the alveolus to collapse. Thus, a poorly ventilated, poorly perfused unit *A* becomes a nonventilated, poorly perfused unit after administration of 100% inspired oxygen. (From Shapiro B.A., Harrison R.A., Walton J.R.: *Clinical Application of Blood Gas,* ed. 3. Chicago, Year Book Medical Publishers, Inc., 1982. Reproduced by permission.)

4. If the patient's minute volume were to increase on a particular low-flow system, the $F_{I_{O_2}}$ would *decrease*. The patient would entrain a larger percentage of room air in the minute volume.
5. If the patient's minute volume were to decrease on a particular low-flow system, the $F_{I_{O_2}}$ would *increase*. The patient would entrain a smaller percentage of room air in the minute volume.
6. The following is an example of the calculations used to *estimate* the $F_{I_{O_2}}$ delivered by low-flow oxygen therapy systems. This calculation is for a cannula at 6 L/min.
   a. Ventilatory variables
      (1) Respiratory rate: 20/min
      (2) Tidal volume: 500 cc
      (3) Inspiratory-expiratory ratio: 1:2
      (4) Inspiratory time: 1 second
      (5) Volume of patient's anatomical reservoir (volume of oral and nasal cavity): 50 cc
   b. Volume delivered by cannula per second
      (1) Flow is 6 L/min, which equals 6,000 ml/min.
      (2) Thus, 100 ml/sec is delivered to patient.
   c. Volume of 100% oxygen inspired per breath
      (1) 100 ml is delivered by cannula in the 1-second inspiratory time.
      (2) A 50 ml volume of oxygen is accumulated in anatomical reservoir prior to inspiration (accumulates during expiratory pause).
      (3) If 150 ml is inspired from 1 and 2 above, then 350 ml of room air would need to be entrained. Since about 20% of room air is oxygen, 70 cc of oxygen is entrained.

$$100 \text{ ml} + 50 \text{ ml} + 70 \text{ ml} = 220 \text{ ml} \qquad (2)$$

   d. Therefore, the inspired oxygen concentration is equal to:

$$\frac{220 \ (O_2)}{500 \ (TV)} = F_{I_{O_2}} \text{ of } 0.44 \qquad (3)$$

   e. *It must be kept in mind that the $F_{I_{O_2}}$ listed for each low-flow system is purely speculative and that the $F_{I_{O_2}}$ is totally dependent on the patient's ventilatory pattern. The values provided should only be used as gross guidelines rather than as the exact $F_{I_{O_2}}$ delivered.*

7. Using calculations similar to those in 6 above, the approximate F_{IO_2} levels for various low-flow systems are listed and discussed below.

  a. *O_2 cannula*

      (1) 1 L/min F_{IO_2}: 0.24

      (2) 2 L/min F_{IO_2}: 0.28

      (3) 3 L/min F_{IO_2}: 0.32

      (4) 4 L/min F_{IO_2}: 0.36

      (5) 5 L/min F_{IO_2}: 0.40

      (6) 6 L/min F_{IO_2}: 0.44

  b. *Simple O_2 mask:* Should be run between 5 and 8 L/min to ensure flushing and prevent CO_2 accumulation in the face mask. This flow will result in an F_{IO_2} between 0.40 and 0.60, *depending on patient's ventilatory pattern.*

  c. *O_2 mask with bag* (partial rebreathing mask): Should be run between 7 and 10 L/min. Flow must be adequate to ensure that bag deflates only about one third during inspiration to prevent CO_2 buildup in system. This flow will result in an F_{IO_2} between 0.70 and 0.80+, *depending on patient's ventilatory pattern.*

  d. *Nonrebreathing mask:* Must be run with sufficient flow to prevent bag from collapsing during inspiration. Nonrebreathing masks are difficult to use properly on patients with a high minute volume. A high-flow cascade setup is more practical for 1.0 F_{IO_2} administration. If a nonrebreathing mask is functioning properly, the F_{IO_2} is 0.90 to 1.0, *depending on patient's ventilatory pattern.*

D. Criteria for use of high- and low-flow oxygen delivery systems.

  1. *Whenever a consistent and predictable F_{IO_2} is required, a high-flow system should be utilized.*

  2. A low-flow system provides relatively stable F_{IO_2} levels if the patient's:

    a. Ventilatory pattern is consistent and regular.

    b. Tidal volume is between 300 and 700 ml.

    c. Respiratory rate is less than 25/min.

E. Monitoring of oxygen therapy

  1. Arterial blood gas analysis

  2. Tidal volume and respiratory rate

  3. Pulse and blood pressure

  4. It is important to evaluate the work of breathing and the work of the myocardium to determine the overall effectiveness of an

increase in the FI_{O_2}. A minor change in the P_{O_2} may be accompanied by a decrease in the work of breathing and the work of the myocardium, indicating the effectiveness of the FI_{O_2} increase.

BIBLIOGRAPHY

Ashton N.: The pathogenesis of retrolental fibroplasia. *Ophthalmology* 86:1695–1699, 1979.

Barber R.E., Lee J., Hamilton W.K.: Oxygen toxicity in man. *N. Engl. J. Med.* 283:1478–1488, 1970.

Bendixen H.H., Egert L.D., Heldey-Whyte J., et al.: *Respiratory Care*. St. Louis, C.V. Mosby Co., 1965.

Block A.J.: Neuropsychological aspects of oxygen therapy. *Respir. Care* 28:885–888, 1983.

Burton G.G., Gee G.N., Hodgkin J.E.: *Respiratory Care: A Guide to Clinical Practice*. Philadelphia, J.B. Lippincott Co., 1977.

Deneke S.M., Fanburg B.L.: Normobaric oxygen toxicity of the lung. *N. Engl. J. Med.* 303:76–86, 1980.

Frank L., Massaro D.: The lung and oxygen toxicity. *Arch. Intern. Med.* 139:347–350, 1979.

Frank L., Massaro D.: Oxygen toxicity. *Am. J. Med.* 69:117–126, 1980.

Gibson R.L., Comer P.B., Beckham R.W., et al.: Actual tracheal oxygen concentration with commonly used oxygen equipment. *Anesthesiology* 44:71–73, 1976.

Harkema J.R., Mauderly J.L., Hahn F.F.: The effects of emphysema on oxygen toxicity in rats. *Am. Rev. Respir. Dis.* 126:1058–1065, 1982.

Hedley-White J., Burgess G.E. III, Feeley T.W., et al.: *Applied Physiology of Respiratory Care*. Boston, Little, Brown & Co., 1976.

Mellemgaard K.: The alveolar-arterial oxygen difference: Its size and components in normal man. *Acta Physiol. Scand.* 67:10–14, 1966.

McPherson S.P.: *Respiratory Therapy Equipment*, ed. 2. St. Louis, C.V. Mosby Co., 1981.

Patz A.: Studies on retinal neovascularization. *Invest. Ophthalmol. Vis. Sci.* 19:1133–1138, 1980.

Redding J.S., McAfee D.D., Parham A.M.: Oxygen concentrations received from commonly used delivery systems. *South. Med. J.* 71:169–172, 1978.

Safar P. (ed.): *Respiratory Therapy*. Philadelphia, F.A. Davis Co., 1965.

Schacter E.W., Littner M.R., Luddy P., et al.: Monitoring of oxygen delivery systems in clinical practice. *Crit. Care Med.* 8:405–409, 1980.

Shapiro B.A., Harrison R.A., Kacmarek R.M., et al.: *Clinical Application of Respiratory Care*, ed. 3. Chicago, Year Book Medical Publishers, Inc., 1985.

Singer M.M., Wright F., Stanley L.K., et al.: Oxygen toxicity in man. *N. Engl. J. Med.* 283:1473–1478, 1970.

Sobini C.A., Grassi V., Solinas E.: Arterial oxygen tension in relation to age in healthy subjects. *Respiration* 25:3–14, 1968.

Spearman C.B., Sheldon R.L., Egan D.F.: *Egan's Fundamentals of Respiratory Therapy*, ed. 4. St. Louis, C.V. Mosby Co., 1982.

Woolner D.F., Larkin J.: An analysis of the performance of a variable venturi-type oxygen mask. *Anesth. Intensive Care* 8:44–51, 1980.

Young J.A., Crocker D.: *Principles and Practice of Respiratory Therapy*, ed. 2. Chicago, Year Book Medical Publishers, Inc., 1976.

25 / Airway Care

I. General Indications for Use of Artificial Airways
   A. To prevent or relieve upper airway obstruction.
   B. To protect the airway from aspiration.
   C. To facilitate tracheal suction.
   D. To provide a sealed, closed system for mechanical ventilation or CPAP.
II. General Classification of Artificial Airways
   A. Oropharyngeal airway
      1. Used to relieve upper airway obstruction by maintaining the base of the tongue off the posterior wall of the oral pharynx.
      2. Used to prevent inadvertent laceration of the tongue in the incoherent or seizuring patient.
      3. Used as a bite block with oral endotracheal tubes.
      4. Poorly tolerated in alert patient due to stimulation of gag reflex.
   B. Nasopharyngeal airway
      1. Used to relieve upper airway obstruction caused by tongue and/or soft palate falling against posterior wall of the pharynx.
      2. Suctioning via this airway is less traumatic than nasal suctioning.
      3. Better tolerated than oropharyngeal airway.
      4. Should be alternated every 24 hours between right and left nares to minimize complications.
      5. Sinusitis, otitis media, and nasal necrosis are possible complications of its use.
   C. Oroendotracheal tube
      1. Advantages when compared to nasotracheal tubes
         a. Easy to insert, the airway of choice in an emergency.
         b. Ideally used for short-term intubation of 24 hours or less.
         c. Tube size inserted can be larger than if a nasotracheal tube were inserted.
         d. Sinusitis and otitis media are not problems.
      2. Problems associated with orotracheal tubes
         a. Poorly tolerated in conscious and semiconscious patients.
         b. Difficult to stabilize.

      c. Inadvertent extubation common.

      d. Bite block necessary to prevent biting of tube.

      e. Vagal stimulation common.

      f. Oral hygiene difficult.

      g. Tip of tube moves when patient's head position changes.

         (1) Extension of head moves tip toward oropharynx (possible extubation).

         (2) Flexion of head moves tip toward carina (possible right endobronchial intubation)

      h. Oral feeding difficult

   D. Nasoendotracheal tube

     1. Advantages over oroendotracheal tube for long-term intubation

      a. Easier to stabilize.

      b. Easier to suction.

      c. Better tolerated.

      d. Safer for equipment attachment.

      e. Easier to maintain oral hygiene.

     2. Problems associated with nasotracheal tubes

      a. Tip of tube moves when patient's head position changes.

      b. Possible pressure necrosis in area of the alae nasi.

      c. Possible obstruction of sinus drainage and acute sinusitis.

      d. Possible obstruction of eustachian tube drainage and otitis media.

      e. Increased incidence of vocal cord damage after 3–7 days (also seen with oroendotracheal tubes).

      f. Possible vagal stimulation, but less frequently than with oroendotracheal tube.

   E. Tracheostomy tube

     1. Advantages over endotracheal tubes

      a. No complications with upper airway or glottis.

      b. Easier to suction.

      c. Easier to stabilize.

      d. Best tolerated of all airways.

     2. Problems associated with tracheostomy tube

      a. Immediate complications

         (1) Bleeding

         (2) Pneumothorax

         (3) Air embolism

         (4) Subcutaneous and mediastinal emphysema

      b. Late complications

         (1) Infection of surgical wound

  (2) Hemorrhage
  (3) Tracheal stenosis
3. Frequent and routine changing of tracheostomy tubes is unnecessary if the airway is functioning properly, is properly humidified, and no infectious process is present in the tracheostomy wound.
4. If stomal infection exists, weekly changing of tracheostomy tubes is recommended.
F. Fenestrated tracheostomy tube (Fig 25–1)
  1. Fenestration is located in outer cannula only.
  2. Inner cannula is similar in design to inner cannula of a normal tracheostomy tube.
  3. Requisites for proper use
    a. Removal of inner cannula
    b. Deflation of cuff
    c. Corking of outer cannula
  4. Patient is forced to ventilate via upper airway through fenestration in outer cannula of tracheostomy tube and around tube.
  5. Problems associated with fenestrated tube
    a. Possible formation of granular tissue at site of fenestration.
    b. Increased resistance to gas flow and work of breathing.
G. Talking tracheostomy tubes (Fig 25–2)

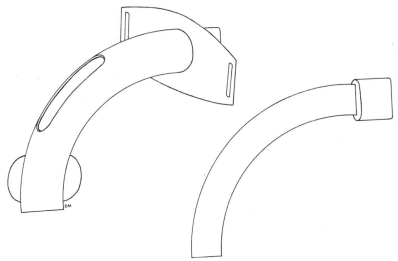

Fig 25–1.—Fenestrated tracheostomy tube. Inner and outer cannulas are depicted.

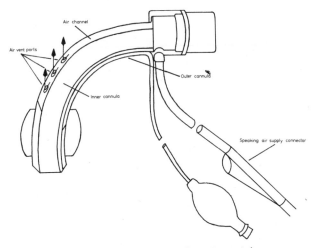

Air channel

Air vent ports

Outer cannula

Inner cannula

Speaking air supply connector

Fig 25–2.—Talking tracheostomy tube.

1. Designed to allow patient to verbalize when cuff is inflated.
2. Functions by directing secondary gas flow through ports in tube above patient's cuff, allowing gas to move past the vocal cords while maintaining ventilation via the airway.
3. Internal diameter of airway smaller than standard tube of same size.

H. Tracheal buttons (Fig 25–3)
   1. Used to maintain patency of tracheal stoma.
   2. Inner lip of button lies on internal anterior tracheal wall, outer lip on tissue of the neck.
   3. Tracheal buttons allow patient to ventilate completely from upper airway without tracheal obstruction.
   4. In an emergency, patient may be suctioned and/or ventilated via the tracheal button.

I. Esophageal obturator (Fig 25–4)

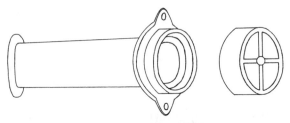

Fig 25–3.—Tracheal button.

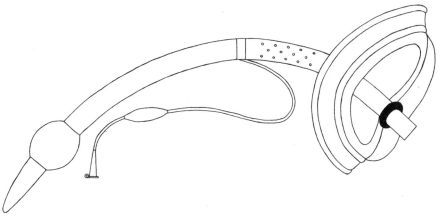

Fig 25–4.—Esophageal obturator.

1. The obturator is used only as an emergency airway.
2. The obturator is a mask attached to a blind endotracheal tube, which has perforations along its length and a cuff at tip of tube.
3. The obturator is inserted into the esophagus and the cuff is inflated.
4. Should only be removed after intubation of the trachea has been performed and cuff inflated.
5. The patient is ventilated by forcing gas into obturator. Gas moves out of perforations in the tube and is forced into the trachea.
6. Problems associated with esophageal obturator
   a. Intubation of trachea during insertion.
   b. Regurgitation on removal of airway.
   c. Rupture of the esophagus.
J. Cricothyroidotomy
   1. Incision through the cricothyroid membrane, located between the cricoid and thyroid cartilages.
   2. Used as an emergency airway if upper airway obstruction prevents oroendotracheal intubation and ventilation.
   3. Advantages:
      a. Rapid establishment of airway.
      b. Easily accomplished during CPR.
   4. Disadvantages:
      a. Perforation of thyroid gland.
      b. Perforation of esophagus.

      c. Mediastinal or subcutaneous emphysema.

      d. Pneumothorax.

      e. Hemorrhage.

      f. Vocal cord damage if performed too high.

      g. Increased airway resistance because of small internal diameter of tube.

III. Laryngotracheal Complications of Endotracheal Intubation

    A. Sore throat and hoarse voice.

    B. Glottic edema.

    C. Subglottic edema.

    D. Ulceration of tracheal mucosa.

    E. Vocal cord ulceration, granuloma, and polyp formation.

    F. Vocal cord paralysis.

    G. Laryngotracheal web.

IV. Postextubation Therapy

    A. Administration of 0.5 ml of 2.25% W/V racemic epinephrine, 1 mg dexamethasone with 4 ml normal saline solution to reverse/prevent glottic and/or subglottic edema.

    B. If symptoms of glottic/subglottic edema persist, reintubation may be necessary.

V. Airway Cuffs

    A. Uses

      1. To mechanically ventilate patient.

      2. To protect airway from aspiration.

    B. Tracheal wall pressures

      1. Intra-arterial pressure approximately 30 mm Hg (42 cm H_2O).

      2. Venous pressures approximately 18 mm Hg (24 cm H_2O).

    C. Lateral tracheal wall pressures of greater than:

      1. 30 mm Hg cause cessation of arterial blood flow.

      2. 18 mm Hg obstruct venous flow.

      3. 5 mm Hg inhibit lymphatic flow.

    D. Cuff pressures must be maintained at less than 20 mm Hg to maintain tracheal capillary blood flow.

    E. Effects of high lateral tracheal wall pressures. Sequence of tracheal changes:

      1. Mucosal ischemia

      2. Mucosal inflammation, hemorrhage, and/or ulceration

        a. Tracheal granuloma formation

      3. Exposure of cartilage

      4. Tracheal ring destruction

        a. Tracheomalacia

        b. Tracheal stenosis

(1) At cuff site

(2) At tip of airway

(3) At stoma in tracheostomies

F. Additional factors predisposing to tracheal damage

1. High peak airway pressure or PEEP requiring higher cuff pressures.

2. Too small or too large a cuff in relation to tracheal size.

3. Noncircular cross-sectional tracheal shape.

4. Cuff material

a. Silicon: requires least inflation pressure

b. Polyvinyl chloride

c. Latex: requires greatest inflation pressure

G. High-volume, low-pressure vs. low-volume, high-pressure cuffs

1. High-volume, low-pressure cuffs are the cuffs of choice for long-term airway maintenance.

a. Advantages

(1) Intracuff pressures lower than with high-pressure cuffs.

(2) Lateral tracheal wall pressure dissipated over large surface area.

b. Disadvantage; may form folds when inflated, allowing aspiration of liquids or entrapment of secretions that cause infection.

H. Special cuffs

1. Kamen-Wilkinson cuff

a. Made of polyurethane foam.

b. Inflated by atmospheric pressure.

c. No positive pressure added to cuff.

d. Minimum pressures normally applied to tracheal wall.

e. Deflation of cuff with syringe before insertion allows reexpansion by atmospheric pressure.

2. Lanz cuff

a. Dynamic cuff theoretically allows only 20 cm H_2O pressure to be developed in cuff.

b. Valve assembly on pilot tube maintains constancy of intracuff pressure by allowing gas movement from pilot balloon to cuff.

I. Cuff inflation techniques

1. Minimal leak technique: Cuff volume maintains seal except at maximum inspiratory pressure.

a. Insertion of enough air into cuff to prevent any leaks.

b. While positive pressure is applied to airway, gas should

be withdrawn from the cuff until a slight leak develops. Leak should not be so great as to overcome purpose of cuff.

2. Minimal occluding volume: Minimal volume of gas required to maintain airway seal at peak positive pressure during inspiration.
   a. Insert enough air to prevent any leak.
   b. Withdraw gas during inspiration until a leak occurs.
   c. Carefully inflate until gas leak is stopped at peak inspiratory pressure.
3. Monitoring of cuff pressures.
   a. A pressure monitor is used to evaluate actual intracuff pressure.
   b. Important to use if high peak airway pressures are necessary or if high levels of PEEP are employed.
   c. If minimal occluding volume technique is used, cuff pressures should be monitored. A 1–2 ml increase in cuff volume can cause a precipitous increase in intracuff pressure.
   Note: Outside the operating room, only high-volume, low-pressure cuffs should be utilized.

VI. Cuff Deflation Technique
   A. Complete suctioning of lower airway.
   B. Complete suctioning above cuff.
   C. Deflation of cuff while positive pressure is applied in order to direct any pooled secretions above cuff up and out of airway.

VII. Artificial Airway Emergencies
   A. Inadvertent extubation
   B. Airway obstruction
      1. Mucous plug
      2. Granuloma tissue
      3. Herniation of cuff over end of tube
   C. Endobronchial intubation
   D. Kinking of airway

VIII. Management of Acute Obstruction of Artificial Airway
   A. Manipulate tube (check for kinks).
   B. Attempt to suction airway.
   C. Deflate cuff.
   D. If all the above fail and tension pneumothorax is ruled out, extubate patient and ventilate with bag and mask.

IX. Airway Suctioning
   A. Complications of airway suctioning
      1. Hypoxemia

2. Arrhythmias
3. Hypotension
4. Lung collapse
5. Cardiac arrest
B. Requisites of suction catheters
  1. Constructed of a material that will cause minimal irritation and trauma to tracheal mucosa.
  2. Minimal frictional resistance when passing through artificial airway is essential.
  3. Sufficiently long to easily pass tip of artificial airway.
  4. Should have smooth, molded ends and side holes to prevent mucosal trauma.
  5. Catheter diameter should be less than one half the internal diameter of the artificial airway
     a. To convert French size to size in millimeters (approximation):

$$\text{mm} = \frac{\text{Fr} - 2}{4} \tag{1}$$

     b. To convert size in millimeters to French size (approximation):

$$\text{Fr} = (4)\,(\text{mm}) + 2 \tag{2}$$

C. Suctioning technique
  1. Use completely sterile technique.
  2. Preoxygenate patient.
  3. Insert catheter without vacuum until an obstruction is met, and then slightly retract catheter.
  4. Apply suction only during removal of the catheter.
  5. Suction catheter should remain in airway no longer than 10–15 seconds.
  6. Reoxygenate and ventilate.
  7. In the event of catheter adherence to wall of airway, release suction, withdraw catheter, and reapply suction.
  8. To minimize airway trauma, use suction pressures of -80 mm Hg to -120 mm Hg.

BIBLIOGRAPHY

Applebaum E.L., Bruce D.L.: *Tracheal Intubation*. Philadelphia, W.B. Saunders Co., 1976.
Bendixen H.H., et al.: *Respiratory Care*. St. Louis, C.V. Mosby Co., 1965.
Burton G.G., Gee G.N., Hodgkin J.E.: *Respiratory Care: A Guide to Clinical Practice*. Philadelphia, J.B. Lippincott Co., 1977.

Conrardy P.A., Goodman L.R., Lainge F., et al.: Alteration of endotracheal tube position, flexion and extension of the neck. *Crit. Care Med.* 4:8–12, 1976.

Demers R.R.: Complications of endotracheal suctioning procedures. *Respir. Care* 27:453–457, 1982.

Dobrin P., Canfield T.: Cuffed endotracheal tubes: Mucosal pressure and tracheal wall blood flow. *Am. J. Surg.* 133:562–568, 1977.

Glover D.W., McCarthy-Glover M.: *Respiratory Therapy-Basics for Nursing and the Allied Health Professions.* St. Louis, C.V. Mosby Co., 1978.

Greisz H., Quarnstrom O., Willen R.: Elective cricothyroidotomy: A clinical and histopathological study. *Crit. Care Med.* 10:387–389, 1982.

Holladay-Skelley F.B., Deeren S.M., Powaser M.M.: The effectiveness of two preoxygenation methods to prevent endotracheal suction-induced hypoxemia. *Heart Lung* 9:316–323, 1980.

Kastanos N., Miro R.E., Perez A.M., et al.: Laryngotracheal injury due to endotracheal intubation: Incidence, evolution, and predisposing factors. A prospective long-term study. *Crit. Care Med.* 11:362–366, 1983.

Kress T.D.: Cricothyroidotomy. *Ann. Emerg. Med.* 11:197–201, 1982.

Langrehe E.A., Washburn S.C., Guthrie M.P.: Oxygen insufflation during endotracheal suctioning. *Heart Lung* 10:1028–1036, 1981.

Lewis F.R., Schlobohm R.M., Thomas A.N.: Prevention of complications from prolonged tracheal intubation. *Am. J. Surg.* 135:452–457, 1978.

MacKenzie C.F.: Compromises in the choice of orotracheal or nasotracheal intubation and tracheostomy. *Heart Lung* 12:485–492, 1983.

McDowell D.E.: Cricothyroidostomy for airway access. *South. Med. J.* 75:282–284, 1982.

Nelson E.J., Morton E.A., Hunter P.M.: *Critical Care Respiratory Therapy—A Laboratory and Clinical Manual.* Boston, Little, Brown & Co., 1983.

Off D., Braun S.R., Tompkins B., et al.: Efficacy of the minimal leak technique of cuff inflation in maintaining proper intracuff pressures for patients with cuffed artificial airways. *Respir. Care* 28:1115–1120, 1983.

Pavlin E.G., Van Nimgegan D., Hornbein T.F.: Failure of a high compliance-low pressure cuff to prevent aspiration. American Standards Association, 1975, vol. 43, p. 216.

Rarey K.P., Youtsey J.W.: *Respiratory Patient Care.* Englewood Cliffs, N.J., Prentice-Hall, Inc., 1981.

Rindfleisch S.H., Tyler M.L.: Duration of suctioning: An important variable, editorial. *Respir. Care* 28:457–458, 1983.

Safer P. (ed.): *Respiratory Therapy.* Philadelphia, F.A. Davis Co., 1965.

Shapiro B.A., Harrison R.A., Kacmarek R.M., et al.: *Clinical Application of Respiratory Care,* ed. 3. Chicago, Year Book Medical Publishers, Inc., 1985.

Spearman C.B., Sheldon R.L., Egan D.F.: *Egan's Fundamentals of Respiratory Care,* ed. 4. St. Louis, C.V. Mosby Co., 1982.

Sinsheimer F.: *Basics of Respiratory Therapy—A Laboratory Manual.* Boston, Little, Brown & Co., 1983.

Stauffer J.L., Olson D.E., Petty T.L.: Complications and consequences of endotracheal intubation and tracheotomy: A prospective study of 150 critically ill adult patients. *Am. J. Surg.* 70:65–76, 1981.

Stauffer J.L., Silvestri R.C.: Complications of endotracheal intubation, tracheostomy, and artificial airways. *Respir. Care* 27:417–434, 1982.

Young J.A., Crocker D.: *Principles and Practice of Respiratory Therapy,* ed. 2. Chicago, Year Book Medical Publishers, Inc., 1976.

26 / Aerosol Therapy

● An aerosol is a suspension of liquid or solid particles in a gas such as smoke or fog.

  I. Stability: Tendency of aerosol particles to remain in suspension. The following factors affect the stability of an aerosol:

  A. Size: The smaller the aerosol particle, the greater the tendency toward stability. The larger the particle, the greater the tendency to rain-out of suspension.

  B. Concentration: The greater the concentration of particles, the greater the tendency for individual particles to coalesce into larger particles and rain-out of suspension.

  C. Humidity: The greater the relative humidity of the gas carrying the aerosol, the greater the stability of the aerosol.

  II. Penetration and Deposition of an Aerosol in the Respiratory Tract

  A. Penetration refers to the depth within the respiratory tract that an aerosol reaches. Deposition is the rain-out of aerosol particles within the respiratory tract.

  B. Depth of penetration and volume of deposition depend on:

    1. Gravity: Gravity decreases penetration and increases premature deposition but has minimal effect on particles in the therapeutic range of 1–5 μ (Table 26–1).

    2. Kinetic energy: The greater the kinetic energy of the gas carrying the particles, the greater the tendency for premature deposition. This is because coalescence and impaction are increased.

    3. Inertial impaction: Deposition of particles is increased at any point of directional change or increased airway resistance. Thus the smaller the airway diameter, the greater the tendency for deposition.

  III. Ventilatory Pattern for Optimal Penetration and Deposition

  A. The patient's ventilatory pattern is the most important variable that can be controlled to ensure maximum penetration and deposition of aerosol particles.

  B. Ideal ventilatory pattern

    1. Large, slowly inspired tidal volume (over 3–4 seconds).

TABLE 26–1.—PENETRATION AND DEPOSITION VS. PARTICLE SIZE

PARTICLE SIZE (μ)	DEPOSITION IN RESPIRATORY TRACT
>100	Do not enter respiratory tract
100–10	Trapped in mouth
100– 5	Trapped in nose
5– 2	Deposited proximal to alveoli
2– 1	Can enter alveoli, 95%–100% of particles 1 μ in size settling
1–0.25	Stable, with minimal settling

    2. During inspiration, the patient's mouth should be opened widely, in order to decrease deposition of the aerosol in the mouth and oropharynx.

    3. After inhalation a 3- to 4-second breath-holding period is advisable to ensure maximum deposition.

    4. With large volume aerosols (ultrasonic nebulizers) a face mask should be used.

    5. With small volume nebulizers, a mouthpiece is normally used. However, the patient's mouth should be opened widely about the mouthpiece.

    6. Exhalation should be relaxed and normal.

    7. Coughing should be encouraged if secretion mobilization occurs and at the completion of treatment.

  C. Attempts should be made to have all patients receiving aerosol therapy assume the ventilatory pattern described.

IV. Clearance of Aerosols: Inhaled particles are removed from the respiratory tract by three mechanisms.

  A. Primary mechanism: Mucociliary escalator, which moves about 100 ml of secretions to the oropharynx per day (see Chap. 3, section I–C).

  B. Normal cough mechanism.

  C. Phagocytosis by type III alveolar cells.

V. Indications for Aerosol Therapy

  A. Retained secretions.

  B. The need for a vehicle to administer bronchodilators and other pharmacologic agents directly on the respiratory mucosa.

  C. Humidification of the inspired gas of patients acutely requiring short-term artificial airways.

  D. Aerosol therapy may be indicated in patients presenting with the following conditions:

    1. Retained secretions

    2. Asthma and other reactive airway diseases

3. Bronchitis/emphysema
4. Cystic fibrosis
5. Severe laryngitis/tracheitis/croup
6. Bronchiectasis
7. Smoke inhalation or chemical trauma to the airways
8. Physical trauma to the upper airway
9. Postextubation therapy to prevent laryngeal edema

E. Aerosol therapy may also be necessary for sputum induction.

VI. General Goals of Aerosol Therapy
A. Improve bronchial hygiene
1. Hydrate dried retained secretions.
2. Improve efficiency of cough mechanism.
3. Restore and maintain normal function of mucociliary escalator.
B. Humidify gases delivered to patients with artificial airways.
C. Deliver medications.

VII. Hazards of Aerosol Therapy
A. Precipitation of bronchoconstriction
1. Most common in asthmatic patients.
2. May follow administration of certain drugs (i.e., acetylcysteine or bland aerosol).
3. May result in hypoxemia.
B. Increased airway obstruction because of swelling of dried retained secretions
1. Usually a problem with ultrasonic nebulizers more frequently than with mechanical aerosols.
2. Seen primarily in debilitated patients with a poor cough mechanism.
3. May result in hypoxemia.
C. Systemic fluid overload
1. Primarily a problem with neonates and infants.
2. Associated with use of ultrasonic nebulizers more frequently than with use of mechanical nebulizers.
D. Cross-contamination
E. When administering bronchodilators, one should be cautious of the side effects associated with bronchodilator therapy (see Chap. 34).

VIII. Mechanical Aerosol Generators
A. These generators use jet mixing (see Chap. 2) to produce an aerosol and entrain a second gas.
B. A system of baffles is utilized to impact large particles out of suspension.

  C. These generators are commonly used in delivery of medications and for humidification of inspired gases.

  D. Heating increases water content of delivered gas.

 IX. Ultrasonic Aerosol Generators

  A. Ultrasonic nebulizers function by transforming standard household current into ultrasonic sound waves.

  B. The frequency range (1–2 megacycles per second) for ultrasonic sound waves of ultrasonic nebulizers is governed by the Federal Commerce Commission. All ultrasonic nebulizers produced and sold in the United States have preset frequencies in this range.

  C. The ultrasonic sound waves are applied to a quartz crystal or ceramic disk, causing it to vibrate at the same frequency as the ultrasonic waves. This is referred to as the piezoelectric quality of the disk.

  D. The crystal or disk transfers its vibratory energy to the fluid to be nebulized, creating an aerosol.

  E. These nebulizers incorporate an amplitude control that varies the intensity of ultrasonic waves, allowing varying aerosol (medication) outputs.

  F. Ultrasonic nebulizers are principally used in maintenance of bronchial hygiene.

 X. Babington (Hydrosphere) Nebulizer

  A. This nebulizer consists of:

   1. A small hollow glass sphere

   2. Medication reservoir

   3. Pneumatic gas source

   4. Baffles

   5. Syphoning system

  B. As pressurized gas enters the unit it:

   1. Activates the syphoning system bringing medication to the area directly above the glass sphere.

   2. The medication then drips over the surface of the sphere, creating a thin film.

   3. The pressurized gas exits the glass sphere via one or two small openings located on the lateral aspect of the sphere.

   4. As the gas exits, it strikes the fluid film, creating an aerosol.

   5. A circular baffle is placed in front of each gas exit port.

   6. Large aerosol particles strike the baffle and return to the medication reservoir.

 XI. Comparison of Nebulizer Output

  A. Mechanical nebulizers: Up to 1–1.5 ml/min.

  B. Ultrasonic nebulizers: Up to 6 ml/min.

    C. Babington nebulizers: Up to 6 ml/min.
XII. Comparison of Nebulizer Particle Size
    A. Mechanical nebulizers: 55% of particles produced fall in therapeutic range of 1–5 μ.
    B. Ultrasonic nebulizers: 97% of particles produced fall in therapeutic range of 1–5 μ.
    C. Babington nebulizers: 50% of the particles produced fall in the therapeutic range of 1–5 μ.

BIBLIOGRAPHY

Bendixen H.H., et al.: *Respiratory Care*. St. Louis, C.V. Mosby Co., 1965.

Brain J.: Aerosol and humidity therapy. *Am. Rev. Respir. Dis.* 122:17–21, 1980.

Brain J., Valberg P.A.: Deposition of aerosol in the respiratory tract. *Am. Rev. Respir. Dis.* 120:1325–1373, 1979.

Brown J.H., Cook K.M., Ney F.G., et al: Influence of particle size upon the retention of particulate matter in the human lung. *Am. J. Public Health* 40:450–458, 1950.

Burton G.G., Gee G.N., Hodgkin J.E.: *Respiratory Care: A Guide to Clinical Practice*. Philadelphia, J.B. Lippincott Co., 1977.

Garrett D., Donaldson W.: *Physical Principles of Respiratory Therapy Equipment*. Madison, Ohio Medical Products, 1978.

Glover D.W., Glover M.M.: *Respiratory Therapy: Basics for Nursing and the Allied Health Professions*. St. Louis, C.V. Mosby Co., 1978.

Jackson E.E.: The administration of respiratory therapy: Aerosol therapy, techniques, and equipment. *J. Am. Assoc. Nurse Anesth.* 44:373–389, 1976.

Klein E., Shah D., Shah N., et al.: Performance characteristics of conventional and prototype humidifiers and nebulizers. *Chest* 64:690–696, 1973.

Krumpe P.E., McNair R.: Successful substitution of aerosol nebulization therapy for IPPB at a veterans administration medical center. *Milit. Med.* 146:689–692, 1981.

Litt M., Swift D.: The Babington nebulizer: A new principle for generation of therapeutic aerosols. *Am. Rev. Respir. Dis.* 105:308–310, 1972.

McPherson S.P.: *Respiratory Therapy Equipment*, ed. 2. St. Louis, C.V. Mosby Co., 1981.

Miller W.: Fundamental principles of aerosol therapy. *Respir. Care* 17:295–302, 1972.

Morrow P.E.: Aerosol characterization and deposition. *Am. Rev. Respir. Dis.* 110:88–99, 1974.

Newhouse M.T.: Principles of aerosol therapy. *Chest* 82 (suppl.):39S–41S, 1982.

Nelson E.J., Morton E.A., Hunter P.M.: *Critical Care Respiratory Therapy: A Laboratory and Clinical Manual*. Boston, Little, Brown & Co., 1983.

Rarey K.P., Youtsey J.W.: *Respiratory Patient Care*. Englewood Cliffs, N.J., Prentice-Hall, Inc., 1981.

Safer P. (ed.): *Respiratory Therapy*. Philadelphia, F.A. Davis Co., 1965.

Shapiro B.A., Harrison R.A., Kacmarek R.M., et al.: *Clinical Application of Respiratory Care*, ed. 3. Chicago, Year Book Medical Publishers, Inc., 1985.

Simonsson B.G.: Anatomical and pathophysiological considerations in aerosol therapy. *Eur. J. Respir. Dis. Suppl.* 63:7–14, 1982.

Spearman C.B., Sheldon R.L., Egan D.F.: *Egan's Fundamentals of Respiratory Therapy*, ed. 4. St. Louis, C.V. Mosby Co., 1982.

Stiksa G.: Indications for continuous aerosol therapy. *Eur. J. Respir. Dis. Suppl.* 63:89–96, 1982.

Swift D.L.: Aerosols and humidity therapy: Generation and respiratory deposition of therapeutic aerosols. *Am. Rev. Respir. Dis.* 122:71–77, 1980.

Tabachnik E., Levison H.: Clinical application of aerosols in pediatrics. *Am. Rev. Respir. Dis.* 122:97–103, 1980.

Young J.A., Crocker D.: *Principles and Practice of Respiratory Therapy*, ed. 2. Chicago, Year Book Medical Publishers, Inc., 1976.

27 / Chest Physiotherapy

I. Chest physiotherapy is a general term used in reference to a number of techniques designed to assist with bronchial hygiene or the mobilization of secretions and prevention or reversal of atelectasis. Specifically, the following modalities are included under this general heading.
  - A. Postural drainage
  - B. Percussion
  - C. Vibration
  - D. Cough assistance
  - E. Breathing instruction and retraining
II. Postural Drainage
  - A. Postural drainage is a method of removing pooled secretions by positioning the patient so as to allow gravity to assist in movement of secretions. Ideally, the patient is placed with the dependent lung segment uppermost and as vertical as possible.
  - B. Indications
    1. Acute or chronic pulmonary diseases in which secretions are poorly mobilized, resulting in excessive retention and accumulation of secretions.
    2. Atelectasis as a postoperative complication or as a result of poor distribution of ventilation.
    3. Prophylactic care of patients in the immediate postoperative period with a history of acute or chronic pulmonary problems and who have undergone an abdominal or thoracic surgical procedure.
  - C. Standard postural drainage positions for each of the lung segments are listed below.
    1. *Apical segments of right and left upper lobes:* Patient in semi-Fowler's position with head of the bed raised 45 degrees (Fig 27–1).
    2. *Anterior segments of both upper lobes:* Patient supine with the bed flat (Fig 27–2).
    3. *Posterior segments of right upper lobe:* Patient one-quarter turn from prone with the right side up, supported by pillows, with head of the bed flat (Fig 27–3).

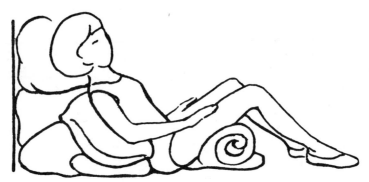

Fig 27–1.—Position for drainage of apical segments of upper lobes.

4. *Apical-posterior segment of left upper lobe:* Patient one-quarter turn from prone with the left side up, supported by pillows, with head of the bed elevated 30 degrees (Fig 27–4).
5. *Medial and lateral segments of right middle lobe:* Patient one-quarter turn from supine with right side up and foot of the bed elevated 12 inches (Fig 27–5).
6. *Superior and inferior segments of lingula:* Patient one-quarter turn from supine with left side up and foot of the bed elevated 12 inches (Fig 27–6).
7. *Superior segments of both lower lobes:* Patient prone with head of the bed flat and pillow under abdominal area (Fig 27–7).
8. *Anteromedial segment of left lower lobe and anterior segment of right lower lobe:* Patient supine, with foot of the bed elevated 20 inches (Fig 27–8).
9. *Lateral segment of right lower lobe:* Patient directly on left side with right side up and foot of the bed elevated 20 inches (Fig 27–9).
10. *Lateral segment of left lower lobe and medial (cardiac) segment of right lower lobe:* Patient directly on right side, with left side up and foot of the bed elevated 20 inches (Fig 27–10).

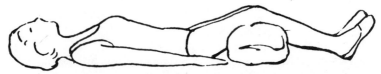

Fig 27–2.—Position for drainage of anterior segments of upper lobes.

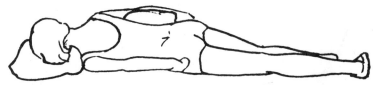

Fig 27–3.—Position for drainage of posterior segment of right upper lobe.

  11. *Posterior segment of both lower lobes:* Patient prone with foot
    of the bed elevated 20 inches (Fig 27–11).
 D. Precautions should be taken when positioning patients with the
  following conditions:
   1. Empyema
   2. Pulmonary embolus
   3. Open wounds, skin grafts, burns
   4. Untreated tension pneumothorax
   5. Flail chest
   6. Frank hemoptysis
   7. Orthopedic procedures
   8. Acute spinal cord injuries
 E. Head-down positioning may be contraindicated in patients with
  the following conditions:
   1. Unstable cardiac status
   2. Hypertension
   3. Head injuries
   4. Thoracic surgery
   5. Abdominal surgery
   6. Diaphragmatic surgery
   7. Tracheoesophageal surgery
   8. COPD
   9. Obesity
   10. Recent meals or tube feeding

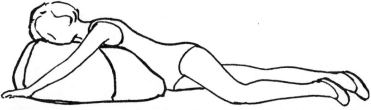

 Fig 27–4.—Position for drainage of apical-posterior segment of left upper
lobe.

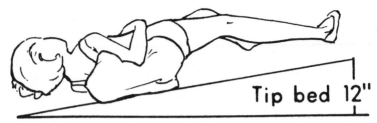

Fig 27–5.—Position for drainage of medial and lateral segments of right middle lobe.

Note: If positioning the patient in the head-down position is necessary, care must be taken to carefully monitor the patient's cardiopulmonary status throughout the procedure.

III. Percussion
  A. Percussion is a technique of rhythmically tapping the chest wall with cupped hands. It is designed to loosen secretions in the area underlying the percussion by the air pressure that is generated by the cupped hand on the chest wall. Percussion is performed during inspiration and expiration.
  B. Indications (same as those for postural drainage, section II-B).
  C. Percussion may be contraindicated in patients with the following conditions:
    1. Cancer with known metastatic changes
    2. Anticoagulant therapy
    3. Tuberculosis
    4. Petechiae
    5. Osteoporotic changes
    6. Empyema
    7. Pulmonary embolus
    8. Wounds, skin grafts, burns
    9. Untreated tension pneumothorax
    10. Flail chest
    11. Frank hemoptysis

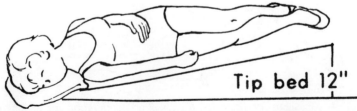

Fig 27–6.—Position for drainage of superior and inferior segments of lingula.

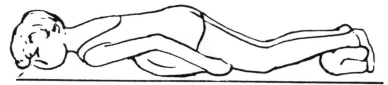

Fig 27–7.—Position for drainage of superior segments of both lower lobes.

    12. Acute spinal cord injuries
    13. Limited patient tolerance
    14. Chest tubes
    15. Unstable cardiac status
    16. Thoracic surgery
    Note: If percussion is performed, care must be taken to carefully monitor the patient's cardiopulmonary status throughout the procedure.
  IV. Vibrations
    A. Vibrations are performed by placing one hand on top of the other over the affected area and tensing the shoulders, keeping the arms straight and applying a vibrating action from shoulder to hand.
    B. Vibrations are intended to move secretions into larger airways.
    C. Vibrations are applied only during exhalation.
    D. Indications (same as those for postural drainage, section II-B).
    E. Possible contraindications are similar to those for percussion (section III-C).
  V. General Hazards and Complications of Postural Drainage, Percussion, and Vibration
    A. Hypoxemia, particularly if patient is positioned with affected areas dependent.

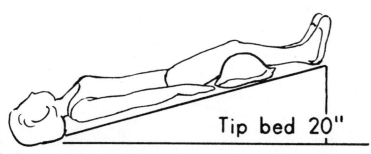

Fig 27–8.—Position for drainage of anteromedial segment of left lower lobe and anterior segment of right lower lobe.

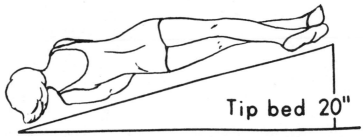

Fig 27–9.—Position for drainage of lateral segment of right lower lobe.

    B. Cardiovascular instability, primarily if patient is positioned head down.

    C. Hemorrhage, hemoptysis.

    D. Fractured ribs, if metastatic cancer is present.

    E. Increased intracranial pressure, principally with head-down positioning.

    F. Dyspnea, particularly if patient is positioned head-down.

VI. Cough Assistance

    A. Sequence of a normal cough

       1. A deep inspiration.

       2. Closure of glottis.

       3. Contraction of abdominal muscles, building up intrapulmonary pressure.

       4. Opening of glottis and a rapid forceful exhalation.

    B. Cough assistance is indicated in the patient who cannot develop a forceful cough.

    C. Cough assistance can be performed by:

       1. Applying pressure to the upper abdominal area during the compression and expiratory phase of the cough.

       2. In patients with an artificial airway, hyperinflating the lung with a manual ventilator, holding gas volume in the lung at

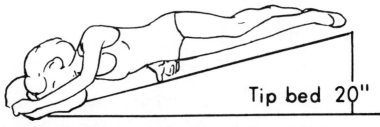

Fig 27–10.—Position for drainage of lateral segment of left lower lobe and medial segment of right lower lobe.

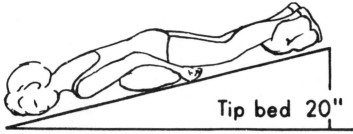

Fig 27–11.—Position for drainage of posterior segments of both lower lobes.

end of inspiration, then rapidly releasing pressure, allowing exhalation, while an associate applies vigorous chest wall compression in an inward and downward fashion. Care should be taken to follow the normal anatomical movement of the chest.

D. "Huffing" (in patients with ineffective cough): Patient is instructed to rapidly expel air through an open glottis. This technique is less painful and less stressful than coughing.

E. "Panting": Patient is instructed to follow normal cough sequence but tongue is kept forward to prevent swallowing of secretions.

VII. Breathing Instruction and Retraining

A. These techniques are designed to assist patients with muscular weakness, postoperative pain, or chronic pulmonary disease to assume an efficient ventilatory pattern and effective cough.

B. Goals
   1. To increase and improve ventilation.
   2. To strengthen respiratory musculature.
   3. To prevent development of atelectasis.
   4. To decrease work of breathing.
   5. To improve the effectiveness of cough.

C. Specific techniques
   1. Diaphragmatic breathing exercises
      a. Therapist and patient locate the xiphoid process. Patient is instructed to "sniff" to determine location of diaphragm.
      b. Patient is relaxed, supported with a pillow and directed to inspire by contracting the diaphragm slowly and completely to allow a normal inspiratory pattern.
         (1) Abdominal expansion.
         (2) Lateral chest expansion.
         (3) Upper chest expansion.

    c. Patient is encouraged to exhale slowly, passively, and completely. Therapist may assist exhalation by exerting a slight inward and upward pressure below the xiphoid process.

  2. Lateral costal expansion exercises

    a. Therapist places hands over patient's lower rib cage with the thumbs just above the xiphoid process.

    b. Patient is encouraged to relax and inspire against a slight pressure exerted by therapist's hands. Patient is instructed to try to expand area located under therapist's hands.

    c. Exhalation should be passive but complete. Therapist can assist exhalation by applying an inward and downward pressure during exhalation.

  3. Localized expansion exercises are designed to direct gas flow to specific area of lung.

    a. Therapist places hands over problem area and instructs patient to inspire against a slight pressure exerted by therapist.

    b. Exhalation should be passive, complete, and assisted by therapist. Therapist exerts an inward and downward force during exhalation, following the natural movement of the rib cage.

BIBLIOGRAPHY

Bartlett R.H., Gazzaniza A.B., Gerahty T.R.: Respiratory maneuvers to prevent postoperative pulmonary complications. *JAMA* 22:1017–1019, 1973.

Bendixen H.H., et al.: *Respiratory Care.* St. Louis, C.V. Mosby Co., 1965.

Breslin E.H.: Prevention and treatment of pulmonary complications in patients after surgery of the upper abdomen. *Heart Lung* 10:511–519, 1981.

Campbell A.H., O'Connell J.M., Wilson F.: The effects of chest physiotherapy upon the FEV, in chronic bronchitis. *Med. J. Aust.* 1:33–35, 1975.

Cherniack R.M.: Physical therapy. *Am. Rev. Respir. Dis.* 122:25–27, 1980.

Connors A.F. Jr., Hammon W.E., Martin R.J., et al.: Chest physical therapy: The immediate effect on oxygenation in acutely ill patients. *Chest* 78:559–564, 1980.

Dhainaut J.-F., Bons J., Bricard C., et al.: Improved oxygenation in patients with extensive unilateral pneumonia using the lateral decubitus position. *Thorax* 35:792–793, 1980.

Gaskell D.V., Webber B.A.: *The Brompton Hospital Guide to Chest Physiotherapy.* Philadelphia, J.B. Lippincott Co., 1974.

Harris J.A., Jerry B.A.: Indications and procedures for segmental bronchial drainage. *Respir. Care* 20:1164–1168, 1975.

Ingwersen U.: *Respiratory Physical Therapy and Pulmonary Care.* New York, John Wiley & Sons, Inc., 1976.

Lewis F.R.: Management of atelectasis and pneumonia. *Surg. Clin. North Am.* 60:1391–1401, 1980.

Oulton J.L., Hobbs G.M., Hicken P.: Incentive breathing devices and chest physiotherapy: A controlled study. *Can. J. Surg.* 24:638–640, 1981.

MacKenzie D.F., Ciesla W., Imle P.C., et al. (eds.): *Chest Physiotherapy in the Intensive Care Unit.* Baltimore, Williams & Wilkins Co., 1981.

MacKenzie C.F., Shin B., McAslan T.C.: Chest physiotherapy: The effect on arterial oxygenation. *Anesth. Analg.* 57:28–30, 1978.

Peters R.M., Turnier E.: Physical therapy indications for and effects in surgical patients. *Am. Rev. Respir. Dis.* 122:147–154, 1980.

Pierce A.K., Robertson J.: Pulmonary complications of general surgery. *Am. Rev. Med.* 28:211–221, 1977.

Rarey K.P., Youtsey J.W.: *Respiratory Patient Care.* Englewood Cliffs, N.J., Prentice-Hall, Inc., 1981.

Rigg J.R.A.: Pulmonary atelectasis after anesthesia: Pathophysiology and management. *Can. Anesth. Soc. J.* 28:305–313, 1981.

Safar P. (ed.): *Respiratory Therapy.* Philadelphia, F.A. Davis Co., 1965.

Schmidt G.B.: Prophylaxis of pulmonary complications following abdominal surgery including atelectasis, ARDS, and pulmonary embolism. *Surgery Annu.* 9:29–73, 1977.

Schuppisser J.P.: Postoperative intermittent positive pressure breathing versus physiotherapy. *Am. J. Surg.* 104:682–686, 1980.

Shapiro B.A., Harrison R.A., Kacmarek R.M., et al.: *Clinical Application of Respiratory Care,* ed. 3. Chicago, Year Book Medical Publishers, Inc., 1985.

Shearer M., Joyce M., Banks B.S.: Lung ventilation during diaphragmatic breathing. *Am. Phys. Ther. Assoc.* 52:139–146, 1972.

Thacker E.W.: *Postural Drainage and Respiratory Control.* Chicago, Year Book Medical Publishers, Inc., 1973.

Tyler M.L.: Complications of positioning and chest physiotherapy. *Respir. Care* 27:458–466, 1982.

Vraciu J.K., Vraciu R.A.: Effectiveness of breathing exercises in preventing pulmonary complications following open heart surgery. *Phys. Ther.* 57:1367–1371, 1977.

Young J.A., Crocker D.: *Principles and Practices of Respiratory Therapy,* ed. 2. Chicago, Year Book Medical Publishers, Inc., 1976.

Zack M.B., Pontoppidantt Kazemi H.: The effect of lateral positions on gas exchange in pulmonary disease: A prospective evaluation. *Am. Rev. Respir. Dis.* 110:49–55, 1974.

28 / Mechanical Aids to Intermittent Lung Expansion

I. Physiologic Basis of Mechanical Aids for Intermittent Lung Inflation in the Treatment or Prevention of Atelectasis
   A. Transpulmonary pressure (alveolar distending pressure) is equal to intra-alveolar pressure minus intrapleural pressure (see Chap. 4).
   B. Increases in lung volumes are accomplished only by increases in transpulmonary pressures.
      1. If intra-alveolar pressure increases more than pleural pressure, transpulmonary pressure increases, as does lung volume. (This occurs during intermittent positive pressure breathing.)
      2. If intrapleural pressure decreases more than intra-alveolar pressure, transpulmonary pressure increases, as does lung volume. (This occurs during incentive spirometry and spontaneous breathing.)
      3. If intrapleural pressure increases the same as intra-alveolar pressure, transpulmonary pressure remains the same, as does lung volume. (This occurs with blow bottles.)
   C. For any lung expansion technique to be successful in overcoming or preventing atelectasis, it must increase transpulmonary pressures, thus increasing lung volume.
   D. This effect is most pronounced if the maneuver sustains inspiratory volume (slow deep breath with inflation hold).
II. Intermittent Positive Pressure Breathing (IPPB)
   A. The delivery of a slow, deep, sustained inspiration by a mechanical device providing a controlled positive pressure breath during inspiration.
   B. Physiologic effects on the respiratory system
      1. Positive pressure breathing reverses the normal intrathoracic and intrapulmonary pressure relationship. With IPPB, the mean intrathoracic pressure is most positive during inspiration and least positive during expiration. Figures 4–3 and 4–4 depict normal intrathoracic and intrapulmonary pressure curves.

These pressure curves are considerably altered during IPPB and may cause decreases in venous return and cardiac output (Fig 28–1).

2. Lung expansion is accomplished by increasing transpulmonary pressure gradients.

3. Work of breathing with properly applied IPPB treatment may be significantly decreased. Since IPPB provides the ventilatory power, the work of the patient's ventilatory muscles is reduced.

    a. This allows the same degree of alveolar ventilation with far less expenditure of muscular energy.

    b. Decreased work of breathing occurs only during therapy, unless significant areas of atelectasis are reversed or a significant volume of secretions is mobilized.

4. Inspiratory-expiratory (I:E) ratios may be manipulated during properly applied IPPB treatment. This is accomplished by restoring a more efficient ventilatory pattern. Under most circumstances, this pattern is maintained only during therapy.

5. The tidal volume (TV) may be increased by three to four times the patient's resting spontaneous tidal exchange during IPPB therapy.

6. Secretions are more effectively mobilized during IPPB treatment. This is accomplished by increasing lung volume and improving distribution of inspired gas.

7. PO_2 normally is increased and PCO_2 normally is decreased *during* IPPB treatment. Improved alveolar ventilation during therapy may result in better gas exchange.

C. Indications for IPPB

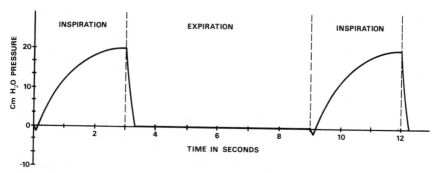

Fig 28–1.—Ideal intrapulmonary pressure curve associated with administration of intermittent positive pressure breathing (IPPB).

1. In general, IPPB is indicated only in patients who cannot voluntarily cough effectively and breathe deeply. Specifically, IPPB *may be* indicated if a patient's vital capacity is *less than* 15 ml/kg of ideal body weight.
   a. Therapeutic
      (1) Atelectasis unresponsive to simple therapy (i.e., incentive spirometry, chest physiotherapy)
      (2) Retained secretions
      (3) Temporary relief of hypoventilation
   b. Prophylactic: Following thoracic or abdominal surgery in patients with chronic or acute pulmonary disease
D. Goals
   1. To provide a significantly deeper breath with more physiologic I:E ratios than patient can produce with spontaneous ventilation
   2. To improve and promote cough mechanism
      a. Optimal peripheral distribution of air through a slow, deep, sustained inspiration with an end-inspiratory pause.
      b. Mechanical provision of necessary power.
   3. To improve distribution of ventilation
      a. In patients with ventilation/perfusion inequalities.
      b. Incidence of postoperative atelectasis and pneumonia is potentially decreased and already atelectatic alveoli may be reexpanded.
   4. To deliver medication
      a. Only if no means other than IPPB (i.e., hand-held nebulizer) can safely and conveniently deliver the medication. The mechanical advantages of IPPB have been overshadowed by its use to deliver medication.
E. Administration
   1. Efficacy of IPPB treatments is greatly dependent on the therapist.
   2. Prerequisites for ideal administration of effective IPPB treatments:
      a. Knowledgeable, well-trained therapist completely familiar with operation, maintenance, and clinical application of equipment.
      b. Relaxed, informed, cooperative patient.
      c. Concise concept of therapeutic goals by physician, therapist, and patient.
      d. Pressure-limited machine.
      e. Appropriate cough and breathing instruction.

    f. Honest appraisal by therapist of benefits from therapy for particular patient.

F. Hazards

  1. Hyperventilation

    a. Incorrect administration of IPPB often causes rapid, deep ventilation leading to acute alveolar hyperventilation with the following possible results:

      (1) Dizziness

      (2) Loss of consciousness

      (3) Tetany

      (4) Paresthesia

    b. Decreased cerebrovascular P_{CO_2} during hyperventilation causes vasoconstriction and decreased cerebral blood flow.

  2. Excessive oxygenation

    a. When driven with oxygen, pneumatically powered, pressure-limited machines give excessively high oxygen concentrations. These high concentrations are potentially harmful to COPD patients who are breathing on a "hypoxic drive."

    b. The high oxygen concentration can be avoided by using machines powered by air compressors or by using a compressed air source.

  3. Increased air trapping

    a. Excessive ventilation of partially obstructed areas in patients with severe COPD.

    b. Post-treatment increase in difficulty of ventilation due to increased FRC.

  4. Decreased cardiac output

    a. Spontaneous ventilation normally facilitates venous return. Increasingly negative intrathoracic pressure on inspiration widens the pressure gradient between abdominal viscera and thoracic cavity. This enhances venous return via inferior vena cava and is called the thoracoabdominal pump.

    b. IPPB ablates the thoracoabdominal pump by causing a less negative or possibly positive mean intrathoracic pressure during inspiration.

    c. Proper I:E ratios in conjunction with minimal airway pressure helps to minimize the above.

    d. Clinical signs of decreased cardiac output

      (1) Systemic hypotension

      (2) Tachycardia

(3) Dyspnea

(4) Distended neck veins

(5) Anxiety

5. Increased intracranial pressure
   a. Cranial venous drainage is potentially impeded by increased mean intrathoracic pressure.
   b. This results in an increase in intracranial pressure, since more blood is contained in the cranium and the volume of the cranium is fixed.

6. Pneumothorax
   a. IPPB mouth pressures of 20 cm H_2O seldom result in excessive alveolar pressures. These pressures by themselves normally are not high enough to cause a "bleb" to rupture.
   b. IPPB may result in better distribution of ventilation and gas entering poorly ventilated lung areas (e.g., a bleb), during IPPB treatment. With a good cough, increased intra-alveolar pressure could rupture a bleb, resulting in pneumothorax.
   c. Possible complaints of chest pain with or after coughing should be anticipated.
   d. If pneumothorax occurs, IPPB should be discontinued until chest decompression is accomplished.

7. Hemoptysis
   a. May occur due to an increase in cough effectiveness that follows IPPB.
   b. Usually the result of bronchial venous bleeding; may be secondary to a tumor or to blood vessel rupture.

8. Gastric distention
   a. The pressure used in IPPB may result in the movement of air into the stomach.
   b. Some patients actually swallow air during IPPB treatments.
   c. The potential for distention increases when administering IPPB to a semialert or comatose patient via mask.

9. Increased airway resistance
   a. IPPB may increase bronchospasm in patients with chronic asthma.

10. Psychological dependence
    a. Patients with COPD receiving IPPB may develop psychological dependence because of the subjective benefit they receive from IPPB.

G. Absolute contraindication

    1. Untreated tension pneumothorax
       a. Tension is increased with positive pressure due to one-way check-valve mechanism.
       b. IPPB treatment should not be initiated until chest decompression is performed.
III. Incentive Spirometry
  A. A technique using visual feedback to encourage patients to take slow, deep, sustained inspirations.
  B. The apparatus acts purely as a visual motivator encouraging patient effort and compliance.
  C. Expansion to a specific lung volume is not guaranteed with the use of an incentive spirometer.
  D. Indications
    1. Treatment of atelectasis
       a. In order for the treatment to be effective the patient must be capable of taking a deep breath.
       b. In general, a vital capacity of greater than 15 ml/kg of ideal body weight is necessary for effective use.
    2. Prevention of atelectasis—Specifically indicated if:
       a. Patient has just undergone thoracic or upper abdominal surgery, and
       b. There is a history of chronic or acute pulmonary disease
  E. For maximum effectiveness the technique should be performed hourly for approximately 10 breaths.
  F. Ideal breathing pattern is a slow, deep, sustained inspiration.
  G. Types of incentive spirometers
    1. Flow-oriented
       a. The patient's inspiratory flow rate causes a float or ball to rise in a cannister. The float or ball remains suspended for a sustained period of time.
       b. The patient should maintain an inspiratory flow that slowly elevates the float.
       c. A rapid inspiration will cause the float to rise quickly but will not maintain it in a suspended position.
       d. Slow inspirations do not generate sufficient flow to raise the float.
    2. Volume-oriented
       a. The patient inspires until a preset volume of gas is inhaled.
       b. Indicators are used to motivate patients and indicate when desired volume is achieved.
       c. Most systems are designed to require a sustained inspiration before the achieved volume indicator is activated.

    H. Possible complications (nondocumented)
        1. Hyperventilation
        2. Barotrauma

VI. Rebreathing Devices
    A. Any tube or cannister designed to increase the depth of breathing by accumulating a patient's exhaled CO_2 and forcing rebreathing.
    B. Normally an increase in respiratory rate is noted with very little increase in tidal volume.
    C. These devices do nothing to control inspiratory flow rates and do not provide for development of an inspiratory pause.
    D. Not effective in reversing alveolar collapse.
    E. Rarely used either prophylactically or therapeutically for the treatment of postoperative pulmonary complications.
    F. No specific indication exists for the use of these devices in modern respiratory care.
    G. Hypoxemia due to small patient tidal volume in relation to the deadspace volume of the device is a common complication that can be prevented by bleeding oxygen into the system.

V. Blow Bottles
    A. Defined as devices in which fluid is moved from one container to another by means of pressure created by the patient during exhalation.
    B. These devices provide a threshold load to exhalation.
    C. Proper use requires a deep inspiration prior to any exhalation.
        1. The deep inspiration is necessary to increase static distending pressures.
        2. If static distending pressures are not increased, no benefit is derived from the use of the device.
        3. The emphasis on exhalation diminishes the likelihood of consistent deep inspirations.
    D. Indications:
        1. Prevention of postoperative atelectasis
        2. Treatment of postoperative atelectasis
    E. Complications:
        1. Atelectasis, if exhalation is started at normal tidal volume and continued to residual volume
        2. Hyperventilation
        3. Barotrauma

BIBLIOGRAPHY

Burton G.G., Gee G.N., Hodgkin J.E.: *Respiratory Care: A Guide to Clinical Practice*. Philadelphia, J.B. Lippincott Co., 1977.

Gale G.D., Sanders D.E.: Incentive spirometry: Its value after cardiac surgery. *Can. Anaesth. Soc. J.* 27:475–480, 1980.

Gale G.D., Sanders D.E.: The Barlett-Edwards incentive spirometer. *Can. Anaesth. Soc. J.* 27:408–416, 1977.

Hudson L.D.: Is IPPB Effective? A controversy in respiratory therapy. *Primary Care* 5:529–542, 1978.

Ingram R.H.: Mechanical aids to lung expansion. *Am. Rev. Respir. Dis.* 123:23–24, 1980.

Iverson L.I.G., Ecker R.R., Fox H.E., et al.: A comparative study of IPPB, the incentive spirometer, and blow bottles: The prevention of atelectasis following cardiac surgery. *Ann. Thorac. Surg.* 25:197–200, 1978.

Jung R., Wight J., Nusser R., et al.: Comparison of three methods of respiratory care following upper abdominal surgery. *Chest* 78:31–35, 1980.

Krastins E.R.B., Corey M.L., McLeod A., et al.: An evaluation of incentive spirometry in the management of pulmonary complications after cardiac surgery in a pediatric population. *Crit. Care Med.* 10:525–528, 1982.

Lewis F.R.: Management of atelectasis and pneumonia. *Surg. Clin. North Am.* 60:1391–1401, 1980.

Martin R.J., Rogers R.M., Gray G.A.: Mechanical aids to lung expansion: The physiologic basis for the use of mechanical aids to lung expansion. *Am. Rev. Respir. Dis.* 122:105–107, 1980.

Murray J.F.: Indications for mechanical aids to assist lung inflation in medical patients. *Am. Rev. Respir. Dis.* 122:121–125, 1980.

Oulton J.L., Hobbs G.M., Hicken P.: Incentive breathing devices and chest physiotherapy: A controlled trial. *Can. J. Surg.* 24:638–640, 1981.

O'Donohue W.J.: Maximum volume IPPB for the management of pulmonary atelectasis. *Chest* 76:683–687, 1976.

Paul W.L., Downs J.B.: Postoperative atelectasis: Intermittent positive pressure breathing, incentive spirometry and face-mask positive end-expiratory pressure. *Arch. Surg.* 116:861–863, 1981.

Pierce A.K., Robertson J.: Pulmonary complications of general surgery. *Annu. Rev. Med.* 28:211–221, 1977.

Pontoppidan H.: Mechanical aids to lung expansion in non-intubated surgical patients. *Am. Rev. Respir. Dis.* 122:109–119, 1980.

Schuppisser J.P., Brandli O., Meili U.: Postoperative intermittent positive pressure breathing versus physiotherapy. *Am. J. Surg.* 104:682–686, 1980.

Shapiro B.A., Harrison R.A., Kacmarek R.M., et al.: *Clinical Application of Respiratory Care*, ed. 3. Chicago, Year Book Medical Publishers, Inc., 1985.

Shapiro B.A., Peterson J., Cane R.D.: Complications of mechanical aids to intermittent lung inflation. *Respir. Care* 27:467–470, 1982.

Spearman C.B., Sheldon R.L., Egan D.F.: *Egan's Fundamentals of Respiratory Therapy*, ed. 4. St. Louis, C.V. Mosby Co., 1982.

Torres G., Lyons H.A., Emerson P.: The effects of intermittent positive pressure breathing on the intrapulmonary distribution of inspired air. *Am. J. Med.* 29:946–954, 1960.

Welch M.A., Shapiro B.J., Mercuiro P., et al.: Methods of intermittent positive pressure breathing. *Chest* 78:463–467, 1980.

29 / Analyzers

I. Oxygen Analyzers
   A. Analyzers that use Pauling's principle of paramagnetic susceptibility of oxygen (Beckman D–2).
      1. The principle of operation is based on the ability of oxygen to be attracted by a magnetic field and cause displacement of nitrogen from the field.
      2. A *dry* gas is drawn into a chamber containing a magnetic field.
         a. The gas is dried by passing through anhydrous (blue) silica gel crystals.
         b. The gas must be dried because water vapor causes interference in the magnetic field and exerts a partial pressure.
      3. Since oxygen is paramagnetic, it is drawn to the strongest portion of the magnetic field. In doing so, oxygen displaces nitrogen, which is diamagnetic, from the field. Displacement occurs by rotation of the nitrogen-filled dumbbell that is suspended by a quartz fiber within the magnetic field.
      4. Attached to the dumbbell is a mirror, which reflects a beam of light that indicates the degree of rotation of the dumbbell.
      5. Degree of rotation is directly related to partial pressure of oxygen in the system and is indicated on a scale in mm Hg P_{O_2} and percentage of oxygen.
      6. Since the analyzer measures partial pressure of oxygen, the mm Hg scale is accurate at all altitudes.
      7. The percent oxygen scale is accurate only at sea level unless it is recalibrated with changes in altitude.
      8. The analyzer accurately measures oxygen partial pressure in all respiratory gas mixtures.
   B. Analyzers that use the thermal conductivity of oxygen
      1. The principle of operation is based on the ability of oxygen to cool an electric wire more so than air.
      2. The cooler the electric wire, the less resistant the wire is to flow of electrons and the greater the current passing through the wire.
      3. The analyzer uses an electric circuit referred to as the *Wheatstone bridge*.

414

4. The Wheatstone bridge has two reference chambers on one side that contain room air. A constant cooling (thermoconductive) effect by the room air maintains current at a specific constant level.
5. On the other side of the bridge is one measuring chamber and a second chamber, which is a calibrating potentiometer.
6. The two sides of the bridge are connected in the middle by a voltmeter (galvanometer), which measures the electrical potentials of each side of the circuit.
7. The potential difference is converted to the percent oxygen of the sample gas.
8. This analyzer actually measures oxygen concentration.
   a. Cooling ability of the sample gas is always compared to the constant thermoconductive effect of room air with about 21% oxygen and 79% nitrogen.
   b. Thus, no matter what the altitude, there is always a comparison to a fixed oxygen-nitrogen ratio.
9. Only oxygen-nitrogen gas mixtures can be analyzed because the cooling effect of sampled gas is always compared to a reference oxygen-nitrogen mixture.
10. In most units gas entering the sample chamber must contain water vapor (some units require a dry sample).
   a. Water vapor is added by using hydrated (pink) silica gel crystals.
   b. The gas is saturated to prevent buildup of a static charge in the system.
11. These analyzers cannot be used with a flammable gas mixture because of the electric circuitry.

C. Analyzers operating on the polarographic principle (Clark electrode) (Figs 29–1 and 29–2)
   1. Basic overall chemical reaction occurring in electrode system is:

$$O_2 + 2H_2O + 4 \text{ electrons} \rightarrow 4OH^- \qquad (1)$$

   2. The analyzer is composed of two electrodes immersed in a potassium chloride electrolyte solution.
      a. At the silver anode, oxidation of chloride ion to silver chloride takes place. This reaction releases electrons, developing a current.
      b. At the platinum cathode, oxygen is reduced to form OH^- ions, thus consuming electrons produced from the anode.

P$_{O_2}$ ELECTRODE:

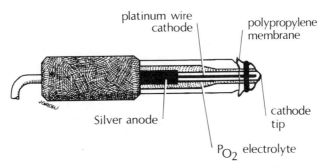

platinum wire
cathode

polypropylene
membrane

Silver anode

cathode
tip

P$_{O_2}$ electrolyte

Fig 29–1.—The Clark electrode. See Figure 29–2 for specifics. (From Shapiro B.A., Harrison R.A., Walton J.R.: *Clinical Application of Arterial Blood Gases*, ed. 3. Chicago, Year Book Medical Publishers, Inc., 1982. Reproduced by permission.)

   3. In solution, the greater the partial pressure of oxygen, the greater the current produced and used.

   4. A -0.6 V polarizing voltage is applied to the anode.

      a. This voltage is needed to maintain direction of current from anode to cathode through the electrolyte solution.

      b. At -0.6 V oxygen is the only respiratory gas that will be readily reduced.

   5. The tip of the Clark electrode is covered with a polypropylene membrane that allows slow diffusion of oxygen from blood or gas being analyzed.

   6. This analyzer type directly measures partial pressure of the gas. For this reason the analyzer must be carefully calibrated at varying altitudes and to changing atmospheric pressures.

   7. The analyzer may be used in all respiratory gas mixtures and is the type incorporated into blood gas analyzer systems.

   8. Measurement of flow of electrons is referred to as an amperometric measurement.

  D. Analyzers using a galvanic cell.

   1. The galvanic cell is similar to a battery cell that utilizes oxygen to create a current between its electrodes.

   2. Current is continually produced if the cell is exposed to oxygen. Thus the life of the cell is dependent on duration and frequency of use.

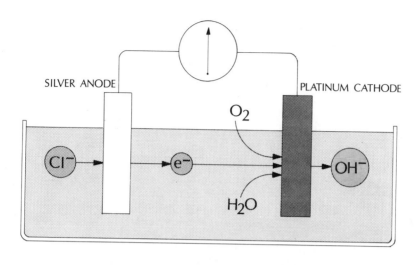

Fig 29–2.—The basic principle of the polarographic electrode. The chloride ion will react with the silver anode to form silver chloride—an oxidation reaction that produces electrons. Oxygen will react with platinum and water, utilizing electrons (a reduction reaction). The flow of electrons can be measured as a current. The greater the concentration of oxygen in solution, the greater the current used. (From Shapiro B.A., Harrison R.A., Walton J.R.: *Clinical Application of Arterial Blood Gases*, ed. 3. Chicago, Year Book Medical Publishers, Inc., 1982. Reproduced by permission.)

3. The analyzer is composed of two electrodes immersed in an alkali metal hydroxide solution. Generally the electrolyte is potassium hydroxide (KOH), but some models use cesium hydroxide (CsOH).
   a. A lead anode, in the presence of oxygen, produces a current as a result of an oxidation reaction with the hydroxide compound.
   b. A gold cathode, in the presence of oxygen, produces the following reaction:

$$O_2 + 2H_2O + 4 \text{ electrons} \rightarrow 4OH^- \qquad (2)$$

   (*Note:* Overall reactions for galvanic cell and polarographic analyzers are the same.)
4. The current is measured from anode to cathode, which allows completion of an electric circuit.
5. The greater the partial pressure of oxygen, the greater the measured current.

6. As with the polarographic analyzer, the galvanic cell measures the partial pressure of oxygen and consequently at varying altitudes and atmospheric pressure.

II. pH (Sanz) Electrode (Figs 29–3 and 29–4)

A. The electrode is composed of two half-cells connected via a potassium chloride electrolyte bridge.

1. A reference half-cell composed of mercury–mercurous chloride (calomel).

2. A measuring half-cell composed of silver–silver chloride.

B. The measuring half-cell has two chambers separated by pH-sensitive glass, which allows measurement of voltage differences across the glass.

1. The enclosed buffer chamber with a buffer of a constant pH surrounds the pH-sensitive glass capillary tube.

2. The sample chamber capillary tube allows blood to be in contact with the pH-sensitive glass.

C. The reference half-cell is immersed in potassium chloride solution, which allows completion of the basic electrical circuit while providing constant reference voltage.

D. As a result of electric activity on the pH-sensitive glass, a potential difference can be measured.

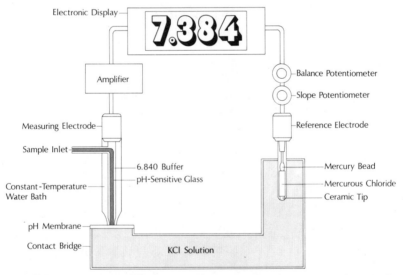

Fig 29–3.—The complete Sanz (pH) electrode. See Figure 29–4 for specifics. (From Shapiro B.A., Harrison R.A., Walton J.R.: *Clinical Application of Arterial Blood Gases,* ed. 3. Chicago, Year Book Medical Publishers, Inc., 1982. Reproduced by permission.)

(a)

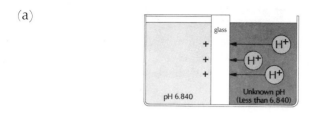

(b)

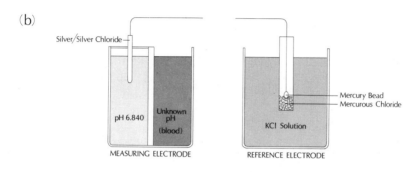

(c)

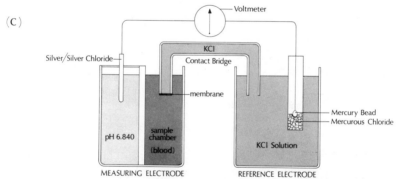

Fig 29–4.—Basic principles of the pH electrode. *a,* voltage is developed across pH-sensitive glass when the hydrogen ion concentration is unequal in the two solutions. *b,* chemical half-cell is used as the measuring electrode and another half-cell is the reference electrode. *c,* the basic principle of the modern pH electrode. (From Shapiro B.A., Harrison R.A., Walton J.R.: *Clinical Application of Arterial Blood Gases,* ed. 3. Chicago, Year Book Medical Publishers, Inc., 1982. Reproduced by permission.)

    E. The potential difference is measured on a voltmeter calibrated in pH units.

    F. This type of system comparing voltage measurements is termed potentiometric.

III. P_{CO_2} (Severinghaus) Electrode (Fig 29–5)

    A. The P_{CO_2} electrode is a modified pH electrode.

    B. P_{CO_2} is measured indirectly by determining change in pH of an $NaHCO_3$ solution.

    C. The electrode is composed of two half-cells, each composed of silver–silver chloride.

    D. Functioning of electrode

      1. Carbon dioxide diffuses across a silicon membrane into an $NaHCO_3$ electrolyte solution.

      2. After entering the solution, carbon dioxide reacts with water to form hydrogen and bicarbonate ions:

$$CO_2 + H_2O \rightarrow H_2CO_3 \rightarrow H^+ + HCO_3^- \tag{3}$$

      3. The H^+ formed sets up a potential difference across the pH-sensitive glass in the measuring half-cell.

    E. All other aspects of the electrode are consistent with the pH electrode.

    F. The potential difference is measured on a voltmeter and reflected as mm Hg carbon dioxide.

    (Note: The PO_2 (Clark) electrode for blood gas analyzers is covered in section I–C.)

IV. Transcutaneous Monitoring (see Chap. 10)

V. Spectrophotometric Analyzers

    A. A spectrophotometer is an apparatus that determines the light absorbence of matter in solution by the quantity of light absorbed in passing through the fluid.

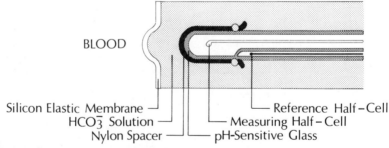

Fig 29–5.—A typical Severinghaus (P_{CO_2}) electrode. (From Shapiro B.A., Harrison R.A., Walton J.R.: *Clinical Application of Arterial Blood Gases,* ed. 3. Chicago, Year Book Medical Publishers, Inc., 1982. Reproduced by permission.)

1. Molecules of a substance in solution can absorb light waves. Various substances absorb differing spectra.
2. Spectrophotometers create light waves specific to the substance to be measured.
3. Light waves of specific spectra are passed through a sample and measured.
4. Since the amount of input light waves is constant, measuring the output waves allows determination of the amount of light absorption by the sample.
5. Finally, according to *Beer's Law*, the absorption of light by a solution is a function of the concentration of the solute and the absorption depth of the solution. The greater the sample absorption, the greater the concentration of the substance being measured since the absorption depth is a constant determined by the sample chamber.

B. Functional components of spectrophotometers
   1. Light source of known intensity
   2. Sample chamber of known depth
   3. Light collector (photomultiplier)
   4. Readout display

C. Types of units commonly used
   1. Oximeter
      a. Spectra specific to oxyhemoglobin. Generally readout is in percent saturation.
      b. Ear oximeter: Noninvasive method of monitoring oxygen saturation in non-critically ill patients.
         (1) Positioned on ear lobe or flat superior aspect of ear.
         (2) Unit heated to greater than body temperature to optimize blood flow to area.
   2. CO-oximeter
      a. Uses light wave spectra specific to:
         (1) Oxyhemoglobin
         (2) Reduced hemoglobin
         (3) Carboxyhemoglobin
         (4) Methemoglobin
      b. In addition, total hemoglobin readout is provided.
   3. Flame photometer
      a. Atomizes blood sample and measures light absorption from a propane flame.
      b. Measures potassium, sodium, and lithium using lithium or cesium as a control.
   4. Capnography

    a. The measurement of the concentration of carbon dioxide in exhaled gas.

    b. A specific infrared spectrum is used.

    c. Exhaled CO_2 levels are compared with ambient CO_2 levels, with the ambient CO_2 acting as a control or reference point.

BIBLIOGRAPHY

Adams A., Hahn C.: *Principles of Blood Gas Analysis*, ed. 2. New York, Churchill-Livingstone, 1982.

Bageant R.: Oxygen analyzers. *Respir. Care* 21:410–416, 1976.

Beyerl D.: Noninvasive measurement of blood oxygen levels. *Am. J. Med. Technol.* 48:355–359, 1982.

Biox Product Literature: *On Ear Oximetry and Biox Ear Oximeter #IIA, #112 M2000 B 7/14/82, 109 M1000 D 6/11/82*. Boulder, Colo., Biox Technology Inc., 1982.

Critikon Product Literature: *Transcutaneous Gas Monitors*. Tampa, Fla., Critikon Inc., 1982.

Degn H., Balsleu I., Brook R. (eds.): *Measurement of Oxygen*. New York, Elsevier Scientific Co., 1976.

Duffin J.: *Physics for Anesthetists*. Springfield, Ill., Bannerstone House Inc., 1976.

Mindt W.: *Skin Sensors for Monitoring Oxygen Tension of Newborns*, product literature. Basel, Switzerland, Hoffmann-LaRoche, 1980.

McPherson S.P.: *Respiratory Therapy Equipment*, ed. 2. St. Louis, C.V. Mosby Co., 1981.

Nuzzo P.: Capnography in infants and children. *Perintol. Neonatol.*, May/June, 1978.

Paloheimo M., Valli M., Ahjopalo H.: *A Guide to CO₂ Monitoring*. Finland, Datex Instumen Tarlum Oy, 1983.

Shapiro B.A., Harrison R.A., Walton J.R.: *Clinical Application of Blood Gases*, ed. 3. Chicago, Year Book Medical Publishers, Inc., 1982.

Spearman C.B., Sheldon R.L., Egan D.F.: *Egan's Fundamentals of Respiratory Therapy*, ed. 4. St. Louis, C.V. Mosby Co., 1982.

Young J.A., Crocker D.: *Principles and Practice of Respiratory Therapy*, ed. 2. Chicago, Year Book Medical Publishers, Inc., 1976.

30 / Fluidics

I. General Characteristics of Fluidic Gas Flow Systems
   A. Fluidic systems possess a basic logic by design.
      1. This basic logic is referred to as the fluidic logic or fluidic element.
      2. The logic determines the direction of gas flow.
   B. These systems normally do not require moving parts for proper function.
   C. Changes in direction of flow are accomplished by:
      1. Backpressure
      2. Subatmospheric (negative inspiratory) pressure
      3. Amplification (cycling pressure)
         a. The control of the direction of a large flow of gas by a small momentary flow of gas (Fig 30–1).
         b. Normally, amplification flow enters the system perpendicular to the main gas flow.
         c. By acting on the main gas flow, the amplification flow causes the main gas flow to alter its direction.
         d. Amplification allows adjustment of sensitivity and cycling pressure.
   D. The basic phenomenon responsible for the overall fluidic mechanism is the *Coanda effect* (Fig 30–2; see also Fig 30–1).
      1. The Coanda effect is based on the fact that a free-flowing gas system creates a subatmospheric pressure at its periphery.
      2. If a wall is placed near the source of gas, the stream of gas adheres to the wall. Adherence is caused by subatmospheric pressure.
      3. When this phenomenon is incorporated in a fluidic system, it is referred to as a wall attachment fluidic element and may be used to alter direction of gas flow.
      4. Once wall attachment has been achieved, a bond between the wall and the gas flow is developed and maintained unless affected by:
         a. Backpressure
         b. Subatmospheric pressure
         c. Amplification

423

5. The creation of the Coanda effect and the strength of its bond are predictable.
   a. The greater the driving pressure the stronger the bond.
   b. The design of the system's logic can strengthen the bond.
      (1) If an "outcropping" (see Fig 30–1) is designed into the system, the Coanda effect is intensified. The outcropping creates an area of low pressure called a vortex. The larger the outcropping, the lower the pressure and the stronger the resulting bond.
      (2) The addition of a *foil* (see Fig 30–2) also strengthens the bond. A foil is a curvilinear narrowing on one wall of the system and acts similar to the wing of an aircraft. As gas moves over the foil, gas velocity increases, creating a negative pressure downstream that enhances wall attachment.

II. Asymmetric Fluidic Logic (Fig 30–3)
   A. Gas powering the logic enters at P_s in Figure 30–3.

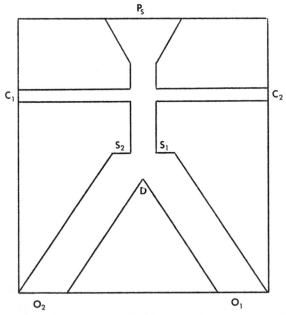

Fig 30–1.—Symmetric bistable fluidic logic. P_s is gas source. S_1 and S_2 are "outcroppings." O_1 and O_2 are exit ports, and D is the separator. A vortex is created at S_2 or S_1. C_1 and C_2 are amplification ports. Momentary gas flow from amplification port C_1 would direct gas flow to exit port O_1. Momentary gas flow from C_2 would direct gas flow to exit port C_1.

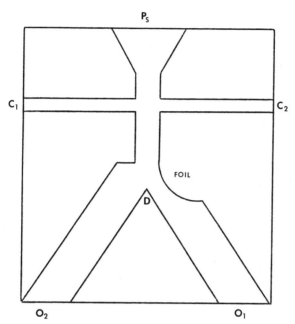

Fig 30–2.—Bistable fluidic logic incorporating a foil. Point *D* is the separator, O_1 and O_2 are exit ports, and C_1 and C_2 are amplification ports. The foil creates a negative pressure, enhancing wall attachment.

      B. Point *A* is a constriction in the gas entry port designed to accelerate gas velocity.

      C. Lateral to point *B* is where the Coanda effect begins to appear.

        D. Outcroppings are represented by S_1 and S_2. Since S_1 is larger than S_2, the wall attachment bond at S_1 would be greater than S_2.

      E. Point *D* is referred to as the separator. The location of the separator determines the type of logic. If the separator is directly midline, the logic is bistable (refer to section III). If the separator is not midline, the system is monostable (refer to section V).

      F. Amplification ports are represented by C_1 and C_2.

III. Symmetric Bistable Fluidic Logic (see Fig 30–1)

      A. Gas entering the element at P_s is stable in either leg (exit port) of the system, O_1 or O_2. Both exit ports in the system are symmetric in design.

      B. Once gas enters a leg of the system, it will remain stable in that leg until acted on by an external force.

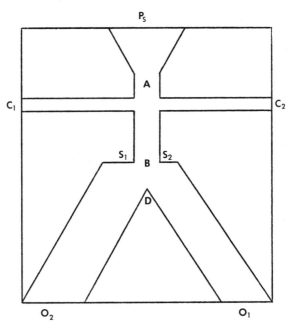

Fig 30–3.—Asymmetric bistable fluidic logic. P_s is a gas source. Point A represents initial constriction of system. Point B indicates location of development of Coanda effect. Point D is the separator. C_1 and C_2 are amplification ports, S_1 and S_2 are outcroppings, and O_1 and O_2 are exit ports. Although the system is bistable, the larger outcropping at S_1 results in a stronger attachment down exit port O_2.

C. Amplification may occur from C_1 (or C_2), causing flow to move from O_2 to O_1 (or O_1 to O_2).

D. A subatmospheric (negative inspiratory) pressure created at O_1 also will cause gas to move in a stable manner down that exit port.

E. As pressure begins to increase at O_1 to a predetermined level (based on design), it will then direct the flow to O_2 and remain stable there until it is acted on by an external force.

F. All bistable logics may be referred to as a *flip-flop valve with a memory.*

IV. Asymmetric Bistable Fluidic Logic (see Fig 30–3)

A. In an asymmetric bistable system the two exit ports of the system (O_1 and O_2) are not designed similarly; however, the separator is midline.

B. As in a symmetric bistable system, once gas flow enters either leg it is stable in that leg unless acted on by an external force.

C. Because of the asymmetric design (S_1 greater in size than S_2) wall attachment is stronger in one leg (O_2) than the other (O_1); however, it is stable in both.

V. Monostable Fluidic Logic (Fig 30–4)
  A. This system is asymmetric in design.
  B. The asymmetric design is a result of positioning one of the system's exit ports off-center. This is accomplished by the location of the separator (point D).
  C. Gas will normally proceed from P_s to O_1 as a result of the separator. Gas flow will be stable in O_1 until an external force causes movement to leg O_2.
  D. As gas moves to O_1, additional gas will be entrained from O_2, thus increasing the volume exiting at O_1. (Air entrainment is possible in any fluidic logic system.)
  E. Gas flow will move to leg O_2 only under the following circumstances:
    1. If backpressure were generated at O_1 great enough to overcome wall attachment.

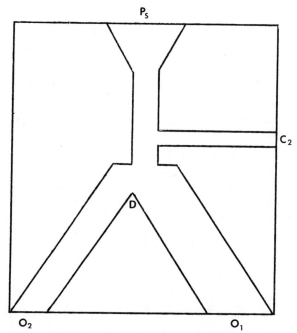

Fig 30–4.—Monostable fluidic logic. P_s is gas source. Point D is the separator. O_1 and O_2 are exit ports and C_2 is an amplification port.

2. If amplification were to occur at point C_2, the main flow of gas would be directed down leg O_2.
   a. The flow from C_2 needs to be directed perpendicular to the main gas flow.
   b. The amplification flow must enter the system on a side opposite to that where it is directing the main gas flow.
 F. Once the backpressure is removed and the amplification flow is stopped, the main flow will return to its original path, O_1.

VI. AND/NAND Fluidic Logic (Fig 30–5 and Table 30–1)
 A. The flow is always stable from P_s to O_2 unless it is acted on by an external force (monostable element).
 B. In order for flow to move from O_2 to O_1, simultaneous amplification must occur from both C_1 and C_3.
 C. If gas were to enter only from C_1, it would exit at C_3 without affecting the main gas flow. The same type of situation occurs if gas enters only from C_3.
 D. Once amplification flow is stopped, flow will revert to O_2 and again remain stable.

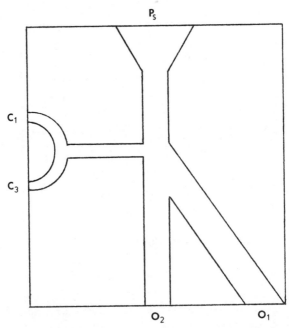

Fig 30–5.—AND/NAND fluidic logic. Flow is normally stable form P_s to O_2. In order for flow to be diverted to O_1, simultaneous amplification must originate from both C_1 and C_3.

TABLE 30–1.—TRUTH TABLE
FOR AND/NAND SYSTEM

LINE	C_1	C_3	O_1	O_2
1	0	0	0	X
2	X	0	0	X
3	0	X	0	X
4	X	X	X	0

E. The truth table (Table 30–1) accompanying Figure 30–5 is used
to explain the direction that flow will take in response to the
forces acting on it.

  1. A zero (0) in Table 30–1 indicates no flow from the particular
  source.

  2. An X in the table indicates flow.

  3. For example, in line 1, there is no flow from C_1 or C_3; thus
  gas only flows to O_2.

VII. OR/NOR Fluidic Logic (Fig 30–6 and Table 30–2)

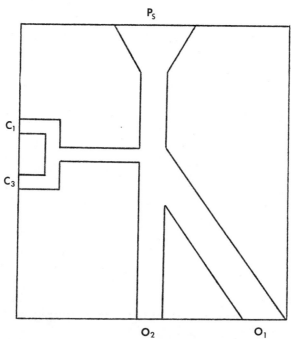

Fig 30–6.—OR/NOR fluidic logic. Flow is normally stable from P_s to O_2. Flow
may be diverted from O_2 to O_1 with amplification from either C_1 or C_3, or both.

TABLE 30–2.—Truth Table
for OR/NOR System

LINE	C_1	C_3	O_1	O_2
1	0	0	0	X
2	X	0	X	0
3	0	X	X	0
4	X	X	X	0

    A. The flow is always stable from P_s to O_2 unless acted on by an external force (monostable logic).

    B. In order for flow to move from O_2 to O_1, amplification must occur from C_1 or C_3, or both.

    C. Once amplification is stopped, flow will revert to O_2 and again remain stable.

VIII. Proportional Amplifier (Fig 30–7)

    A. This is basically a symmetric bistable logic system in which directional flow change occurs by amplification alone.

    B. Flow always enters the system from C_1 and C_2.

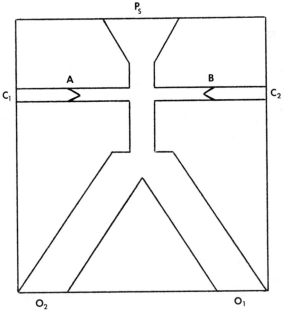

Fig 30–7.—Proportional amplifier. P_s is gas source. A and B are adjustable valves. C_1 and C_2 are amplification ports, and O_1 and O_2 are exit ports.

C. Gas moves toward O_1 or O_2, depending upon whether amplification is greater at C_1 or C_2.

D. Points A and B are adjustable valves. These valves may be incorporated and used to function as sensitivity or pressure cycling regulators.

    1. If a patient were connected at point O_1, valve A would act as a sensitivity control. Thus, gas flow from O_2 to O_1 would depend on amplification from A and patient subatmospheric pressure at O_1.

    2. In the situation described, B would act as a peak pressure (cycling pressure) control. Gas movement from O_1 to O_2 would depend on backpressure at O_1 and amplification at C_2.

IX. Backpressure Switch (Fig 30–8)

A. This is a modified monostable logic. Gas is stable in leg O_2.

B. As gas enters the system, a portion of it is shunted through X because of the restriction at point E.

C. The gas entering X moves through the restriction at point G and out C_1.

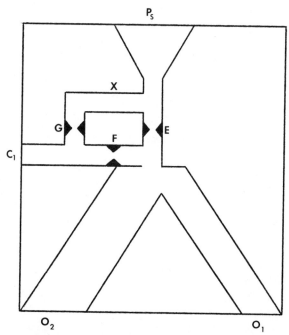

Fig 30–8.—Backpressure switch. P_s is gas source. Points E, F, and G are restrictors. X is shunt for main flow gas. C_1 is an amplification port, and O_1 and O_2 are exit ports.

   D. If C_1 is blocked, gas from X moves through the restriction at
      point F and acts as amplification on the system. As a result, gas
      is forced from O_2 to O_1.
   E. Opening and closing of C_1 can be governed by a microprocessor-
      controlled solenoid switch.
   F. If a patient were connected at point O_1, the opening and closing
      of C_1 would act as a time cycling mechanism that is determining
      the amount of time gas would flow to O_1.
X. Ventilators Incorporating Fluidic Logics
   A. Retec X70/IPPB
   B. Mine Safety Appliance IPPB
   C. Ohio 550
   D. Monaghan 225
   E. Sechrist IV-100B

BIBLIOGRAPHY

Angrist S.: Fluid control devices. *Sci. Am.* 211:80, 1964.
Garrett D.F.: *Physical Principles of Respiratory Therapy Equipment.* Madison, Wis., Ohio Medical Products, 1978.
McPherson S.P.: *Respiratory Therapy Equipment*, ed. 2. St. Louis, C.V. Mosby Co., 1981.
Monaghan Product Information: *Fluidics and Monaghan Volume Ventilators.* Schaumburg, Ill., Monaghan Co., A Division of Sandoz, Inc., 1973.
Mushin W.W.: *Automatic Ventilation of the Lungs*, ed. 3. Oxford, Blackwell Scientific Publications, 1980.
Reba I.: Application of the Coanda effect. *Sci. Am.* 214:84, 1966.
Respiratory Products Bulletin, Retec X70/IPPB. Portland, Ore., Retec Development Laboratory, 1975.
Spearman C.P., Sheldon R.L., Egan D.F.: *Egan's Fundamentals of Respiratory Therapy*, ed. 4. St. Louis, C.V. Mosby Co., 1982.

31 / Technical Aspects of Mechanical Ventilators

I. Classification of Mechanical Ventilators

This chapter discusses the technical characteristics of mechanical ventilators. In order to present this material in a logical manner, the following 12-point system is used to classify ventilators.

A. Positive or negative pressure
   1. Positive pressure ventilators make use of a supra-atmospheric pressure applied to the airway to deliver tidal volumes.
   2. Negative pressure ventilators make use of a subatmospheric pressure applied to the thorax to deliver tidal volumes.

B. Powering mechanism
   1. Physical energy source that provides the power for ventilator function.
   2. Available powering mechanisms.
      a. Electric: Normally uses 120-volt electrical current.
      b. Pneumatic: Normally uses a 40–60 psi gas source.
      c. Combined electric/pneumatic: Both must be activated for proper machine function.

C. Driving mechanism
   1. Provides the mechanical force that produces the flow of gas necessary for delivery of tidal volumes.
   2. Characteristic types of driving systems
      a. Pneumatic systems: Driven by a compressed gas source (either internal or external to ventilator) regulated by electronic, fluidic, or mechanical devices inside the ventilator.
         (1) Pneumatic clutches and valves
         (2) Electronic servo mechanisms
         (3) Electronic and mechanical solenoids
         (4) Preset and adjustable regulators
         (5) Fluidic regulation
      b. Piston systems: Driven by devices exhibiting
         (1) Linear motion
         (2) Rotary motion (i.e., exponential or logarithmic acceleration/deceleration)

433

    c. Bellows systems: Driven by a compressed gas source (either internal or external to ventilator) generated by a:

      (1) Compressor (e.g., turbine)

      (2) Fluidic system

      (3) Pneumatic system

D. Maintenance of gas flow pattern

  1. The ability of a ventilator to maintain a consistent gas flow pattern is dependent on the driving mechanism of the ventilator and the total patient resistance to ventilation.

  2. If the maximum pressure generated by the driving force of a ventilator is at least five times the highest system pressure developed during gas delivery, the ventilator is considered a *flow generator*. These machines can maintain their gas flow patterns despite increasing backpressure.

  3. If the driving mechanism generates a force considerably less than five times the highest system pressure, the ventilator is referred to as a *pressure generator*. These ventilators demonstrate significant variations in gas flow patterns as resistance to ventilation changes (e.g., increased airway resistance and/or decreased compliance).

  4. Constant flow vs. constant pressure generators.

    a. Constant flow generators: Driving pressures maintained are greater than 4,000 cm H_2O. *There is little or no variation in gas flow pattern.*

    b. Non-constant flow generators: Driving pressures are normally greater than 4,000 cm H_2O and there is a reproducible gas flow pattern that does not vary with alterations in patient resistance to ventilation. *Although the pattern of gas flow is the same breath after breath, the rate of gas delivery during each breath varies.*

    c. Modified constant flow generators: Driving pressures are considerably less than 4,000 cm H_2O. *Gas flow patterns may change significantly with changes in resistance to ventilation.*

    d. Constant pressure generators: Driving pressures are less than 100 cm H_2O. *There may be a continual modification of gas flow pattern during the inspiratory phase in response to changes in resistance to ventilation.*

E. Number of circuits

  1. A circuit is the path the gas flow follows inside the ventilator.

  2. A single circuit ventilator has one pressurized gas volume. This pressurized gas volume is the same as that delivered to

the patient (i.e., the same gas flow that is produced by the ventilator's driving mechanism is delivered to the patient).

    3. A double circuit ventilator has two separate pressurized gas volumes. One gas volume is used to compress the second gas. This latter compressed gas is the volume delivered to the patient (i.e., one gas powers the driving mechanism and the other gas is delivered to the patient). Two distinct gas flow systems are involved in tidal volume delivery.

F. Gas flow and airway pressure patterns

    1. The gas flow pattern developed during inspiration is dependent on the driving mechanism employed and the ability of the machine to maintain flow despite increasing backpressure.

    2. The pressure pattern is dependent on the gas flow pattern and total resistance to ventilation (pressure = gas flow × resistance).

    3. Specific pressure patterns are always associated with a particular gas flow pattern. However, this may not hold true if the patient fights the ventilator.

    4. Characteristic gas flow and pressure patterns

       a. Square wave flow and rectilinear pressure patterns: A constant flow is maintained throughout the inspiratory phase. This tends to result in a constant pressure change per unit of time, or a rectilinear pressure pattern (Fig 31–1). However, few ventilators are capable of maintaining a constant flow. The dotted lines in Figure 31–1 demonstrate the effect of backpressure on flow rate and pressure patterns. If this flow taper effect (decelerating flow pattern) develops,

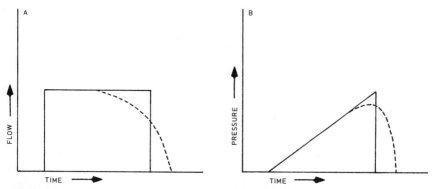

Fig 31–1.—**A,** square wave flow pattern. *Dotted line* represents normal flow tapering. **B,** rectilinear pressure pattern. *Dotted line* represents the effect of a flow taper.

inspiratory time is lengthened. These flow and pressure patterns are characteristic of modified constant flow generators.

b. Sine wave flow and sigmoidal pressure patterns: Normally produced by logarithmically accelerating/decelerating (rotary) piston-driving mechanisms. Flow begins slowly, then accelerates until the middle of inspiration, then decreases toward the end of inspiration. One half of a sine wave is produced, resulting in a sigmoidal pressure pattern (Fig 31–2). This is the most common example of a non-constant flow generator.

c. Accelerating flow and nonlinearly increasing pressure patterns: Flow progressively increases during inspiration until a preset limit is reached, at which time the flow plateaus to a square wave (Fig 31–3). A nonlinearly increasing pressure pattern develops. These curves are produced by non-constant flow generators.

d. Decelerating flow and parabolic pressure patterns. Gas flow begins at a maximum and at some preset point during the inspiratory phase the flow rate begins to decrease until the end of inspiration. Two basic patterns exist, a flow taper (Fig 31–4) and a decaying flow pattern (Fig 31–5). These flow patterns result in parabolic pressure patterns that may be initially linear but terminally the rate of pressure change diminishes. Figure 31–4 is an example of a modified constant flow generator and Figure 31–5 is an example of a constant pressure generator.

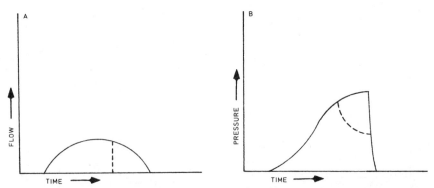

Fig 31–2.—A, sine wave flow pattern. *Dotted line* represents a modified sine wave flow pattern. **B,** sigmoidal pressure pattern. *Dotted line* represents the pressure curve seen with a modified sine wave flow pattern.

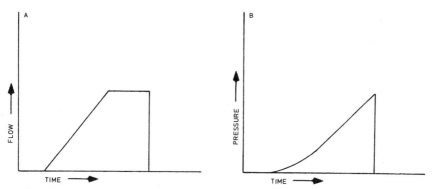

Fig 31–3.—A, accelerating flow pattern. **B,** nonlinearly increasing pressure pattern.

G. Cycling parameter
   1. The physical parameter that, when reached, will result in termination of the mechanical inspiratory phase.
   2. Four basic parameters are involved in the delivery of gas to any patient. One (or more) of these is always the cycling parameter.
      a. Volume
      b. Pressure
      c. Time
      d. Flow
   3. A primary cycling parameter that has been attained does *not* activate an audiovisual or audio alarm.

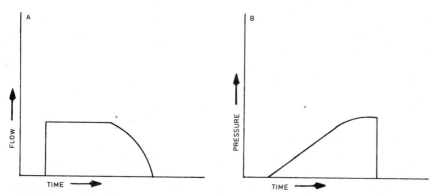

Fig 31–4.—A, square wave flow with flow taper (decelerating flow). **B,** parabolic pressure pattern.

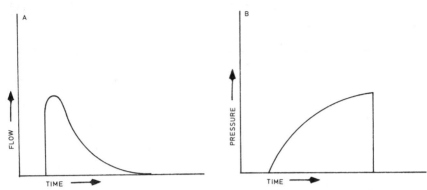

Fig 31–5.—A, decaying flow pattern (decelerating flow). **B,** parabolic pressure pattern.

  a. An alarm being activated with each inspiration normally indicates an inappropriate condition for continuous mechanical ventilation.
  b. Limiting parameters (see below) may function as secondary cycling mechanisms. When attained, these parameters normally activate an alarm.

H. Limit
  1. A limit is a physical parameter (flow, time, pressure, volume) that cannot be exceeded but is not the primary cycling mechanism. Limiting parameters may be divided into three categories.
    a. Limits that are preset but adjustable. *Examples:*
      (1) Peak flow control on the MA-1
      (2) Normal pressure limit control on the Bourns Bear I
      (3) Pressure relief on the Emerson Post-Op
    b. Limits that are the result of two preset adjustable parameters. *Examples:*
    (1) Inspiratory time on the MA-1,

$$\text{Inspiratory Time} = \frac{\text{TV}}{\text{flow}}$$

    (2) Volume on the Veriflo CV 2000,

$$\text{Tidal Volume} = \frac{\text{flow}}{\text{inspiratory time}}$$

    c. Some limits also may serve as a secondary means of ending inspiration. All limiting factors that end inspiration should have simultaneous audio or audiovisual alarms. *Examples:*
      (1) Pressure limit on the MA-1
      (2) I:E ratio limit on the Bourns Bear I

I. Modes of ventilation. The term mode is used to represent the manner in which gas is delivered, regardless of whether the tidal volume is pressurized or not.

  1. Control: The machine is responsible for initiation and delivery of each tidal volume.

  2. Assist: The patient is totally responsible for initiation of the inspiratory phase, but the ventilator delivers the tidal volume.

  3. Assist/control: The machine functions in the assist mode unless the patient's respiratory rate falls below a present level, at which time the machine converts to the control mode.

  4. Intermittent Mandatory Ventilation (IMV): The patient is allowed to breathe spontaneously from an external high-flow system or from the ventilator via a demand valve, and at preset intervals the machine functions in the control mode.

  5. Synchronized Intermittent Mandatory Ventilation (SIMV): The patient is allowed to breathe spontaneously from the ventilator via a demand valve, and at preset intervals the machine functions in the assist/control mode.

  6. Extended Mandatory Minute Volume (EMMV): A minimum minute volume delivery is set on the machine. The patient may receive this volume (1) breathing totally spontaneously, (2) while being mechanically ventilated, or (3) a combination of 1 and 2. If the patient's spontaneous minute volume falls below the minimum level, mandatory positive pressure breaths make up the difference.

  7. Continuous Positive Airway Pressure (CPAP): The patient breathes spontaneously via a demand valve or high-flow system, (no positive pressure breaths are delivered.) PEEP can be maintained at any level.

  8. Pressure support: During spontaneous ventilation, the ventilator functions as a constant pressure generator.
    a. Pressure develops rapidly in the ventilator system and remains at that level until spontaneous inspiratory flow rates decrease to 25% of peak inspiratory flow.
    b. The mode may be used:
      (1) Independently

       (2) In conjunction with CPAP
       (3) In conjunction with SIMV
   9. Inspiratory assist: During spontaneous ventilation, the ventilator functions as a modified constant pressure generator.
     a. Pressure develops slowly in the ventilator system up to a preset limit. When the patient's spontaneous inspiratory flow rate decreases to a preset level, the inspiratory assist is ended.
     b. This mode may be used:
       (1) Independently
       (2) In conjunction with CPAP
       (3) In conjunction with SIMV
     Note: The clinical applications of each of the described modes are presented in Chapter 32, "Principles of Mechanical Ventilation."
  J. Inspiratory airway maneuvers. (A discussion of the physiologic effects and clinical use of these maneuvers is found in Chapter 32.)
   1. Sigh: The periodic delivery of a mechanical tidal volume that is greater (commonly 50%) than the patient's set mechanical tidal volume.
   2. Inflation hold (inspiratory hold, inspiratory pause): The incorporation of a static phase at the end of inspiration. This can be achieved by holding the delivered tidal volume within the patient's airway or by maintaining a constant pressure at the patient's airway.
   3. Flow taper: The gradual reduction of delivered flow rate during inspiration. Flow tapers may be adjusted to modify flow, beginning at any point during inspiration.
  K. Expiratory airway maneuvers. (A discussion of the physiologic effects and clinical use of these maneuvers is found in Chapter 32.)
   1. Expiratory retard: Establishment of a resistance to exhalation, decreasing expiratory gas flow and hence lengthening the time it takes peak airway pressure to reach baseline.
   2. Positive End-Expiratory Pressure (PEEP): The maintenance of airway pressure above atmospheric at end-exhalation.
   3. Negative End-Expiratory Pressure (NEEP): The maintenance of airway pressure below atmospheric at end-exhalation.
  L. Ventilator alarm systems: Standard alarms incorporated into the ventilation system that indicate malfunction in gas delivery, oxygen concentration, machine function, or patient status.
II. Specific Mechanical Ventilators: The following commonly used ventilators are classified according to the 12-point classification scheme pre-

sented above, in their factory-delivered stock condition. Many can be significantly modified from that which is presented.

A. Bird Mark 7 and 8
1. Pressure: Positive
2. Powering mechanism: Pneumatic
3. Driving mechanism: Pneumatic system regulated by a Venturi device with a pneumatic clutch and peak flow needle valve
4. Maintenance of gas flow pattern: Modified constant pressure generator
5. Circuit: Single
6. Gas flow and airway pressure patterns:
   a. Airmix setting: Decelerating flow and parabolic pressure pattern
   b. 100% setting: Square wave flow and rectilinear pressure pattern
7. Cycling parameter: Pressure
8. Limit: Flow (preset)
9. Modes
   a. Assist
   b. Assist/control
   c. Control
10. Inspiratory airway maneuvers: None
11. Expiratory airway maneuvers: Mark 7, none; Mark 8, negative end-expiratory pressure
12. Alarms: None standard

B. Bennett PR series
1. Pressure: Positive
2. Powering mechanism: Pneumatic
3. Driving mechanism: Pneumatic system regulated by pressure-reducing valve (diluter-regulator)
4. Maintenance of gas flow pattern: Modified constant pressure generator
5. Circuit: Single
6. Gas flow and airway pressure patterns: Decelerating flow and parabolic pressure patterns
7. Cycling parameters
   a. Flow (primary)
   b. Time
8. Limit: Pressure (preset)
9. Modes
   a. Assist
   b. Assist/control

      10. Inspiratory airway maneuvers: None
      11. Expiratory airway maneuvers: NEEP (PR-2 only)
      12. Alarms: None standard

C. Emerson 3-PV Post-Operative
      1. Pressure: Positive
      2. Powering mechanism: Electric
      3. Driving mechanism: Rotary piston system driven by electric motor
      4. Maintenance of gas flow pattern: Non-constant flow generator
      5. Circuit: Single
      6. Gas flow and airway pressure patterns: Sine wave and sigmoidal pressure patterns
      7. Cycling parameter: Time
      8. Limits (preset):
        a. Volume (preset)
        b. Pressure (relief/pop-off)
        c. Flow (resultant of time and volume)
      9. Mode: Control
      10. Inspiratory airway maneuvers: Sigh (optional)
      11. Expiratory airway maneuvers: PEEP
      12. Alarms: None standard

D. Emerson 3-MV (IMV ventilator)
      1. Pressure: Positive
      2. Powering mechanism: Electric/pneumatic (pneumatic source required for spontaneous breathing in IMV mode)
      3. Driving mechanism: Rotary piston system driven by an electric motor
      4. Maintenance of gas flow pattern: Non-constant flow generator
      5. Circuit: Single
      6. Gas flow and airway pressure patterns: Sine wave flow and sigmoidal pressure patterns
      7. Cycling parameter: Time
      8. Limits (preset)
        a. Pressure (relief/pop-off)
        b. Volume (preset)
        c. Flow (result of time and volume)
      9. Modes
        a. Control
        b. IMV
      10. Inspiratory airway maneuvers: None
      11. Expiratory airway maneuvers: PEEP
      12. Alarms: None standard

E. Bennett MA-1
  1. Pressure: Positive
  2. Powering mechanism: Electric
  3. Driving mechanism: Bellows system driven by gas from electric compressor
  4. Maintenance of gas flow pattern: Modified constant flow generator
  5. Circuit: Double
  6. Gas flow and airway pressure patterns: Square wave flow with taper; rectilinear to parabolic pressure pattern
  7. Cycling parameters
     a. Volume (primary)
     b. Pressure
  8. Limits
     a. Flow (preset)
     b. Pressure (preset)
     c. Time (result of volume and flow)
  9. Modes
     a. Control
     b. Assist/control
     c. Assist
     d. IMV (option)
     e. SIMV (option)
     f. CPAP (option)
  10. Inspiratory airway maneuvers: Sigh
  11. Expiratory airway maneuvers
     a. PEEP (option)
     b. NEEP (option)
     c. Expiratory retard
  12. Alarms
     a. Patient alarms
        (1) High inspiratory pressure
        (2) Low exhaled tidal volume and/or disconnect
        (3) I:E ratio
     b. Machine alarms
        (1) Oxygen system failure
F. Bennett MA-2, MA-2+2
  1. Pressure: Positive
  2. Powering mechanism: Electric
  3. Driving mechanism: Bellows system driven by gas from an electric compressor
  4. Maintenance of gas flow pattern: Modified constant flow generator

5. Circuit: Double
6. Gas flow and airway pressure patterns: Square wave flow with taper; rectilinear to parabolic pressure pattern
7. Cycling parameters
   a. Volume (primary)
   b. Pressure
8. Limits
   a. Pressure (preset)
   b. Flow (preset)
   c. Time (result of volume and flow)
9. Modes
   a. Control
   b. Assist
   c. Assist/control
   d. IMV (option)
   e. SIMV
   f. CPAP
10. Inspiratory airway maneuvers
    a. Sigh
    b. Inflation hold
11. Expiratory airway maneuvers
    a. PEEP
12. Alarms
    a. Patient alarms
       (1) High airway pressure
       (2) Low inspiratory pressure
       (3) Loss of pressure
       (4) Low PEEP/CPAP
       (5) Low exhaled tidal volume
       (6) I:E ratio
       (7) Fail to cycle
    b. Machine alarms
       (1) Oxygen/compressed air system failure
       (2) High gas temperature
       (3) High/low F_{IO_2} (option)
G. Bear I
   1. Pressure: Positive
   2. Powering mechanism: Electric
   3. Driving mechanism: Pneumatic system regulated by solenoids and regulators

  4. Maintenance of gas flow pattern: Modified constant flow generator
  5. Circuit: Single
  6. Gas flow and airway pressure patterns: Square wave flow with taper; rectilinear to parabolic pressure pattern
  7. Cycling parameters
     a. Volume (primary)
     b. Pressure
     c. Time (via I:E ratio limit)
  8. Limits
     a. Pressure (preset)
     b. Flow (preset)
     c. Time (result of volume and flow)
  9. Modes
     a. Control
     b. Assist/control
     c. SIMV
     d. CPAP
 10. Inspiratory airway maneuvers
     a. Sigh
     b. Inflation hold
     c. Flow taper
 11. Expiratory airway maneuvers: PEEP
 12. Alarms
     a. Patient alarms
        (1) High/low inspiratory airway pressure
        (2) Low PEEP/CPAP
        (3) Low exhaled tidal volume
        (4) I:E ratio
        (5) Apnea
     b. Machine alarms
        (1) Oxygen/compressed air system failure
        (2) Ventilator inoperative
        (3) Electric failure
H. Bear II
  1. Pressure: Positive
  2. Powering mechanism: Electric
  3. Driving mechanism: Pneumatic system operated by solenoids and regulators
  4. Maintenance of gas flow pattern: Modified constant flow pattern

   5. Circuit: Single
   6. Gas flow and airway pressure patterns: Square wave flow with taper; rectilinear to parabolic pressure pattern
   7. Cycling parameters
      a. Volume (primary)
      b. Pressure
      c. Time (via I:E ratio limit)
   8. Limits
      a. Pressure (preset)
      b. Flow (preset)
      c. Time (result of volume and flow)
   9. Modes
      a. Control
      b. Assist/control
      c. SIMV
      d. CPAP
  10. Inspiratory airway maneuvers
      a. Sigh
      b. Inflation hold
      c. Flow taper
  11. Expiratory airway maneuvers: PEEP
  12. Alarms
      a. Patient alarms
         (1) High/low inspiratory pressure
         (2) Low PEEP/CPAP
         (3) Low exhaled tidal volume
         (4) I:E ratio
         (5) Apnea
         (6) High respiratory rate
      b. Machine alarms
         (1) Oxygen/compressed air system failure
         (2) Ventilator inoperative
         (3) High gas temperature
         (4) Electric failure
I. Veriflo CV 2000
   1. Pressure: Positive
   2. Powering mechanism: Pneumatic
   3. Driving mechanism: Pneumatic system regulated by pneumatic relays and balanced diaphragm mechanism
   4. Maintenance of gas flow pattern: Constant flow generator
   5. Circuit: Single

6. Gas flow and airway pressure patterns: Square wave flow and rectilinear pressure patterns
7. Cycling parameter: Time
8. Limits
   a. Pressure (relief/pop-off)
   b. Flow (preset)
   c. Volume (result of time and flow)
9. Modes
   a. Control
   b. Assist/control
   c. SIMV
   d. CPAP
10. Inspiratory airway maneuvers: Sigh
11. Expiratory airway maneuvers: PEEP
12. Alarms
    a. Patient alarms: High/low inspiratory pressure
    b. Machine alarms: Oxygen/compressed air system failure
J. Servo 900, 900B, 900C
   1. Pressure: Positive
   2. Powering mechanism: Combined electric/pneumatic
   3. Driving mechanism: Pneumatic system regulated by servo-mechanisms
   4. Maintenance of gas flow pattern: Modified constant flow and non-constant flow generator
   5. Circuit: Single
   6. Gas flow and pressure patterns
      a. Square wave flow with taper; rectilinear to parabolic pressure pattern (modified constant flow)
      b. Accelerating flow and nonlinearly increasing pressure pattern (non-constant flow)
   7. Cycling parameters
      a. Time (primary)
      b. Pressure
   8. Limits
      a. Pressure (preset)
      b. Volume (preset)
      c. Volume (result of time and volume)
   9. Modes
      a. Control
      b. Assist/control
      c. SIMV (900B and 900C)

    d. CPAP

    e. Pressure support (900C only)

    f. Pressure control (900C only). The ventilator functions as a time-cycled pressure-limited unit. Sufficient flow is provided to allow pressure to be reached rapidly and held for the remainder of the inspiratory time. In this mode the unit functions as a near-constant pressure generator.

10. Inspiratory airway maneuvers

    a. Sigh

    b. Inflation hold (pause time %)

    c. Accelerating flow pattern

11. Expiratory airway maneuvers

    a. PEEP

    b. NEEP (option)

    c. Expiratory retard

12. Alarms

    a. Patient alarms

      (1) High inspiratory pressure

      (2) High/low expired minute volume

      (3) Apnea (900C only)

    b. Machine alarms

      (1) Power failure

      (2) Oxygen/compressed air system failure (900C only)

      (3) Ventilator inoperative (900C only)

      (4) High/low O_2% (900C only)

K. Engström ER300

1. Pressure: Positive

2. Powering mechanism: Electric

3. Driving mechanism: Piston system driven via rotary motion by electric motor

4. Maintenance of gas flow pattern: Non-constant flow generator

5. Circuit: Double

6. Gas flow and pressure pattern: Modified sine wave flow and modified sigmoidal pressure patterns

7. Cycling parameter: Time (fixed I:E ratio, 1:2)

8. Limits (preset)

    a. Pressure (relief/pop-off)

    b. Volume

9. Modes

    a. Control

    b. IMV (option)

10. Inspiratory airway maneuvers: Inflation hold, variable but mandatory
11. Expiratory airway maneuvers
    a. PEEP
    b. NEEP
    c. Expiratory retard
12. Alarms
    a. Patient alarms: Low inspiratory pressure
    b. Machine alarms: Power failure
L. Engström Erica
1. Pressure: Positive
2. Powering mechanism: Combined electric/pneumatic
3. Driving mechanism: Modified bellows system driven by electronically regulated compressed gases
4. Maintenance of gas flow pattern: Constant and non-constant flow generator
5. Circuit: Double
6. Gas flow and pressure pattern:
    a. Square wave flow and rectilinear pressure pattern (constant flow)
    b. Accelerating flow and nonlinearly increasing pressure patterns (non-constant flow)
    c. Decelerating flow and parabolic pressure patterns (non-constant flow)
7. Cycling parameters
    a. Volume (primary)
    b. Time
    c. Pressure
8. Limits (preset)
    a. Time
    b. Pressure
    c. Flow
9. Modes
    a. Control
    b. Assist/control
    c. SIMV
    d. EMMV
    e. Pressure assist
    f. CPAP
10. Inspiratory airway maneuvers
    a. Sigh

    b. Inflation hold
    c. Flow taper
  11. Expiratory airway maneuvers: PEEP
  12. Alarms
    a. Patient alarms
      (1) High/low inspiratory pressure
      (2) High/low minute volume
      (3) Apnea
    b. Machine alarms
      (1) Oxygen/compressed air system failure
      (2) Electrical failure
M. Monaghan 225 and 225/SIMV
  1. Pressure: Positive
  2. Powering mechanism: Pneumatic
  3. Driving mechanism: Bellows system driven by compressed gas source
  4. Maintenance of gas flow pattern: Constant flow generator
  5. Circuit: Double
  6. Gas flow and pressure pattern: Square wave flow and rectilinear pressure patterns
  7. Cycling parameters
    a. Volume (primary)
    b. Pressure
    c. Time
  8. Limits (preset)
    a. Pressure
    b. Time
    c. Flow
  9. Modes
    a. Control
    b. Assist
    c. Assist/control
    d. SIMV
    e. CPAP
  10. Inspiratory airway maneuvers: None
  11. Expiratory airway maneuvers: PEEP
  12. Alarms (visual only)
    a. Patient alarms
      (1) High inspiratory pressure
      (2) I:E ratio
    b. Machine alarms: None
N. Biomed Devices IC-5

1. Pressure: Positive
2. Powering mechanism: Combined electric/pneumatic
3. Driving mechanism: Microprocessor controlled pneumatic system
4. Maintenance of gas flow pattern: Constant flow generator
5. Circuit: Single
6. Gas flow and pressure patterns: Square wave flow and rectilinear pressure patterns
7. Cycling parameters
   a. Time (primary)
   b. Pressure
8. Limits (preset)
   a. Pressure
   b. Volume
   c. Flow
9. Modes
   a. Assist/control
   b. SIMV
   c. CPAP
10. Inspiratory airway maneuvers
    a. Sigh
    b. Inflation hold
11. Expiratory airway maneuvers: PEEP
12. Alarms
    a. Patient alarms
       (1) High/low inspiratory pressure
       (2) High/low mean airway pressure
       (3) High/low PEEP
       (4) High/low tidal volume
       (5) High/low minute volume
       (6) High/low $F_{I_{O_2}}$
    b. Machine alarms
       (1) Oxygen/compressed air system failure
       (2) Fail to cycle
       (3) High/low gas temperature
O. Baby Bird
   1. Pressure: Positive
   2. Powering mechanism: Pneumatic
   3. Driving mechanism: Pneumatic system adjustable reducing valve
   4. Maintenance of gas flow pattern: Constant flow generator
   5. Circuit: Single

6. Gas flow and pressure patterns: Square wave flow and rectilinear pressure patterns
7. Cycling parameter: Time
8. Limits (preset)
    a. Pressure (does not cycle)
    b. Flow
9. Modes
    a. IMV
    b. CPAP
10. Inspiratory airway maneuvers: Inflation hold (via pressure limit setting)
11. Expiratory airway maneuvers
    a. PEEP
    b. NEEP
12. Alarms
    a. Patient alarms: Inspiratory time
    b. Machine alarms
        (1) Low source gas pressure
        (2) Oxygen/compressed air system failure

Note: When used as a pressure-limited, time cycled unit, the machine functions essentially as a constant pressure generator.

P. Baby Bird 2A
1. Pressure: Positive
2. Powering mechanism: Combined electric/pneumatic
3. Driving mechanism: Pneumatic system regulated by a microprocessor
4. Maintenance of gas flow pattern: Constant flow generator
5. Circuit: Single
6. Gas flow and pressure patterns: Square wave flow and rectilinear pressure patterns
7. Cycling parameter: Time
8. Limits (preset)
    a. Pressure (does not cycle)
    b. Flow
9. Modes
    a. IMV
    b. CPAP
10. Inspiratory airway maneuvers: Inflation hold (via pressure limit)
11. Expiratory airway maneuvers: PEEP
12. Alarms
    a. Patient alarms
        (1) Short expiratory time

(2) Long inspiratory time
  b. Machine alarms
    (1) Low source gas pressure (air/O$_2$)
    (2) Power failure
Note: When used as a pressure-limited, time cycled unit, the machine functions essentially as a constant pressure generator.
Q. Bourns LS 104-150
  1. Pressure: Positive
  2. Powering mechanism: Electric
  3. Driving mechanism: Linear motion piston system driven by electric motor
  4. Maintenance of gas flow pattern: Constant flow generator
  5. Circuit: Single
  6. Gas flow and pressure patterns: Square wave flow and rectilinear pressure patterns
  7. Cycling parameters
    a. Volume (primary)
    b. Pressure
  8. Limits
    a. Flow (preset)
    b. Pressure (relief/pop-off or ends inspiration)
    c. Time (resultant of volume and flow)
  9. Modes
    a. Control
    b. IMV
    c. Assist/control
    d. Assist
  10. Inspiratory airway maneuvers: None
  11. Expiratory airway maneuvers: PEEP
  12. Alarms: Machine alarms
    a. Low airway pressure
    b. High airway pressure
    c. Apnea
R. Bourns BP200
  1. Pressure: Positive
  2. Powering mechanism: Combined electric/pneumatic
  3. Driving mechanism: Pneumatic system regulated by solenoids and regulators
  4. Maintenance of gas flow pattern: Constant flow generator
  5. Circuit: Single
  6. Gas flow and pressure pattern: Square wave flow and rectilinear pressure pattern
  7. Cycling parameters: Time

8. Limits (preset)
    a. Pressure (does not cycle)
    b. Flow
9. Modes
    a. IMV
    b. CPAP
10. Inspiratory airway maneuvers: Inflation hold (via pressure limit)
11. Expiratory airway maneuvers: PEEP
12. Alarms
    a. Patient alarms: Insufficient expiratory time
    b. Machine alarms
       (1) Low source gas pressure (air/O_2)
       (2) Power failure

Note: When used as a pressure-limited, time-cycled unit, the machine functions essentially as a constant pressure generator.

S. Bear Cub Infant Ventilator BP 2001
1. Pressure: Positive
2. Powering mechanism: Combined electric/pneumatic
3. Driving mechanism: Servo-operated pneumatic system
4. Maintenance of gas flow pattern: Constant flow generator
5. Circuit: Single
6. Gas flow and pressure pattern: Square wave flow and rectilinear pressure pattern
7. Cycling parameter: Time
8. Limits (preset)
    a. Pressure (does not cycle)
    b. Flow
9. Modes
    a. IMV
    b. CPAP
10. Inspiratory airway maneuvers: Inflation hold (via pressure limit)
11. Expiratory airway maneuvers: PEEP
12. Alarms
    a. Patient alarms
       (1) Low inspiratory pressure
       (2) Low PEEP/CPAP
       (3) I:E ratio
       (4) High pressure
    b. Machine alarms
       (1) Low source gas pressure (air/O_2)

  (2) Ventilator inoperative
  (3) Electrical failure or disconnect
  (4) Rate/time incompatibility (expiratory time must be at least 0.25 second)

Note: When used as a pressure-limited, time-cycled unit, the machine functions essentially as a constant pressure generator.

T. Sechrist IV-100B (infant/pediatric)
  1. Pressure: Positive
  2. Powering mechanism: Combined electric/pneumatic
  3. Driving mechanism: Pneumatic, controlled by a microprocessor and fluidic system
  4. Maintenance of gas flow pattern: Constant flow generator
  5. Circuit: Single
  6. Gas flow and pressure pattern: Square wave flow and rectilinear pressure pattern
  7. Cycling parameter: Time
  8. Limits (preset)
    a. Pressure (does not cycle)
    b. Flow
  9. Modes
    a. IMV
    b. CPAP
  10. Inspiratory airway maneuvers: Inflation hold (via pressure limit)
  11. Expiratory airway maneuvers: PEEP
  12. Alarms
    a. Patient alarms
      (1) Low airway pressure
      (2) Prolonged inspiratory time or expiratory time
      (3) Apnea
    b. Machine alarms: Ventilator disconnect

Note: When used as a pressure-limited, time-cycled unit, the machine functions essentially as a constant pressure generator.

U. Healthdyne 105 (infant/pediatric)
  1. Pressure: Positive
  2. Powering mechanism: Combined electric/pneumatic
  3. Driving mechanism: Pneumatic system regulated by microprocessors
  4. Maintenance of gas flow pattern: Constant flow generator
  5. Circuit: Single
  6. Gas flow and pressure pattern: Square wave flow and rectilinear pressure pattern

7. Cycling parameter: Time
8. Limits (preset)
   a. Pressure (does not cycle)
   b. Flow
9. Modes
   a. IMV
   b. CPAP
10. Inspiratory airway maneuvers: Inflation hold (via pressure limit)
11. Expiratory airway maneuvers: PEEP
12. Alarms
    a. Patient alarms
       (1) High/low inspiratory pressure
       (2) I:E ratio
       (3) Short expiratory time
       (4) Disconnect
    b. Machine alarms
       (1) Low source gas pressure (air/O_2)
       (2) Electrical failure

Note: When used as a pressure-limited, time-cycled unit, the machine functions essentially as a constant pressure generator.

V. McGaw CV200 (neonatal/pediatric)
   1. Pressure: Positive
   2. Powering mechanism: Pneumatic
   3. Driving mechanism: Pneumatic system regulated by relays and a balanced diaphragm
   4. Maintenance of gas flow pattern: Constant flow generator
   5. Circuit: Single
   6. Gas flow and pressure pattern: Square wave flow and rectilinear pressure pattern
   7. Cycling parameter: Time
   8. Limits (preset)
      a. Pressure (does not cycle)
      b. Flow
   9. Modes
      a. Control
      b. Assist/control
      c. IMV
      d. CPAP
   10. Inspiratory airway maneuvers: Inflation hold (via pressure limit)
   11. Expiratory airway maneuvers

        a. PEEP
        b. NEEP
   12. Alarms
        a. Patient alarms
           (1) High/low inspiratory pressure
           (2) Low PEEP/CPAP
           (3) Apnea
           (4) Patient disconnect
        b. Machine alarms
           (1) Oxygen/compressed air system failure
           (2) Power failure
W. Sechrist volume ventilator
   1. Pressure: Positive
   2. Powering mechanism: Electric
   3. Driving mechanism: Piston driven by microprocessor in a linear or nonlinear fashion
   4. Maintenance of gas flow pattern: Selectable constant or nonconstant flow generator
   5. Circuit: Single
   6. Gas flow and pressure patterns: Capable of consistently producing square wave, square wave and taper, accelerating and square or sine wave flow patterns producing rectilinear, rectilinear and parabolic, accelerating and rectilinear, or sigmoidal pressure patterns, respectively.
   7. Cycling parameters
        a. Time (primary)
        b. Pressure
   8. Limits (preset)
        a. Pressure (relief/pop-off)
        b. Volume
        c. Flow
   9. Modes
        a. Control
        b. Assist/control
        c. SIMV
        d. MMV (mandatory minute ventilation, same as EMMV)
        e. CPAP
  10. Inspiratory airway maneuvers
        a. Sigh
        b. Inflation hold
        c. Selectable flow wave forms:
           (1) Square

         (2) Square to taper

         (3) Accelerate to square

         (4) Sine wave

  11. Expiratory airway maneuver: PEEP

  12. Alarms

     a. Patient alarms

         (1) High/low tidal volume

         (2) High/low minute volume

         (3) High/low pressure

         (4) High/low respiratory rate

     b. Machine alarms

         (1) Low source gas pressures (O_2/air)

         (2) Electrical disconnect

         (3) High temperature

X. Puritan-Bennett 7200

  1. Pressure: Positive

  2. Powering mechanism: Electric

  3. Driving mechanism: Pneumatic sources regulated by microprocessors operating proportional solenoid valves

  4. Maintenance of gas flow patterns: Constant or non-constant flow generator

  5. Circuit: Single

  6. Gas flow and pressure patterns: Capable of producing consistently square, tapered, or sine wave flow patterns which produce rectilinear, parabolic or sigmoidal pressure patterns, respectively

  7. Cycling parameters:

     a. Volume (primary)

     b. Pressure

  8. Limits (preset)

     a. Pressure

     b. Flow

     c. Time (resultant of flow pattern and volume)

  9. Modes

     a. Control

     b. Assist/control

     c. SIMV

     d. CPAP

     e. Pressure support (option)

     f. MMV (option) (same as EMMV).

  10. Inspiratory airway maneuvers

     a. Sigh

    b. Inflation hold

    c. Selectable flow wave forms

       (1) Square

       (2) Tapered

       (3) Sine

11. Expiratory airway maneuvers: PEEP

12. Alarms

    a. Patient alarms:

       (1) High/low pressure

       (2) Low tidal volume

       (3) Low minute volume

       (4) Low PEEP/CPAP pressure

       (5) High respiratory rate

       (6) Apnea

       (7) I:E ratio

    b. Machine alarms

       (1) Low source gas pressure (O_2/air)

       (2) Low battery

       (3) Exhalation valve leak during inspiration

       (4) Ventilator inoperative

Y. Ohio CPU-1

  1. Pressure: Positive

  2. Power mechanism: Combined electric/pneumatic

  3. Driving mechanism: Pneumatic source controlled by microprocessor operated valves

  4. Maintenance of gas flow patterns: Constant flow generator

  5. Circuit: Single

  6. Gas flow and pressure patterns: Square wave flow and rectilinear pressure pattern

  7. Cycling parameters

    a. Time (primary)

    b. Pressure (primary)

  8. Limits (preset)

    a. Volume (result of flow and inspiratory time)

    b. Flow

  9. Modes

    a. IMV

    b. SIMV

    c. MMV (same as EMMV)

    d. Pressure-cycled IMV

    e. Pressure-cycled SIMV

    f. CPAP

   10. Inspiratory airway maneuver: Sigh
   11. Expiratory airway maneuver: PEEP
   12. Alarms
     a. Patient alarms
       (1) High pressure
       (2) Low tidal volume
       (3) I : E ratio
       (4) Apnea
       (5) Circuit disconnect and leaks
     b. Machine alarms
       (1) Source gas disconnect
       (2) Electrical disconnect or failure
       (3) Flow transducer failure
       (4) Microprocessor failure

BIBLIOGRAPHY

Air-Shields: *Manufacturer's Literature: Healthdyne Model 105 Infant/Pediatric Ventilator.* Hatboro, Penna., Healthdyne Inc.

Bear Medical Systems, Inc.: *Instruction Manual: Bear 1 Adult Volume Ventilator.* Riverside, Calif., Bear Medical Systems, Inc.

Bear Medical Systems, Inc.: *Instruction Manual: Bear 2 Adult Volume Ventilator.* Riverside, Calif., Bear Medical Systems, Inc.

Bear Medical Systems, Inc.: *Instruction Manual: Bear Cub Infant Ventilator Model BP2001.* Riverside, Calif., Bear Medical Systems, Inc.

Bear Medical Systems, Inc.: *Instruction Manual: Infant Ventilator Model BP200.* Riverside, Calif., Bear Medical Systems, Inc.

Bennett Medical Equipment. *Operating Instructions: Bennett Model PR1 Respiration Unit.* Los Angeles, Puritan-Bennett Corporation.

Bennett Medical Equipment: *Operating Instructions: Bennett Model PR-2 Respiration Unit.* Los Angeles, Puritan-Bennett Corporation.

Bio-med Devices Inc.: *Instruction Manual: Bio-med Devices 1C-5 Ventilator.* Stamford, Conn., Bio-med Devices Inc.

Bird Products/3M: *Manufacturer's Literature: Baby Bird.* St. Paul, Minn., Bird Products/3M.

Bird Products/3M: *Manufacturer's Literature: Baby Bird 2A.* St. Paul, Minn., Bird Products/3M.

Bird Corporation: *Instruction Manual: Bird Mark 7 Respirator.* Palm Springs, Calif., Bird Corporation/3M.

Bourns Medical Systems, Inc.: *Instruction Manual: Bourns LS 104-150D Ventilator.* Riverside, Calif., Bourns Medical System, Inc.

J.H. Emerson Company: *Manufacturer's Literature: Emerson IMV 3MV Ventilator.* Cambridge, Mass., J.H. Emerson Company.

J.H. Emerson Company: *Manufacturer's Literature: Emerson Post-Op 3PV Volume Ventilator.* Cambridge, Mass., J.H. Emerson Company.

Engström Medical AB: *Manufacturer's Literature: Engström 300 Ventilator.* Bromma, Sweden, Engström Medical AB.

Engström Medical AB: *Reference Manual: Engström Erica.* Bromma, Sweden, Engström Medical AB.

Life Products Inc.: *Operation Manual: Model LP5 Volume Ventilator.* Boulder, Colo., Life Products Inc.

McGaw Respiratory Therapy: *Manufacturer's Literature: CV200 Neonatal Ventilator.* Carlsbad, Calif., AHSC/International Export.

McGaw Respiratory Therapy: *Manufacturer's Literature: Monaghan 225/SIMV Volume Ventilator.* Plattsburgh, N.Y., Monaghan Medical Corporation.

McPherson S.P.: *Respiratory Therapy Equipment,* ed. 3. St. Louis, C.V. Mosby Co., 1985.

Mushin W.W., et al.: *Automatic Ventilation of the Lungs,* ed. 3. Oxford, Blackwell Scientific Publications, 1980.

Newport Medical Instruments Inc.: *Manufacturer's Literature: The E100 Ventilator.* Newport Beach, Calif., Newport Medical Instruments Inc.

Ohio Medical Products: *Manufacturer's Literature: CPU1 Ventilator.* Madison, Wis., Ohio Medical Products.

Puritan-Bennett Corporation: *Operating Instructions: MA-1 Ventilator.* Kansas City, Mo., Puritan-Bennett Corporation.

Puritan-Bennett Corporation: *Operating Instructions: MA2 and MA2+2 Ventilators.* Kansas City, Mo., Puritan-Bennett Corporation.

Puritan-Bennett Corporation: *Manufacturer's Literature: 7200 Microprocessor Ventilator.* Kansas City, Mo., Puritan-Bennett Corporation.

Sechrist Industries Inc.: *Operational Instructions Manual: Model IV-100B Infant Ventilator.* Anaheim, Calif., Sechrist Industries Inc., Medical Products Division.

Sechrist Industries Inc.: *Operational Instructions Manual: Sechrist Volume Ventilator.* Anaheim, Calif., Sechrist Industries Inc., Medical Products Division.

Siemens-Elema AB: *Operating Manual: Servo Ventilator 900/900B.* Solona, Sweden, Siemens-Elema AB.

Siemens-Elema AB: *Training Instructions: Servo Ventilator 900C.* Solona, Sweden, Siemens-Elema AB.

32 / Continuous Mechanical Ventilation

I. Physiologic Effects of Positive Pressure in Relation to Continuous Mechanical Ventilation
   A. Increased mean airway pressure
      1. Normally mean airway pressure is about zero (or atmospheric) (see Fig 4–4).
      2. Since positive pressure ablates the normal mechanisms for gas movement, intrapulmonary pressures are always supra-atmospheric (see Fig 28–1).
      3. The extent that intrapulmonary pressure is increased is dependent on:
         a. Tidal volume
         b. Inspiratory time
         c. Respiratory rate
         d. Airway resistance
         e. Pulmonary and thoracic compliance.
   B. Increased mean intrathoracic pressure (Fig 32–1)
      1. Transmission of intrapulmonary pressure to the intrathoracic space is dependent on pulmonary and thoracic compliance. In general, the stiffer the lung, the lower the amount of pressure transmitted from the intrapulmonary to the intrathoracic space. In contrast, the stiffer the thorax, the greater the amount of pressure transmitted to the intrathoracic space.
      2. In most patients requiring mechanical ventilation, *the mean intrathoracic pressure changes from negative to positive.*
   C. Decreased venous return (see Fig 32–1)
      1. Since intrathoracic pressures become positive with the application of mechanical ventilation, the thoracic pump mechanism assisting venous return is eliminated.
      2. As a result the pressure gradient favoring venous flow to the right heart is decreased and right ventricular filling is impaired.
      3. Frequently the decreased transmural pressure across the

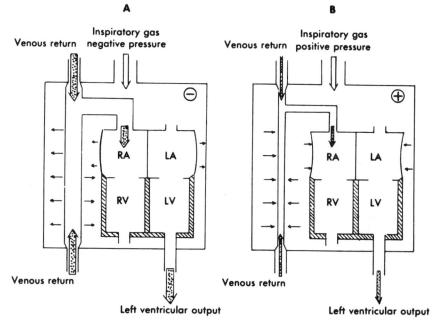

Fig 32–1.—A, effect of spontaneous ventilation or negative pressure ventilation on intrathoracic pressure and cardiac output. **B,** effect of positive pressure on intrathoracic pressure and cardiac output. (From Spearman C.B., Sheldon R.L., Egan D.F.: *Egan's Fundamentals of Respiratory Therapy,* ed. 4. St. Louis, C.V. Mosby Co., 1982. Reproduced by permission.)

vena cava is large enough to require fluid therapy in order to maintain appropriate right ventricular filling.

4. Most patients are hypoxemic, acidotic, and hypercarbic prior to the institution of mechanical ventilation, which causes an increased sympathetic tone. The normalization of acid-base balance, the relief of hypoxemia, and the decrease in work of breathing results in a marked decrease in sympathetic tone. This may result in:
   a. Decreased vascular tone and relative hypovolemia.
   b. Decreased heart rate.
   c. Decreased force of myocardial contraction.

D. Decreased cardiac output
   1. Since venous return and sympathetic tone are decreased, there is some decrease in cardiac output.
   2. With appropriate fluid therapy and/or pharmacologic support adequate cardiac output can be maintained.

E. Increased intracranial pressure
    1. Since venous return is decreased, blood will pool in the periphery and in the cranium.
    2. The increased volume of blood in the cranium will increase intracranial pressure.
F. Decreased urinary output
    1. Decreased cardiac output results in decreased renal blood flow, which alters renal filtration pressures and diminishes urine formation.
    2. Decreased venous return and decreased right atrial pressures are interpreted as a decrease in overall blood volume. As a result, antidiuretic hormone levels are increased and urine formation is decreased (see Chaps. 9 and 15).
G. Decreased work of breathing
    1. Since the force necessary to ventilate is provided by the ventilator, the patient's work of breathing decreases.
    2. The amount of work performed by the ventilator and the amount performed by the patient vary, depending on the approach used to ventilate (see Ventilator Modes, section IV).
H. Mechanical bronchodilation
    1. Positive pressure causes a mechanical dilation of all conducting airways.
    2. The transmural pressure gradients affecting the airways are always greater than during normal spontaneous ventilation.
I. Increased deadspace ventilation
    1. Since positive pressure distends conducting airways and inhibits venous return, the portion of the tidal volume that is deadspace increases.
    2. In addition there is an alteration of normal distribution of ventilation. A greater percentage of ventilation goes to the apices and less to the bases than in spontaneous ventilation.
    3. Normal deadspace to tidal volume ratios are 0.20–0.40; however, mechanical ventilation will cause these ratios to increase to 0.40–0.60 in the normal individual.
J. Increased intrapulmonary shunt
    1. With positive pressure ventilation gas distribution and pulmonary perfusion are altered.
    2. Ventilation to the most gravity-dependent aspects of the lung is decreased, while blood flow to these areas is increased.

3. Normal intrapulmonary shunts are about 2.0%–5.0%; however, mechanical ventilation may increase the shunt fraction to about 10% in the normal individual.

4. Allowing some level of spontaneous ventilation, (partial ventilatory support, see Ventricular Modes, section IV.) minimizes the $\dot{V}/\dot{Q}$ mismatch.

K. Manipulation of level of ventilation. Hyperventilation or hypoventilation may be induced by inappropriate setting of parameters.

L. Respiratory rate, tidal volume, inspiratory time, and flow rate may all be manipulated.

M. Effect on gastrointestinal tract. The stress produced by positive pressure ventilation may lead to increased gastric secretion, resulting in the development of stress ulcers.

N. Effect on psychological status. The continued stress associated with mechanical ventilation may result in:

1. Insomnia
2. Anxiety
3. Frustration
4. Depression
5. Apprehension
6. Fear

II. Indications for Mechanical Ventilation. Numerous pathophysiologic conditions may necessitate mechanical ventilation. However, each may be categorized into one of the following general indications:

A. Apnea: The cessation of breathing.

B. Acute ventilatory failure: A P_{CO_2} of more than 50 mm Hg along with a pH less than 7.30.

C. Impending acute ventilatory failure

1. A clinical prognosis based on serial laboratory data and clinical findings indicating that the patient is progressing toward ventilatory failure.

2. Clinical problems frequently resulting in impending acute ventilatory failure may be categorized as:

   a. Primary pulmonary abnormalities, such as:
      (1) Respiratory distress syndrome
      (2) Pneumonia
      (3) Pulmonary emboli
   b. Abnormalities associated with the mechanical ability of the lung to move air, such as:
      (1) Fatigue
      (2) Nutritional deficiencies

      (3) Chest injury
      (4) Thoracic abnormalities
      (5) Pleural disease
      (6) Myoneural disease
      (7) Neurologic disease
3. Clinical evaluation of the patient in impending acute ventilatory failure.
    a. Vital signs: With increased cardiopulmonary stress, pulse and blood pressure typically increase. If bacterial infection is present, temperature also increases.
    b. Ventilatory parameters: As work of breathing increases,
      (1) Tidal volume decreases.
      (2) Respiratory rate increases.
      (3) Accessory muscle use increases.
    c. Paradoxical breathing may occur.
    d. Retractions may be noted.
    e. Ventilatory reserve is decreased.
      (1) If vital capacity decreases acutely below 10 ml/kg of ideal body weight, ventilatory failure may be imminent.
      (2) If negative (maximum) inspiratory force less negative than -20 cm H_2O in 20 seconds, ventilatory failure may be imminent.
      (3) As TV becomes a greater percentage of VC, the likelihood of the development of ventilatory failure increases.
    f. Progression of disease state, for example:
      (1) Progressive muscle weakness in patients with neuromuscular or neurologic diseases.
      (2) Continued progress of pulmonary or pleural infections.
      (3) *Increasing fatigue* associated with any cardiorespiratory disease. *Fatigue* can be the primary factor precipitating impending acute ventilatory failure in any disease state.
      (4) Serial blood gases demonstrating a trend toward acute ventilatory failure. For example:

	9 A.M.	10 A.M.	11 A.M.	12 P.M.
pH	7.58	7.53	7.46	7.38
PCO_2	22	28	35	42
HCO_3^-	21	22	23	24
PO_2	60	55	50	43

Along with these results, the patient's respiratory rate, heart rate, and blood pressure continued to increase while the tidal volume decreased.

(a) Without intervention to break this trend, a blood gas value measured at 1 P.M. may show a pH of 7.33 and a P_{CO_2} of 48 mm Hg, while at 2 P.M. the pH may be 7.28 and the P_{CO_2} 53 mm Hg.

(b) As a result, the decision may be made at 12 noon to institute mechanical ventilation because the patient is in impending acute ventilatory failure.

Note: None of the material presented above discussed oxygenation, because oxygenation is not a direct indication for ventilation. However, the increased work of breathing associated with attempting to maintain a normal oxygenation state may precipitate impending acute ventilatory failure. *It is ventilatory problems that require mechanical ventilation, not oxygenation problems.* Oxygenation problems are treated with oxygen therapy, PEEP, or cardiovascular stabilization.

III. Ventilator Commitment

A. Ventilation with bag and mask followed by establishment of an artificial airway.

B. Manually supported ventilation
1. Reverse hypercarbia and acidosis
2. Decrease work of breathing
3. Slowly alter patient's ventilatory pattern to pattern desired during mechanical ventilation.

C. Stabilize cardiovascular system
1. Prior to manual ventilation, the patient's sympathetic tone is pronounced because of:
a. Hypercarbia
b. Acidosis
c. Hypoxemia
d. Generalized increased stress
2. Since manual ventilation and mechanical ventilation inhibit venous return and theoretically reverse hypercarbia, acidosis, and hypoxemia, a decreased sympathetic tone results. *This may result in hypotension when manual or mechanical ventilation is instituted.*
3. The use of narcotics may also add to the hypotensive state.
4. Fluid therapy may be essential during ventilator commitment (see Chap. 15).
5. In addition, some patients may require the use of sympathomimetics for beta one effects (see Chapter 34).

    D. Record baseline values for:
        1. Vital signs
        2. Blood gases
    E. Institute appropriate cardiovascular and pulmonary monitors
        1. ECG
        2. Arterial line
        3. Central venous line
        4. Pulmonary artery line
    F. Determine settings on the ventilator (see section IV)
    G. Sedate and/or paralyze patient, if indicated.
    H. Attach patient to ventilator. Transition should be smooth, orderly, and controlled.
IV. Determination of Settings on the Mechanical Ventilator
    A. Modes (technical)
        1. Control (Fig 32–2)
            a. Patient is unable to control any aspect of gas delivery.
            b. All work of breathing is taken over by the ventilator.
            c. Sedation is typically required.
        2. Assist (Fig 32–3)
            a. Patient is able to control ventilatory rate.
            b. Machine performs vast majority of the work of breathing.
            c. *This mode should not be used for continuous ventilation because if the patient becomes apneic, ventilation stops.*
        3. Assist/control (Fig 32–4)

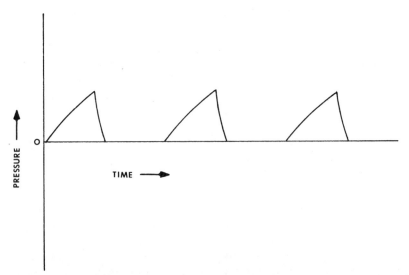

Fig 32–2.—Ventilator system pressure curve developed during control mode ventilation. No negative deflections should be noted.

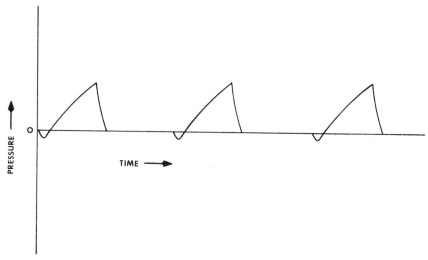

Fig 32–3.—Ventilator system pressure curve developed during assist mode ventilation. The negative deflection prior to inspiration is the patient triggering the breath.

    a. Patient is able to control ventilatory rate as long as spontaneous rate is greater than machine backup rate; if not, machine goes into control mode.

    b. Machine performs vast majority of the work of breathing.

    c. Because patient controls ventilatory rate, wide swings in acid-base status may occur. This is particularly true with CNS disturbances and bulbar involvement.

    d. As the patient-initiated ventilatory rate increases, mean intrapulmonary pressure increases and normally results in an increased mean intrathoracic pressure and a decrease in venous return.

    e. Sedation is frequently required.

4. Intermittent mandatory ventilation (IMV) (Fig 32–5)

    a. Positive pressure ventilation is provided by a control mode breath on a periodic basis.

    b. In between positive pressure breaths, the patient breathes spontaneously.

    c. Gas flow during spontaneous ventilation is provided by an external continuous gas flow system or an internal demand valve.

        (1) Because of poor responsiveness or resistance to gas flow resulting in increased work of breathing, demand valve IMV systems *are not recommended.*

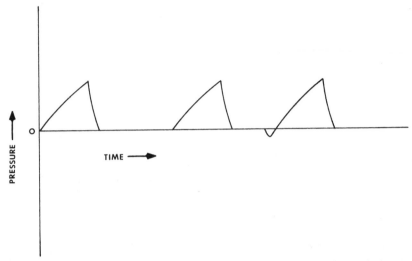

Fig 32–4.—Ventilatory system pressure curve developed during assist/control mode ventilation. Assist breaths are mixed with control breaths. The negative deflection prior to inspiration is the patient triggering the assist breath.

(2) Continuous gas flow systems should always be of the *closed rather than the open type* (Fig 32–6).

    (a) At least 4 times the patient's measured spontaneous minute volume should be entering the system (30 to 90 lpm).

    (b) Throughout the spontaneous breathing phase, gas should be continuously leaving the exhalation valve.

    (c) A 3- to 5-L reservoir attached proximal to the system humidifier should be used.

d. Sedation may be necessary.

5. Synchronized intermittent mandatory ventilation (SIMV) (Fig 32–7).

    a. Positive pressure ventilation is provided by a periodic assist/control breath.

    b. In between positive pressure breaths, the patient is allowed to breathe spontaneously.

    c. Gas flow during spontaneous ventilation is provided by a demand valve (Fig 32–8). If the system is a true SIMV system, a demand valve must be used. Continuous flow would interfere with the patient's triggering of the positive pressure breath.

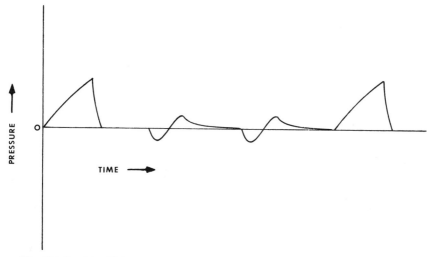

PRESSURE

TIME

Fig 32–5.—Ventilator system pressure curve developed during IMV mode ventilation. The positive pressure breaths are always control breaths.

Note: Because many of the demand valves respond poorly and cause an increased work of breathing, it is not advisable to use the SIMV mode at rates of 4 breaths per minute or less or to use the CPAP mode on these ventilators. Under these circumstances the system should be transformed to or replaced by an IMV system or a continuous flow CPAP system (see Chap. 33).

6. Pressure support (Fig 32–9)
   a. The ventilator functions as a constant low-pressure generator during the spontaneous breathing phase.
     (1) A positive pressure is set.
     (2) Once the patient initiates inspiration, a predetermined pressure is rapidly established and held at the patient's airway.
   b. The patient ventilates spontaneously, establishing his own rate, and inspires the tidal volume he feels is appropriate.
   c. When inspiratory flow rates decrease to a designated level the positive pressure returns to baseline, allowing the patient to exhale or complete inspiration without the pressure support.
   d. Pressure support can be used independently or in conjunction with CPAP or SIMV.

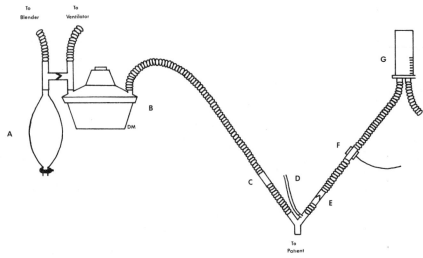

Fig 32–6.—Continuous flow IMV circuit. *A,* 5-L reservoir attached to ventilator's inspiratory limb via one-way valve; *B,* large-volume humidifier; *C,* temperature probe; *D,* proximal system pressure manometer attachment; *E,* optional one-way valve in expiratory limb; *F,* exhalation valve; *G,* Emerson water column PEEP valve.

    7. Inspiratory assist (Fig 32–10)
       a. The ventilator provides a low level of positive pressure during spontaneous inspiration.
       b. The ventilator functions as a modified constant flow generator.
       c. System pressure gradually increases to the preset level.
       d. When inspiratory flow rate decreases to a preset level, the inspiratory assist stops, pressure returns to baseline, and the patient may continue to inspire or exhale.
       e. Inspiratory assist can be used independently or in conjunction with CPAP and SIMV.
    8. Extended mandatory minute ventilation (EMMV) (Fig 32–11)
       a. A desired minute volume is set on the machine.
       b. The patient may receive this volume:
         (1) Entirely as positive pressure minute volume.
         (2) Entirely as spontaneous minute volume.
         (3) As a combination of spontaneous and positive pressure minute volume.
   B. Modes (clinical)

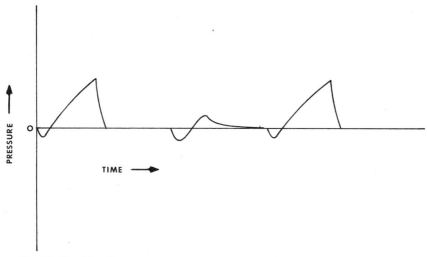

Fig 32–7.—Ventilator system pressure curve developed during SIMV mode ventilation. The positive pressure breaths are normally assist breaths.

1. Full ventilatory support
   a. The ventilator provides the vast majority of the work of breathing.
   b. Defined *arbitrarily* as a positive pressure rate of 8/minute or more.
   c. Can be accomplished in the following modes:
      (1) Control
      (2) Assist/control
      (3) IMV
      (4) SIMV
      (5) EMMV
   d. Most patients require full ventilatory support for the first 24–48 hours of ventilatory support.
   e. Regardless of mode chosen, the need for sedation usually exists.
2. Partial ventilatory support
   a. The patient performs a significant portion of the work of breathing.
   b. Defined *arbitrarily* as a positive pressure rate of 7/minute or less.
   c. Can only be accomplished in the following modes:
      (1) IMV
      (2) SIMV

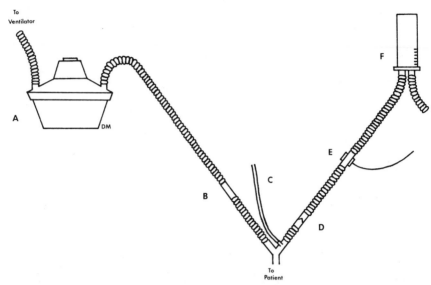

To
Ventilator

A

DM

B

C

E

F

D

To
Patient

Fig 32–8.—SIMV circuit. *A,* large-volume humidifier; *B,* temperature probe; *C,* proximal demand valve probe attachment; *D,* one-way valve expiratory limb; *E,* exhalation valve; *F,* Emerson water column PEEP valve.

           (3) Extended mandatory minute ventilation

           (4) Pressure support

           (5) Inspiratory assist

      d. Partial ventilatory support may be indicated in the majority of patients after 24–48 hours of ventilatory support.

      e. Advantages of partial ventilatory support:

           (1) Ventilation is provided in a more normal physiologic manner.

           (2) Mean intrathoracic pressures are lower than with full ventilatory support.

           (3) Distribution of gas is more normal than with full ventilatory support.

           (4) Efficacy of PEEP is increased.

  C. Tidal volume and ventilatory rate

      1. Large tidal volumes with slow ventilatory rates are used in preference to small tidal volumes and rapid rates because:

      a. Alveolar ventilation is increased.

      b. Distribution of inspired gas is improved.

      c. Mean intrathoracic pressure is reduced.

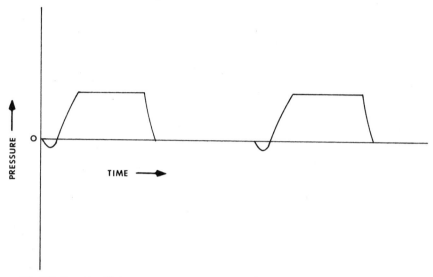

Fig 32–9.—Ventilator system pressure curve developed during pressure support. The negative deflection indicates patient triggering.

    2. Tidal volume settings in adults range between 10 and 20 ml/ kg of *ideal* body weight. Normally, initial tidal volumes are calculated at 12–15 ml/kg of ideal body weight.
    3. Ventilatory rates in adults normally range between 4 and 12/min. However, patients with very stiff lungs may require much higher rates.
    4. This tidal volume-ventilatory rate relationship is indicated in all patients except those with severe chronic restrictive pulmonary disease.
       a. In these patients small volumes and rapid rates are used because of the decrease in lung volumes associated with the disease.
       b. TV values in the range of 5–10 ml/kg of ideal body weight and RR of 20–30 or more per minute may be necessary.
D. Inspiratory time (IT)
    1. In most adults inspiratory times are maintained between 0.5 and 1.5 seconds.
    2. An estimate of IT can be made by using the following formula:

$$IT = \frac{TV}{flow} \tag{1}$$

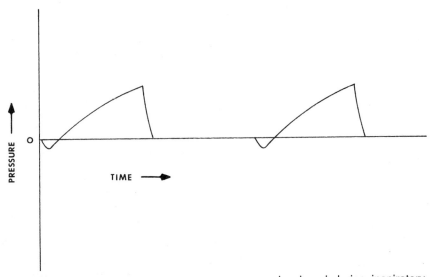

Fig 32–10.—Ventilator system pressure curve developed during inspiratory assist. The negative deflection indicates patient triggering.

where IT is in seconds, TV is in liters, and flow is in liters/second.

Thus, if the TV were 1.0 L and the flow rate 60 L/minute, or 1 L/second, the inspiratory time would be 1 second:

$$IT = \frac{1.0 \text{ L}}{1 \text{ L/sec}} = 1 \text{ second}$$

    a. This estimate may be on the low side because most ventilators are incapable of maintaining a constant flow.

    b. This estimate can only be used if the ventilator is designed to deliver a square wave flow pattern.

    c. If the flow pattern is nonconstant a stopwatch may be used to estimate inspiratory time.

3. Many patients fight positive pressure breaths because the time over which the breath is delivered is too lengthy. Decreasing the IT within the 0.5- to 1.5-second range will partially correct this problem.

4. Inspiratory time is of concern because of its effect on mean intrathoracic pressure. The greater the inspiratory time, the higher the mean intrathoracic pressure. This is usually true even if the peak airway pressure is increased when the in-

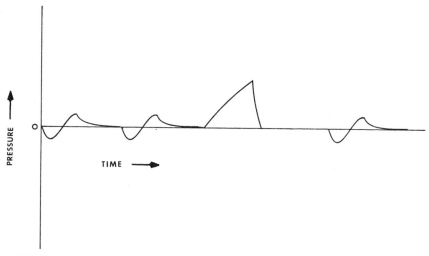

Fig 32–11.—Ventilator system pressure curve developed during EMMV. Positive pressure breaths are delivered only if the patient's spontaneous minute volume is not at or above the mandatory level.

spiratory time is decreased. The length of time pressure is applied to the airway has a greater effect on mean airway pressure than does peak airway pressure.

   E. Flow rate
      1. In most adult patients flow rate settings are between 30 and 70 L/minute.
      2. The flow rate settings used are dependent on the desired inspiratory time and the tidal volume, as in equation 1.
      3. Most ventilators that are designed to provide a square wave flow pattern are actually incapable of maintaining a constant flow throughout inspiration. That is, the flow rate tapers toward the end of inspiration.
      4. A flow taper setting is available on many ventilators. Activation of the flow taper setting is used to improve the distribution of inspired gas.
   F. IMV system, continuous flow:
      1. At least four times the patient's measured minute volume should enter the system (30 to 90 L/minute).
      2. Gas should leave the system throughout the patient's spontaneous ventilatory cycle. Flow should be measurable leaving the exhalation valve during peak spontaneous inspiration.

3. If flows are not sufficient to meet the patient's peak inspiratory demands, the work of breathing may markedly increase.
G. Inflation hold (Fig 32–12)
   1. The maintenance of the delivered tidal volume or of a fixed pressure in the airway at the terminal portion of inspiration.
   2. It improves the distribution of inspired gas in situations where regional variations in airway resistance and compliance cause ventilation/perfusion mismatch.
   3. The length of time an inflation hold is activated is normally between 0.1 and 1.0 second.
   4. When an inflation hold is used, it extends the *total inspiratory time* and thus may adversely affect mean intrathoracic pressure.
   5. If an inflation hold is used, an increase in flow rate may be necessary in order to keep total inspiratory time between 0.5 and 1.5 second.
H. Expiratory retard (Fig 32–13)
   1. The application of a fixed resistance during exhalation.
   2. This increases the length of time it takes for peak airway pressure to return to baseline during exhalation.
   3. Expiratory retard is used to prevent premature closure of small airways during exhalation.
   4. This maneuver is used primarily with obstructive pulmonary disease.

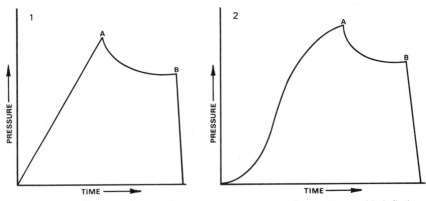

Fig 32–12.—Ideal pressure curves for square wave flow pattern with inflation hold *(1)* and sine wave flow pattern with inflation hold *(2)*. The pressure drop from A to B indicates equilibrium between mouth and alveolar pressure during inflation hold period.

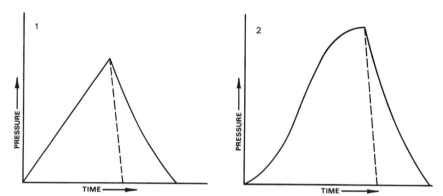

Fig 32–13.—Ideal pressure curves for square wave flow pattern with expiratory retard *(1)* and sine wave flow pattern with expiratory retard *(2). Dotted line* denotes "normal" return of pressure to baseline.

      5. The extent that expiratory retard is used is dependent on the severity of air trapping.

      6. Mean intrathoracic pressure may be increased.

I. PEEP (see Chap. 33).

J. NEEP (negative end-expiratory pressure) (Fig 32–14)

      1. The maintenance of a subatmospheric airway pressure at end exhalation.

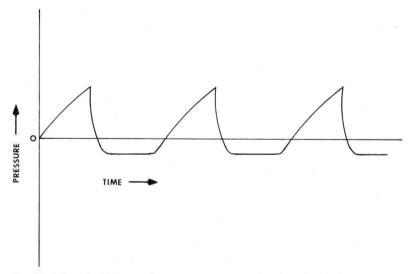

Fig 32–14.—Ventilator system pressure curve developed with the use of negative end-expiratory pressure in the control mode.

2. Theoretically used to prevent a significant increase in mean intrathoracic pressure.
3. This maneuver is not recommended because it promotes air trapping and pulmonary edema, and has not been demonstrated to clinically affect intrathoracic pressure.

K. Sigh
1. The periodic delivery of a tidal volume approximately 1.5 times the set tidal volume.
2. A sigh breath is used to prevent the patchy microatelectasis that may develop during continuous control or assist/control ventilation with small tidal volumes.
3. The use of large tidal volumes and the development of IMV and SIMV have eliminated the need for sigh breaths. However, some recommend its use in the control and assist/control modes of ventilation.

V. Monitoring the Patient/Ventilator System
A. Monitoring the functions of the system should be performed as frequently as the clinical situation dictates. In general, most patient/ventilator systems should be evaluated every 2 hours. However, the highly unstable patient may require hourly evaluation, whereas the chronic ventilator patient may only require evaluation every 4 hours.
1. Drain all system tubing of condensate.
2. Verify ventilator parameters are set as ordered.
3. Independently measure exhaled tidal volumes to verify volumes ordered are actually delivered.
   a. Exhaled tidal volumes (ETV) are measured because inhaled tidal volumes may not indicate the volume of gas the patient is actually receiving, especially if a system leak is present.
   b. Correcting the exhaled tidal volume for compressible volume loss can also be done.
      (1) Compressible volume loss is the quantity of gas compressed in the system that is not delivered to the patient.
      (2) For most systems, this is about 3–4 ml/cm H_2O peak airway pressure. However, individual system values should be determined for each system used.
      (3) The use of this correction in determining exhaled tidal volume is not essential in adults because the magnitude of the compressible volume will be relatively consistent with every evaluation.

(4) If correction is to be done, it should be done consistently, or conflicting exhaled tidal volumes will be recorded.
4. Time the ventilator rate to ensure appropriate calibration.
5. Time the inspiratory phase as accurately as possible.
6. Independently analyze the delivered FI_{O_2}.
7. Measure the IMV continuous flow and the FI_{O_2} delivered by this system.
8. Check the temperature and function of the humidifying system.
9. Evaluate the function of the cuff on the artificial airway.

B. The patient's response to mechanical ventilation should be monitored at the same time the technical function of the machine is evaluated.
1. Determine spontaneous respiratory rate and heart rate.
2. Measure blood pressure.
3. If hemodynamic monitoring is being utilized, record all available parameters.
4. Record peak and plateau pressures (Fig 32–15).
5. Measure spontaneous tidal volume. Ideally, measure for 10 breaths and calculate average.
6. Measure and record vital capacity and negative inspiratory force once per shift.

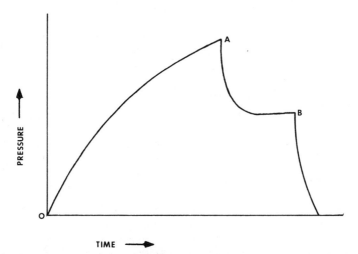

Fig 32–15.—*A*, peak airway pressure; *B*, plateau pressure. *A* − *B*, approximate pressure necessary to overcome airway resistance. *B*, approximate pressure necessary to overcome total patient/ventilator system compliance.

7. Determine patient/ventilator system compliance
   a. Patient/ventilator system compliance is referred to as *effective static compliance* (C_{ES}) to differentiate it from true compliance calculated in the pulmonary function laboratory.
   b. C_{ES} is determined by dividing the ETV by the plateau pressure (P_{plat}) minus PEEP (see Fig 32–15). Ideally, plateau pressure should be measured as close to the patient's airway as possible:

   $$C_{ES} = \frac{ETV}{P_{plat} - PEEP} \qquad (2)$$

   (1) ETV is used because it most closely reflects the volume of gas in the airway at end inspiration.
       (a) The ETV can be corrected for the patient/system compressible volume loss.
       (b) This correction, however, is not necessary because the same level of error is included in each determination and specific C_{ES} values are not as important as the change in this variable over time.
   (2) P_{plat} is used because it is an equilibration pressure that reflects the airway pressure under the most static conditions attainable in the patient/ventilator system.
   (3) Peak airway pressure is not used because it reflects the amount of pressure necessary to overcome airway resistance as well as elastic resistance.
   (4) PEEP levels *must* be subtracted from the P_{plat} because the amount of pressure necessary to maintain the tidal volume in the patient's airway is the increase in pressure from baseline levels. When PEEP is used, the PEEP level becomes the new baseline level.

   Example:

   ETV = 1,000 ml
   P_{plat} = 35 cm H_2O
   PEEP = 10 cm H_2O

   $$C_{ES} = \frac{1,000 \text{ ml}}{35 \text{ cm } H_2O - 10 \text{ cm } H_2O} = 40 \text{ ml/cm } H_2O$$

   c. C_{ES} in most adults is much lower than C_{tot} because of existing disease and the crude conditions under which the determination is made.

   d. Normal C_{ES} for most adults is about 40–60 ml/cm H_2O.

   e. The use of C_{ES} is limited by the ability to obtain a true static plateau pressure.

      (1) If the patient is ventilating spontaneously, inspiratory efforts will prevent a true plateau pressure from being obtained.

      (2) However, with conscious patient cooperation or control mode ventilation, P_{plat} can generally be obtained.

   f. C_{ES} reflects the "stiffness" of the lung-thorax/ventilator system.

8. Determination of airway resistance (R) (see Fig 32–15)

   a. An estimate of airway resistance can be obtained by dividing the difference between the peak pressure (P_{peak}) and P_{plat} by the flow rate ($\dot{V}$) in liters per second or liters per minute.

$$R = \frac{P_{peak} - P_{plat}}{\dot{V}} \qquad (3)$$

      (1) Since P_{peak} is the maximum pressure developed in the system and P_{plat} is the static system pressure, the difference between these two values reflects the amount of pressure necessary to maintain gas flow.

      (2) In order for a reasonable estimate of R to be made, $\dot{V}$ should be constant (square wave flow pattern).

      Example:

$$P_{peak} = 60 \text{ cm } H_2O$$
$$P_{plat} = 40 \text{ cm } H_2O$$
$$\dot{V} = 60 \text{ L/min or } 1 \text{ L/sec}$$

$$R = \frac{(60 \text{ cm } H_2O) - (40 \text{ cm } H_2O)}{60 \text{ L/min}}$$

$$R = 0.33 \text{ cm } H_2O/L/min$$

or

$$R = \frac{(60 \text{ cm } H_2O) - (40 \text{ cm } H_2O)}{1 \text{ L/sec}}$$

$$R = 20 \text{ cm } H_2O/L/sec$$

b. In spontaneously ventilating patients, the accuracy of the
P_{plat} determination and the stability of the P_{peak} limit the
accuracy of R determinations.

C. Arterial blood gas analysis should be performed whenever *a
change in the patient's clinical status or ventilator settings occur.*
   1. Ideally, critically ill patients should have an arterial line in
   place to permit rapid access to arterial blood.
   2. Routine blood gas analysis is usually necessary only on an 8-
   hour basis in critically ill patients and less frequently as the
   patient's condition improves.

D. Determination of intrapulmonary shunt on a daily basis provides
information on the extent of the patient's pulmonary pathophysiology (see Chap. 12).

E. Hemodynamic monitoring on a regular basis is crucial to the care
of critically ill mechanically ventilated patients. The data should
be tabulated with other patient/ventilator system data to ensure
the unwanted cardiovascular changes associated with ventilator
adjustments or changes are identified.

F. Careful monitoring of fluid and electrolyte balance is also essential to the overall care of the ventilator patient (see Chap. 15).

VI. Ventilator Alarm Systems
   A. Every volume ventilator must incorporate at least the following
   ventilator alarm systems for safe function:
      1. Patient/system leak or disconnect. This alarm may be either:
         a. Low exhaled tidal volume
         b. Low system pressure
      2. High inspiratory pressure
      3. If PEEP is used, a low system pressure alarm is necessary.
   B. All alarms incorporated into the ventilator should be continu-
   ously activated (see Chap. 31 for a listing of the alarms available
   on specific ventilators).

VII. Ventilator Maintenance
   A. Eucapneic ventilation
      1. All patients who are mechanically ventilated should be
      maintained at a P_{CO_2} within a range of *their normal values.*
         a. For most patients, that is a Pa_{CO_2} between 30 to 50
         mm Hg.
         b. In COPD patients who retain CO_2, Pa_{CO_2} should be
         maintained in a range which provides a normal acid-base
         status resulting in a pH between 7.35 and 7.45. If a pre-
         vious baseline Pa_{CO_2} is known, Pa_{CO_2} should be main-
         tained at that level.

2. In patients with increased intracranial pressure (ICP), Pa_{CO_2} is frequently maintained at the lower limits of acceptable, 30–35 mm Hg.
   a. When ICP is acutely increased, the patient should be further hyperventilated. This constricts cerebral vasculature and decreases cerebral vascular volume, resulting in a decreased ICP.
      (1) Constant hyperventilation is effective in decreasing ICP only for short periods of time (approximately 12–24 hours).
      (2) After this period cerebral vascular tone and blood volume return toward normal despite continued hyperventilation.
      (3) For this reason, hyperventilation is encouraged during initial stabilization but not for prolonged periods of time. If low to normal Pa_{CO_2} values are maintained, the patient can be easily hyperventilated if ICP should spike acutely.
3. Chronic hyperventilation results in:
   a. Electrolyte imbalances, decreased HCO_3^-, K^+, and Cl^-.
   b. Increased potential for cardiac arrhythmias.
   c. Altered hepatorenal function.
   d. Decreased cerebral blood volume.
   e. Altered autonomic receptor response to pharmacologic agents.
4. *The ventilator should never be used to correct metabolic acid/base disturbances.*
   a. The source of the disturbances should be identified and appropriately treated.
   b. If mechanical hypoventilation or hyperventilation is used to normalize a metabolic acid-base disturbance, when the metabolic disturbance is finally corrected, the patient is frequently in a state of chronic respiratory acidosis or alkalosis.
   c. In addition, mechanical hypoventilation or hyperventilation will mask the metabolic problem and may interfere with its identification and final resolution.
B. Fighting the ventilator
1. Patients generally fight the ventilator or ventilate out of phase with the ventilator secondary to technical and/or clinically related inadequacies.

    2. The most common cause is the *technical* setup of the ventilator system.
      a. Inadequate IMV system flow
      b. Insensitive demand valves
      c. Lengthy inspiratory times as a result of inadequate positive pressure inspiratory flow rates.
    3. If the problem is not technical, an assessment of the patient's clinical status should be made.
      a. Level of ventilation
      b. Level of oxygenation
      c. Cardiovascular stability
      d. Metabolic rate
      e. Electrolyte imbalance
      f. Breath sounds
    4. If the cause of the problem can be identified, it should be corrected. If a cause is not immediately identifiable or the patient is simply agitated, sedation and/or paralysis may be indicated.
  C. Pharmacologic support (refer to Chap. 34 for details)
    1. Most patients require some level of pharmacologic support during the initial phase of mechanical ventilation.
    2. If a patient is fighting the ventilator, pharmacologic intervention may be indicated.
    3. When patients are maintained on *full ventilatory support*, pharmacologic support is needed if the control mode is used and is frequently necessary if the assist/control, IMV, or SIMV mode is used.
    4. The ideal pharmacologic agent for use in maintaining patients receiving ventilatory support must:
      a. Be a potent CNS depressant
      b. Have minimal cardiovascular side effects
      c. Be a potent euphoric
      d. Be a strong analgesic
      e. Be *totally reversible*
    5. Morphine sulfate most closely fits the description of the ideal agent.
      a. It is a potent CNS depressant.
      b. It does cause some hypotension because of:
        (1) Decreased venous tone
        (2) Histamine release
      c. The hypotension is usually easily correctable with fluid therapy.

    d. It is a potent euphoric and analgesic.

    e. It is totally reversible with naloxone hydrochloride (Narcan).

    f. Initial morphinizing dosage is 0.2–0.3 mg/kg.

    g. Maintenance dosage is 0.05–0.1 mg/kg every hour.

    h. Hypotensive side effects are greatly minimized if patients are kept totally sedated. In patients in whom sedation is allowed to "wear off," hypotension may develop with each morphinizing dose.

6. Diazepam (Valium)

    a. Has minimal cardiovascular side effects.

    b. It is a euphoric.

    c. It is *not* an analgesic.

    d. It has variable and unpredictable CNS depressant effects.

    e. It is *not* reversible.

7. Paralyzing agents

    a. For ventilator maintenance, nondepolarizing neuromuscular blocking agents are the drugs of choice.

       (1) *d*-Tubocurarine (Curare)

       (2) Pancuronium bromide (Pavulon)

    b. Since these agents do not affect a patient's mental state, morphine sulfate or some other sedative should *always be used* in conjunction with paralyzing agents.

D. Bronchial hygiene

1. Many patients requiring mechanical ventilation also require bronchial hygiene therapy.

2. Aerosol therapy may be provided in-line with the ventilator circuit.

3. Postural drainage, chest percussion, and chest vibration may be performed.

4. Fiberoptic bronchoscopy may also be indicated.

5. Frequent tracheal suctioning.

6. Manual ventilation (hyperinflation).

7. Aerosolized bronchodilator therapy.

E. Adjustment of ventilator settings

1. In general, one ventilator parameter should be adjusted at a time, followed by cardiovascular assessment and arterial blood gas measurement in 10–15 minutes.

2. Simultaneous adjustment of ventilator parameters is only encouraged when significant and detrimental variations from expected blood gas values exist.

Example:

Blood gas results are

pH	7.28	HCO_3^-	26
Pa_{CO_2}	56	Pa_{O_2}	40

    a. Clearly this patient is being mechanically hypoventilated and is severely hypoxemic.

    b. Because of the severity of the abnormality, both ventilation and FI_{O_2} or PEEP should be increased as rapidly as possible.

  3. When parameters are adjusted simultaneously, it is occasionally difficult to determine a precise cause-and-effect relationship if expected outcomes are not realized.

F. Approaches to maintaining proper Pa_{CO_2} levels

  1. In general, all adjustments in level of ventilation should only be made after careful consideration of the cardiovascular consequence of each adjustment.

  2. The adjustment of choice is generally the one resulting in the least cardiovascular embarrassment.

  3. Use of mechanical deadspace is appropriate only if a patient is being ventilated in the control mode.

    a. Increasing deadspace will increase Pa_{CO_2}.

    b. Decreasing deadspace will decrease Pa_{CO_2}.

    c. In the control mode mechanical deadspace is recommended only when very large mechanical tidal volumes are required to satisfy a patient's sense that he/she is being adequately ventilated. Typically, patients mechanically ventilated for nonpulmonary disease require the use of deadspace.

      (1) Neuromuscular diseases

      (2) Neurologic diseases

    d. If deadspace is used in other modes, it simply increases the patient's ventilatory drive, increasing the work of breathing.

  4. Control mode

    a. To correct increased Pa_{CO_2}:

      (1) Increase tidal volume (first)

      (2) Increase rate

    b. To correct decreased Pa_{CO_2}:

      (1) Decrease rate (first)

      (2) Decrease tidal volume

  5. Assist/control mode

  a. To correct increased Pa_{CO_2}:
    (1) Increase tidal volume (first)
    (2) Increase rate
  b. To correct decreased Pa_{CO_2}:
    (1) Because the patient has control over the frequency of ventilation, decreasing the machine rate or the tidal volume may have no effect on the level of ventilation.
    (2) Patients mechanically hyperventilating in the assist/control mode frequently require pharmacologic intervention to decrease the ventilatory drive.
6. IMV/SIMV modes
  a. To correct increased Pa_{CO_2}:
    (1) Increase tidal volume (first)
    (2) Increase rate
  b. To correct decreased Pa_{CO_2}:
    (1) Decrease rate (first)
    (2) Decrease tidal volume
7. Extended mandatory minute ventilation
  a. To correct increased Pa_{CO_2}, increase mandatory minute ventilation.
  b. To correct decreased Pa_{CO_2}, decrease mandatory minute ventilation.
8. Pressure support or inspiratory assist
  a. To correct increased Pa_{CO_2}:
    (1) Increase pressure support level.
    (2) Implement SIMV breaths if not already being used or increase the number of SIMV breaths.
    (3) Change to some other mode guaranteeing a specific level of ventilation.
  b. To correct decreased Pa_{CO_2}, decrease pressure support level.
9. When considering changes in tidal volume, remember that for most patients, tidal volume should remain in the 10–20 ml/kg range. Ideally, tidal volumes are about 12–15 ml/kg.
10. Changes in the rate should be considered in connection with changes in the tidal volume.
    Example A:

Pa_{CO_2}:	52	Rate:	4/min
Mode:	IMV	TV:	15 ml/kg

In this situation the rate should be increased because the tidal volume is large but greater ventilation is required and the rate is slow.

Example B:

Pa_{CO_2}:	52	Rate:	10/min
Mode:	Control	TV:	10 ml/kg

Here, the tidal volume should be increased because the rate is adequate, yet increased ventilation is required and the tidal volume is relatively small. Always make the change that will correct hypoventilation but also cause the least increase in mean intrathoracic pressure.

G. Approaches to maintaining proper arterial oxygenation
1. The most crucial variable determining oxygen *content* is the hemoglobin value, which should be maintained as close to normal as possible.
2. If hemoglobin is normal, a Pa_{O_2} of 60 mm Hg will normally result in a HbO_2 %sat. of 90%.
3. If hypoxemia is primarily responsive, alter the FI_{O_2} to keep the Pa_{O_2} above 60 mm Hg.
4. If the responsive hypoxemia is a result of noncardiogenic pulmonary edema, 5–15 cm H_2O PEEP may be helpful.
5. If the hypoxemia is refractory, higher levels of PEEP therapy may be indicated (see Chap. 34).
6. Tissue oxygenation is also dependent on:
   a. Acid-base status
   b. Tissue perfusion
7. Patients that fight the ventilator increase their oxygen consumption and may develop hypoxemia.

VIII. Ventilator Discontinuance
A. Criteria for ventilator discontinuance
1. *Reversal of pathophysiologic condition necessitating ventilatory support.*
2. No active acute pulmonary disease process.
3. Stable vital signs
   a. Fever even if not of pulmonary origin:
      (1) Increases oxygen consumption
      (2) Increases carbon dioxide production
   b. Tachycardia and hypertension are indicative of increased level of stress.
   c. Bradycardia and hypotension may indicate lack of myocardial reserves and poor peripheral perfusion.
4. Optimal nutritional status
   a. This is of particular concern if patients have been ventilated for a lengthy period of time and have a chronic underlying disease process.

b. If a patient is receiving hyperalimentation, it may be
preferable to delay ventilator discontinuance until hyperalimentation is complete.
  (1) This is particularly true if all nonprotein calories are
  administered as carbohydrates.
  (2) When lipids are not administered, the respiratory
  quotient for the conversion of carbohydrates to lipids
  is greater than 8.0.
  (3) As a result, the patient's carbon dioxide production is
  markedly increased.
  (4) Patients with marginal cardiopulmonary reserves may
  not be able to meet the demands of ventilator discontinuance when coupled with an increased carbon
  dioxide load.
5. Adequate cardiovascular reserves
  a. Normal pulse and blood pressure
  b. No arrhythmias
  c. Good peripheral perfusion
  d. If a pulmonary artery catheter is in place
    (1) Stable and relatively normal hemodynamic values
    (2) Normal cardiac output
    (3) Normal $P\bar{v}_{O_2}$ and $a-\bar{v}DO_2$
6. Normal renal function
7. Intact CNS
8. Normally functioning gastrointestinal tract
9. Proper electrolyte and fluid balance (see Chap. 15)
  a. Electrolyte abnormalities may result in muscular weakness. Specifically, the following electrolytes should be
  normal:
    (1) K^+
    (2) Cl^-
    (3) Ca^{+2}
    (4) PO_4^{-3}
    (5) Mg^{+2}
Note: Any electrolyte, fluid, or major organ system malfunction results in an increase in physiologic stress. This, coupled with the added stress of spontaneous ventilation, may
be enough to cause a patient to fail and require ventilatory
support.
10. Adequate gas exchange capabilities
  a. Acceptable arterial blood gas values
    (1) Pa_{CO_2} at patient's normal level.
      (a) For most patients, this is about 40 mm Hg.

(b) For COPD patients, it may be at some elevated Pa_{CO_2} level.

(2) Normal pH.

(3) Pa_{O_2} greater than 60 mm Hg but not above normal level.

b. Intrapulmonary shunt fraction less than 20%–25%.

c. No indication of increased deadspace.

11. Adequate ventilatory capability. Even if all the above variables are acceptable, if the patient's ventilatory capabilities are diminished he or she may not be able to sustain spontaneous ventilation.

   a. Vital capacity greater than or equal to 10–15 ml/kg of ideal body weight.

   b. If the vital capacity cannot be determined, there should be a negative inspiratory force of at least -20 to -25 cm H_2O in 20 seconds.

   c. Spontaneous tidal volume of 2–3 ml/kg of ideal body weight.

   d. Spontaneous respiratory rate less than 25/minute.

   Note: If patients have been maintained on full ventilatory support, their stimulus to ventilate spontaneously may be diminished. As a result, when evaluating ventilatory capabilities, values below the levels indicated may be obtained. If this occurs, a well-monitored trial off the ventilator may produce the stimulus necessary for the patient to exhibit acceptable ventilatory abilities. A trial of this type is referred to as a *CO₂* challenge.

B. Psychological preparation

   1. The transition from mechanical ventilation to spontaneous ventilation produces a great deal of anxiety in most patients. This is particularly evident in patients ventilated for more than several days.

   2. To relieve some of this anxiety, the following steps should be followed:

      a. Carefully explain the procedure in detail.

      b. Attempt to develop the patient's confidence by reinforcing the improvement noted in the disease process.

      c. Assure patients that they will be continually monitored throughout the time they are ventilating spontaneously and that you will stay with them.

      d. *Do not tell patients they will never need the ventilator again.*

(1) If this is done and ventilatory support must be reestablished, it is not uncommon for the patient to lose confidence in himself and the medical team that is caring for him.

(2) It is more appropriate to inform patients that their capability of ventilating spontaneously is going to be evaluated. If they are ventilating adequately, they will be allowed to continue; however, if they deteriorate clinically, mechanical ventilation will be reinstituted.

C. Complete discontinuance

1. In some 80%–90% of patients maintained on ventilatory support, support can be totally discontinued without a gradual weaning phase if:

   a. Physiologic preparation is adequate.

   b. The ventilatory course was short.

   c. There is no need for psychological support.

2. Discontinuance procedure

   a. Manually ventilate with a high FI_{O_2} (0.70+)

      (1) This allows a gradual transition from ventilatory support to spontaneous ventilation.

      (2) The FI_{O_2} is increased in order to avoid any increased stress from an inappropriate oxygenation status.

      (3) However, patients functioning on a hypoxic drive must be maintained at their maintenance FI_{O_2}.

   b. Over a 5- to 10-minute period, gradually allow the patient to assume a greater role in ventilation.

   c. After the transition is complete, administer an aerosol via a Briggs T piece at an FI_{O_2} 0.10 higher than the ventilator FI_{O_2}. (Do not elevate the FI_{O_2} in patients functioning on a hypoxic drive.) Ensure a high flow system is used (see Chap. 24).

   d. Monitor patient's clinical presentation, vital signs, and work of breathing.

   e. Obtain an arterial blood gas in 10–15 minutes.

   f. Normal Pa_{CO_2} rise during initial discontinuance period.

      (1) If a patient is apneic with a normal metabolic rate, the arterial Pa_{CO_2} will increase about 6 mm Hg in the first minute and about 3 mm Hg every minute thereafter.

      (2) An increased Pa_{CO_2} is expected during the first 10–15 minutes in order to establish a stimulus to main-

tain spontaneous ventilation. After this the Pa_{CO_2} should return to the patient's normal level.

  (3) In general a 5–10 mm Hg increase in Pa_{CO_2} may occur in the initial period.

    (a) If this increase is *not* accompanied by significant cardiovascular and pulmonary stress, allow spontaneous ventilation to continue.

    (b) If pulse, blood pressure, and respiratory rate are markedly elevated, arrhythmias develop, the patient becomes diaphoretic and makes extensive use of accessory muscles, reinstitute mechanical ventilation.

  g. Reassess blood gases and clinical status 15 minutes later. If the patient is stable, continue.

  h. Repeat frequent reassessment of status.

  i. Once the patient is stabilized, return $F_{I_{O_2}}$ to an appropriate level.

  j. When satisfied ventilatory support will not need to be reinstituted, evaluate for extubation (see Chap. 25).

D. Gradually decreasing IMV or SIMV rate

  1. About 7%–10% of patients receiving mechanical ventilation require a gradual discontinuance of ventilatory support.

  2. In the majority of these patients ventilatory support can be discontinued over 6–8 hours.

  3. If the process is extended over days, the patient's ventilatory capabilities should be reevaluated.

  4. A gradual decrease in IMV/SIMV rate is necessary if:

    a. Physiologic preparation is questionable.

    b. Ventilatory course is prolonged.

    c. An underlying chronic disease exists in any organ system.

    d. Psychological support is necessary.

  5. Procedure

    a. Convert to IMV or SIMV mode, rate of 8–10 breaths per minute.

    b. Evaluate cardiopulmonary status.

    c. If tolerated, decrease rate by 2 breaths per minute every 1 to 2 hours, followed by evaluation of cardiopulmonary status.

    d. Discontinue support when rate is decreased to 2 breaths per minute. Follow procedure outlined in section C–2 above.

E. Use of extended mandatory minute ventilation (EMMV) and pressure support and inspiratory assist modes.
   1. These three modes may prove to be beneficial adjuncts to IMV/SIMV when ventilatory support is to be gradually decreased.
   2. Each allows the patient to assume an increasingly greater role in the processes of spontaneous ventilation.
   3. However, insufficient data are available to define protocols for the use of either EMMV, pressure support, or inspiratory assist modes.
F. Periodic discontinuance
   1. A small population of patients (approximately 1%–2%) require a very lengthy weaning phase.
   2. Most patients in this group have severe COPD.
   3. This approach gradually increases the patient's physiologic and psychological assets but also permits their ventilatory muscles to rest while they are being ventilated.
   4. The procedure is begun with a 5- to 10-minute trial off the ventilator with appropriate oxygenation and monitoring.
   5. After this trial, the patient is returned to full ventilatory support.
   6. This process is continued on an hourly or 2-hourly basis.
   7. The time off the ventilator is gradually increased over a few days until the patient requires the ventilator only at night.
   8. If possible, the ventilator is then discontinued at night.
G. The difficult-to-wean patient
   1. There is always an underlying reason why ventilatory support cannot be discontinued in a patient.
   2. Many such patients have pathophysiologic conditions that prevent them from ventilating spontaneously and as a result become chronic ventilator patients.
   3. However, many are not prepared to assume the increased stress associated with spontaneous ventilation.
   4. If support cannot be discontinued, the protocol given below may be followed:
      a. Evaluate the technical setup used during the discontinuance phase.
         (1) The work required to activate demand systems may be excessive.
         (2) The gas flow through the high-flow system used may be inadequate.

    b. Reassess the patient's physiologic preparation for discontinuance, paying particular attention to:

      (1) Acid-base status

      (2) Oxygenation status

      (3) Nutritional status

      (4) Fluid and electrolyte balance

    c. Determine if a psychological dependence has developed.

      (1) If this occurs it may be necessary to transfer the patient to another institution where the patient's confidence in the medical staff is not a factor.

5. Most patients within this group are:

    a. Improperly maintained patients, either from a ventilatory or a general medical perspective.

    b. COPD patients with:

      (1) Poor physiologic preparation

      (2) Psychological dependence on the ventilator

    c. Patients with spinal cord injuries.

6. Many of these patients end up as chronic ventilator patients.

BIBLIOGRAPHY

Agusti A.G.N., Torres A., Estopa R., et al.: Hypophosphatemia as a cause of failed weaning: The importance of metabolic factors. *Crit. Care Med.* 12:142–143, 1982.

Benzer H.: The value of intermittent mandatory ventilation, editorial. *Intensive Care Med.* 8:267–268, 1982.

Berry A.J.: Respiratory support and renal failure. *Anesthesiology* 55:655–667, 1981.

Bone R.C.: Complications of mechanical ventilation and positive end-expiratory pressure. *Respir. Care* 27:402–407, 1982.

Burton G.G., Hodgkin J.E.: *Respiratory Care: A Guide to Clinical Practice*, ed. 2. Philadelphia, J.B. Lippincott, 1984.

Cartwright D.W., Willis M.M., Gregory G.A.: Functional residual capacity and lung mechanics at different levels of mechanical ventilation. *Crit. Care Med.* 12:422–427, 1984.

Civetta J.M.: Intermittent mandatory ventilation and positive end-expiratory pressure in acute ventilatory insufficiency. *Int. Anesthesiol. Clin.* 18:123–141, 1980.

Civetta J.M., Banner M.: Nursing assessment of intermittent mandatory ventilation. *Int. Anesthesiol. Clin.* 18:143–177, 1980.

Dhingra S., Solven F., Wilson A., et al.: Hypomagnesemia and respiratory muscle power. *Am. Rev. Respir. Dis.* 129:497–498, 1984.

Downs J.B., Douglas M.E.: Intermittent mandatory ventilation and weaning. *Int. Anesthesiol. Clin.* 18:81–95, 1980.

Eross B., Powner D., Greenvik A.: Common ventilatory modes: Terminology. *Int. Anesthesiol. Clin.* 18:11–22, 1980.

Fairley H.G.: Critique of intermittent mandatory ventilation. *Int. Anesthesiol. Clin.* 18:179–189, 1980.

Fernandez A., de la Cal M.A., Esteban A., et al.: Simplified method for measuring physiologic V_D/V_T in patients on mechanical ventilation. *Crit. Care Med.* 11:823, 1983.

Gibney R.T.N., Wilson R.S., Pontoppidan H.: Comparison of work of breathing on high gas flow and demand valve continuous positive airway pressure systems. *Chest* 82:692–695, 1982.

Gjerde G.E., Katz J.A., Kraemer R.W.: Inspiratory work and airway pressure with continuous positive airway pressure delivery systems, abstract. *Crit. Care Med.* 12:272, 1984.

Graybar G.B., Smith R.A.: Apparatus and techniques for intermittent mandatory ventilation. *Int. Anesthesiol. Clin.* 18:53–79, 1980.

Henry W.C., West G.A., Wilson R.S.: A comparison of the oxygen cost of breathing between a continuous-flow CPAP system and a demand-flow CPAP system. *Respir. Care* 28:1273–1281, 1983.

Hylkema B.S., Barkmeijer-Degenhart P., van der Mark T.W., et al.: Central venous versus esophageal pressure changes for calculation of lung compliance during mechanical ventilation. *Crit. Care Med.* 11:271–275, 1983.

Kacmarek R.M., Dimas S., Reynolds J., et al.: Technical aspects of positive end-expiratory pressure (PEEP): Part II. PEEP with positive-pressure ventilation. *Respir. Care* 27:1490–1504, 1982.

Lindahl S.: Influence of an end inspiratory pause on pulmonary ventilation, gas distribution and lung perfusion during artificial ventilation. *Crit. Care Med.* 7:540–546, 1979.

Marquez J.M., Douglas M.E., Downs J.B., et al.: Renal function and cardiovascular responses during positive airway pressure. *Anesthesiology* 50:393–398, 1979.

Mathru M., Venus B.: Ventilator-induced barotrauma in controlled mechanical ventilation versus intermittent mandatory ventilation. *Crit. Care Med.* 11:359–361, 1983.

Millbern S.M., Downs J.B., Jumper L.C., et al.: Evaluation of criteria for discontinuing mechanical ventilatory support. *Arch. Surg.* 113:1441–1443, 1978.

Nishimura M., Tabnaka N., Takezawa J., et al.: Oxygen cost of breathing and inspiratory work of breathing as weaning monitor in critically ill. *Crit. Care Med.* 12:2–58, 1984.

Rasanen J., Nikki P., Heikkila J.: Acute myocardial infarction complicated by respiratory failure: The effects of mechanical ventilation. *Chest* 85:21–28, 1984.

Rau J.L.: Continuous mechanical ventilation: Part I. *Crit. Care Update* 8:10–29, 1981.

Rau J.L.: Continuous mechanical ventilation: Part II. *Crit. Care Update* 8:5–19, 1981.

Rivara D., Artucio H., Arcos J., et al.: Positional hypoxemia during artificial ventilation. *Crit. Care Med.* 12:436–438, 1984.

Robotham J.L., Cherry D., Mitzner W., et al.: A re-evaluation of the hemodynamic consequences of intermittent positive pressure ventilation. *Crit. Care Med.* 11:783–793, 1983.

Schachter E.N., Tucker D., Beck G.L.: Does intermittent mandatory ventilation accelerate weaning? *JAMA* 246:1210–1214, 1981.

Shapiro B.A., Harrison R.A., Kacmarek R.M., et al.: *Clinical Application of Respiratory Care,* ed. 3. Chicago, Year Book Medical Publishers, 1985.

Spearman C.B., Sheldon R.L., Egan D.L.: *Egan's Fundamentals of Respiratory Therapy,* ed. 4. St. Louis, C.V. Mosby Co., 1982.

Weisman I.M., Rinaldo J.E., Rogers R.M., et al.: Intermittent mandatory ventilation. *Am. Rev. Respir. Dis.* 127:641–647, 1983.

33 / Positive End-Expiratory Pressure

I. Definition of Terms
   A. PEEP: Positive End-Expiratory Pressure. The establishment and maintenance of a preset airway pressure greater than ambient at end exhalation.
   B. CPAP: Continuous Positive Airway Pressure. The application of PEEP therapy to the spontaneously breathing patient. Both inspiratory and expiratory airway pressures are supra-atmospheric.
   C. CPPV: Continuous Positive Pressure Ventilation. The application of PEEP therapy to a patient receiving positive pressure ventilation. CPPV is applied regardless of mode of ventilation used on the ventilator (control, assist/control, IMV, etc.).
   D. Additional terminology
      1. IMV + CPAP: The application of PEEP therapy to the patient being ventilated in the IMV mode.
      2. SIMV + CPAP: The application of PEEP therapy to the patient being ventilated in the SIMV mode.
      3. EPAP: Expiratory Positive Airway Pressure. The application of PEEP therapy to the spontaneously breathing patient. Positive pressure is maintained only during exhalation; a subatmospheric pressure must be developed during inspiration.
         a. This approach of applying PEEP to the spontaneously breathing patient parallels the development of CPAP.
         b. However, it has been demonstrated that the work of breathing with EPAP may be *four times* as great as when CPAP is delivered via a continuous flow system at the same PEEP level.
         c. This technical approach of applying PEEP *is not recommended.*
II. Physiologic Effects of PEEP
   A. Effects on intrapulmonary pressures
      1. Figure 33–1 indicates the intrapulmonary pressure curves during spontaneous breathing, CPAP, EPAP, CPPV, IMV or SIMV with CPAP, and IMV or SIMV with EPAP.
      2. With CPAP, CPPV, and IMV or SIMV with CPAP, the shape of the curve is not altered, only the baseline pressure

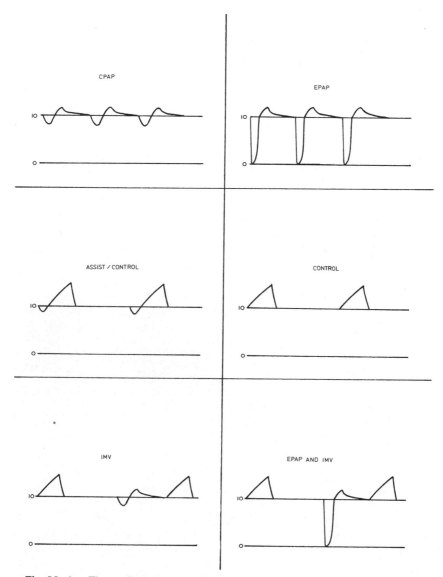

Fig 33–1.—Theoretical airway pressure curves with the application of PEEP to various modes of ventilation.

from which the patient is ventilated changes. Therefore the dynamics of air movement are not directly affected.

3. With EPAP and IMV or EPAP and SIMV there is a significant alteration in the airway pressure curve during spontaneous ventilation. Therefore the dynamics of gas movement are grossly affected, causing large increases in the work of breathing.

B. Effects on intrapleural (intrathoracic) pressures
   1. PEEP increases intrapleural pressures.
   2. The extent of the increase is determined by:
      a. The amount of PEEP applied.
      b. The stiffness of the individual's lung
         (1) The greater the individual's pulmonary compliance, the greater the transmission of PEEP to the intrapleural space and the greater the increase in intrapleural pressure.
         (2) In patients with normal lungs, PEEP therapy causes a significant increase in intrapleural pressure.
         (3) In patients with a generalized diffuse pulmonary disease process resulting in decreased compliance, a given level of PEEP may not cause a significant increase in intrapleural pressure.
         (4) Patients with localized pulmonary disease (e.g., pneumonia, atelectasis) demonstrate a similar increase in intrapleural pressure as patients with normal pulmonary compliance.
      c. Changes in thoracic compliance also affect transmission of pressure to the intrapleural space.
         (1) If thoracic compliance is decreased, more pressure than normal will be transmitted to the intrapleural space because overall expansion of the lung-thorax system is inhibited.
         (2) An increase in thoracic compliance will allow the system to expand and usually results in less of an increase in intrapleural pressure when compared to normal.

C. Effects on functional residual capacity (FRC)
   1. PEEP therapy causes an increase in FRC regardless of the condition of the lung at the time of application.
   2. FRC is increased by:
      a. Increasing the transpulmonary pressure gradient (Fig 33–2). This occurs in all individuals.
      b. Recruiting collapsed alveoli.

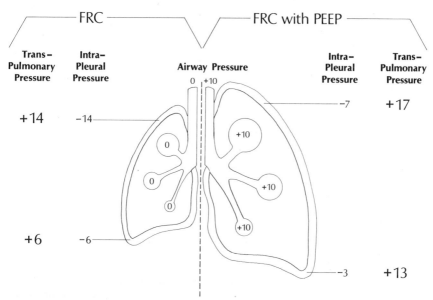

Fig 33–2.—Transpulmonary pressure gradients vary from the apex to the base of the lung. In ARDS the magnitude of these gradients increase because of the increased elastance of the lung. Applying PEEP increases the FRC by increasing the transpulmonary pressure gradient. Note that the gradient is normally increased most in the most gravity-dependent area of the lung. (From Shapiro B.A., Harrison R.A., Kacmarek R.A., et al.: *Clinical Application of Respiratory Care,* ed. 3. Chicago, Year Book Medical Publishers, Inc., 1985. Reproduced by permission.)

(1) In patients with a decreased FRC as a result of alveolar collapse due to surfactant instability, PEEP maintains alveoli inflated.

(2) This is accomplished by PEEP maintaining a back-pressure exceeding the force of surface tension and lung elastance, which tend to collapse alveoli.

(3) The actual reexpansion of alveoli is accomplished by the force of normal inspiration or positive pressure. PEEP simply maintains the alveoli open once they are reexpanded.

D. Effect on pulmonary compliance

1. Since PEEP therapy increases FRC, it may alter pulmonary compliance.

2. In the normal lung the increased FRC may move alveoli from the steep portion to the flat portion of their compliance curve, thus decreasing compliance (Fig 33–3).

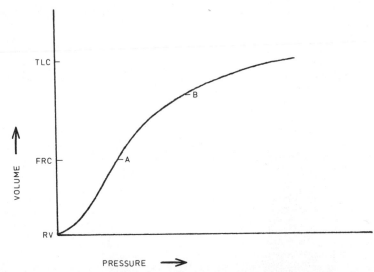

Fig 33–3.—Total compliance curve of the lung-thorax system. *A*, normal pressure-volume point (FRC) in a healthy individual. *B*, the application of PEEP in the normal lung increases the FRC and may move the pressure-volume point at FRC to the steep portion of the curve, decreasing total compliance.

3. In patients with adult respiratory distress syndrome (ARDS), the application of PEEP therapy increases compliance (Fig 33–4).
   a. As ARDS develops, the compliance curve shifts to the right and downward.
   b. As PEEP therapy is applied, the compliance curve shifts upward and to the left.
   c. With appropriate application of PEEP, a near-normal compliance curve can be reestablished.
4. The monitoring of effective static compliance (see Chap. 32) can be used to determine "best" or optimal PEEP level.
   a. The highest compliance is thought to coincide with the most appropriate PEEP level.
   b. The major problem associated with the use of compliance as a means of determining "optimal" PEEP is the difficulty in determining compliance in patients ventilated in anything but the control mode. With other modes, a reliable measurement of effective static compliance is often difficult.
E. Effect of PEEP on the cardiovascular system

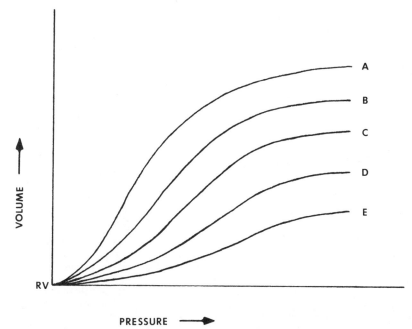

Fig 33–4.—*A,* normal total compliance curve. *B* through *E,* total compliance curves with increasing acute restrictive lung disease (ARDS). The application of PEEP, by recruiting alveoli and increasing transpulmonary pressure gradients, can alter the compliance curve, moving the curve from *E* to *D* or from *D* to *B,* and ideally returning the pressure-volume relationship back to normal *(A).*

1. Since PEEP therapy increases intrapleural pressure, it can decrease venous return and thus decrease cardiac output.
2. The greater the increase in intrapleural pressure, the greater the potential detrimental effect on cardiac output.
3. PEEP therapy causes a decrease in cardiac output by:
   a. Decreasing venous return (decreased preload).
   b. Increasing right ventricular afterload.
   c. Decreasing left ventricular distensibility (intraventricular septal shift).
4. When evaluating the effect of PEEP on cardiac output it is important to place the decreased cardiac output into proper perspective. Following are two examples of the effect of PEEP on cardiac output. In example A, the patient is young and has excellent cardiovascular reserves, while in example B, the patient is older and has very limited cardiovascular reserves.

Example A:

A 25-year-old man with ARDS:

Pa_{O_2}	48	Pulse	130/min
pH	7.53	BP	160/100
Pa_{CO_2}	27	CO	13.5 L/min
HCO_3^-	22	CI	7.7 L/min/m^2
Spon. RR	35	FI_{O_2}	0.8
TV	350	No mech. vent. support	

(CO is cardiac output, CI is cardiac index.)

With the application of PEEP, the following data are obtained:

Pa_{O_2}	75	Pulse	85/min
pH	7.43	BP	130/80
Pa_{CO_2}	38	CO	6.6 L/min
HCO_3^-	24	CI	3.7 L/min/m^2
Spon. RR	20	FI_{O_2}	0.8
TV	350	CPAP at 10 cm H_2O	

In this example the patient's cardiac output dropped 7 L but his cardiac index returned to normal. This occurred because the original cardiac output of 13.5 L/min was a result of cardiopulmonary stress. With the application of PEEP, oxygenation improved and cardiopulmonary stress decreased. Thus the cardiac output and cardiac index returned to normal. This reduction in cardiac output, and cardiac index is both dramatic and desirable.

Example B:

A 60-year-old man with ARDS:

Pa_{O_2}	48	Pulse	130/min
pH	7.48	BP	140/90
Pa_{CO_2}	32	CO	5.5 L/min
HCO_3^-	23	CI	3.6 L/min/m^2
Spon. RR	35	FI_{O_2}	0.6
TV	300	No mech. vent. support	

With the application of PEEP, the following data are obtained:

Pa_{O_2}	68	Pulse	150/min
pH	7.47	BP	90/60
Pa_{CO_2}	33	CO	3.5 L/min

HCO_3^-	23	CI	2.3 L/min/m^2
Spon. RR	28	FI_{O_2}	0.6
TV	300	CPAP at 10 cm H_2O	

In this example the patient's cardiac output dropped only 2 L/min but the cardiac index is now well below normal. A cardiac output of 3.5 L/min is clearly inappropriately low for this patient, and either fluid therapy or pharmacologic support is required to return the cardiac output to an acceptable level. The reduction in cardiac output is small but places the patient at increased risk.

   a. The drop in cardiac output was appropriate in example A but clearly inappropriate in example B.
   b. The patient's complete clinical presentation must be evaluated in order to determine if PEEP therapy had a detrimental effect on cardiac output.

5. Hemodynamic effects of PEEP therapy (see Chap. 14)
   a. Since PEEP therapy decreases venous return and cardiac output, a decrease in systemic blood pressure is normally noted as PEEP is applied.
      (1) Usually the decrease is minimal or moves the blood pressure to a more acceptable level.
      (2) However, with PEEP levels that significantly interfere with cardiac output, systemic blood pressure may drop precipitously.
   b. As PEEP therapy increases intrapleural pressure, it abates the thoracic pump mechanism. As a result, the pressure gradient distending intrathoracic blood vessels decreases, thereby increasing resistance to blood flow. This causes:
      (1) A decrease in the volume of blood returning to the right ventricle.
      (2) An alteration in pressure measured within the intrathoracic vessels.
   c. If the increased intrapleural pressure *does not significantly* alter flow, hemodynamic readings taken within the thoracic cavity *will increase slightly*.
      (1) ↑ CVP
      (2) ↑ PAP
      (3) ↑ PWP
   d. If, on the other hand, the increased intrapleural pressure *does significantly* alter flow, hemodynamic readings taken within the thoracic cavity *will decrease*. The extent

of the decrease is a result of the interrelationship among myocardial capabilities, vascular volume, and intra-pleural pressure.

(1) ↓ CVP
(2) ↓ $\overline{PAP}$
(3) ↓ PWP

e. If pulmonary hemodynamic values drop with the appli-cation of PEEP, then fluid therapy, pharmacologic sup-port, or a decrease in PEEP level is indicated.

f. The following example is designed to illustrate the effects of PEEP on hemodynamics values.

No PEEP

Pulse	160/min	CVP	12 cm H_2O
BP	150/100	$\overline{PAP}$	26 mm Hg
		PWP	10 mm Hg

5 cm H_2O PEEP

Pulse	158/min	CVP	13 cm H_2O
BP	148/92	$\overline{PAP}$	27 mm Hg
		PWP	11 mm Hg

10 cm H_2O PEEP

Pulse	140/min	CVP	15 cm H_2O
BP	142/96	$\overline{PAP}$	29 mm Hg
		PWP	13 mm Hg

15 cm H_2O PEEP

Pulse	126/min	CVP	16 cm H_2O
BP	130/84	$\overline{PAP}$	30 mm Hg
		PWP	14 mm Hg

20 cm H_2O PEEP

Pulse	154/min	CVP	6 cm H_2O
BP	90/60	$\overline{PAP}$	22 mm Hg
		PWP	5 mm Hg

The application of 5, 10, and 15 cm H_2O PEEP was ap-propriately tolerated from a hemodynamic perspective. However, with the application of 20 cm H_2O PEEP, the hemodynamic values decreased sharply, indicating in-ability of the cardiovascular system to tolerate 20 cm H_2O PEEP at its present status. If this patient receives proper fluid therapy and/or pharmacologic support the following profile may be achieved.

20 cm H_2O PEEP

Pulse	124/min	CVP	18 cm H_2O
BP	120/84	PAP	32 mm Hg
		PWP	16 mm Hg

Note: In actual clinical practice hemodynamic values should also be correlated with the patient's clinical presentation, signs of adequate tissue perfusion (e.g., urinary output, sensorium, skin temperature, etc.), and cardiac output.

F. Effect of PEEP therapy on Pa_{O_2}

1. Since PEEP therapy causes a minor increase in the partial pressure of oxygen in the lung, a small increase in Pa_{O_2} may be noted even in the healthy lung.

2. In the patient with ARDS, Pa_{O_2} levels also demonstrate only a small increase as the PEEP level is increased and will not markedly rise until a significant number of alveoli have been recruited. When appropriate numbers of alveoli have been recruited, Pa_{O_2} values may increase 20–40 mm Hg or more. The examples below illustrate how Pa_{O_2} may change as PEEP is applied:

PEEP	Pa_{O_2}
0 cm H_2O	45 mm Hg
5 cm H_2O	48 mm Hg
10 cm H_2O	53 mm Hg
15 cm H_2O	56 mm Hg
20 cm H_2O	110 mm Hg

3. Pa_{O_2} values may continue to increase slightly, remain the same, or decrease if PEEP levels inhibit cardiac output.

   a. A continual increase in PEEP will eventually affect cardiac output. However, the blood that is capable of perfusing the lung will still be oxygenated and its oxygenation state may continue to improve slightly as cardiac output decreases.

   b. When monitoring appropriateness of PEEP therapy, Pa_{O_2} must be evaluated; however, Pa_{O_2} provides no indication of the adequacy of cardiovascular function or of systemic oxygen delivery (see section II–J).

G. Effects on intrapulmonary shunt
   1. Increasing PEEP levels result in a decrease in intrapulmonary shunt.
   2. As alveoli are recruited, ventilation/perfusion matching improves and shunting decreases.
   3. As with Pa_{O_2}, intrapulmonary shunt may continue to decrease even when cardiac output is significantly decreased.
      a. This occurs because any blood that is presented to the lung may be better oxygenated.
      b. When monitoring appropriateness of PEEP therapy, intrapulmonary shunt should be evaluated; however, the intrapulmonary shunt provides no indication of adequacy of cardiovascular function or systemic oxygen delivery (see section II–J).
H. Mixed venous Po_2 $(P\bar{v}_{O_2})$ (see Chap. 14)
   1. $P\bar{v}_{O_2}$ is a variable affected by:
      a. Cardiac output
      b. Tissue perfusion
      c. Oxygen content
      d. Metabolic rate
   2. A decreased cardiac output, a decrease in oxygen content, an increase in tissue perfusion, or an increase in metabolic rate can cause a decrease in $P\bar{v}_{O_2}$.
   3. In cardiopulmonary stressed patients with ARDS, the $P\bar{v}_{O_2}$ is normally decreased.
      a. The extent of this decrease is *most* dependent on the cardiovascular reserves of the patient.
      b. In patients with good cardiovascular reserves, the $P\bar{v}_{O_2}$ will only be decreased slightly (35–40 mm Hg) because these patients can increase their cardiac outputs significantly in response to stress.
      c. However, in patients with limited cardiovascular reserves, the $P\bar{v}_{O_2}$ may be significantly decreased (30–35 mm Hg or lower) because these patients cannot increase their cardiac outputs in response to stress.
   4. As PEEP therapy is applied, the $P\bar{v}_{O_2}$ should increase if the cardiac output is not adversely affected. This occurs because oxygen delivery increases.
   5. If excessive PEEP is applied, the $P\bar{v}_{O_2}$ will decrease because of the effect of PEEP on cardiac output, thus decreasing oxygen delivery:

PEEP	$P\bar{v}_{O_2}$	CO
0 cm H_2O	36 mm Hg	12.5 L/min
5 cm H_2O	36 mm Hg	12.3 L/min
10 cm H_2O	38 mm Hg	9.6 L/min
15 cm H_2O	40 mm Hg	8.9 L/min
20 cm H_2O	43 mm Hg	7.2 L/min
25 cm H_2O	35 mm Hg	4.8 L/min

At PEEP levels from 5 to 20 cm H_2O, the $P\bar{v}_{O_2}$ increased appropriately, but at 25 cm H_2O the PEEP inhibited cardiac output significantly, resulting in a drop in the $P\bar{v}_{O_2}$. Fluid therapy, pharmacologic support, or a decrease in PEEP level is indicated to support cardiovascular function and optimize $P\bar{v}_{O_2}$.

I. Arteriovenous oxygen content difference $a - \bar{v}DO_2$ (see Chap. 14)
   1. $a - \bar{v}DO_2$ is dependent on:
     a. Arterial oxygen content
     b. Venous oxygen content
     c. Metabolic rate
     d. Cardiac output
   2. In patients with ARDS, $a - \bar{v}DO_2$ varies from normal, depending on the cardiovascular reserves of the patient.
   3. In the patient with good cardiovascular reserves, decreased arterial oxygen content results in an increase in cardiac output.
     a. If the patient's metabolic rate is constant and cardiac output is increased, the volume of oxygen extracted per volume of blood decreases.
       (1) As a result the venous oxygen content of the patient will not be significantly decreased, and
       (2) $a - \bar{v}DO_2$ will decrease.
       (3) Since the tissue is extracting less oxygen per given volume of blood, the difference between the arterial and venous contents becomes smaller, regardless of the actual contents of each.
   4. In patients with poor cardiovascular reserves, a decrease in arterial oxygen content may not affect cardiac output.
     a. If the patient's metabolic rate and cardiac output are constant but arterial oxygen content is decreased, then $a - \bar{v}DO_2$ will stay the same.

510ESSENTIALS OF RESPIRATORY THERAPY

b. If the patient's metabolic rate is constant and the cardiac output and arterial oxygen content are decreased, then $a-\bar{v}DO_2$ will increase.
5. With the appropriate application of PEEP, the $a-\bar{v}DO_2$ should return toward normal levels.
   a. If PEEP is applied and $a-\bar{v}DO_2$ levels increase beyond acceptable limits, cardiovascular reserves are questionable. Fluid therapy or pharmacologic support may be indicated.
   b. If, with the application of PEEP, $a-\bar{v}DO_2$ values increase appropriately but then exceed upper limits, PEEP therapy is beginning to adversely affect cardiac output. Fluid therapy, pharmacologic support, or a decrease in PEEP level may be indicated:

PEEP	$a-\bar{v}DO_2$	CO
0 cm H_2O	2.8 vol%	12.2 L/min
5 cm H_2O	3.0 vol%	10.5 L/min
10 cm H_2O	3.3 vol%	9.0 L/min
15 cm H_2O	3.6 vol%	7.5 L/min
20 cm H_2O	4.0 vol%	6.0 L/min
25 cm H_2O	5.6 vol%	3.5 L/min

In the above table it is assumed the patient's cardiovascular reserves are good. The application of 5–20 cm H_2O PEEP resulted in appropriate increases in $a-\bar{v}DO_2$. However, with the application of 25 cm H_2O PEEP, cardiac output was adversely affected, causing $a-\bar{v}DO_2$ to increase significantly toward the upper limits of normal. Fluid therapy, pharmacologic support, or decreasing PEEP is indicated.
J. Effect of PEEP on oxygen transport
   1. Oxygen transport is defined as cardiac output times arterial oxygen content:

$$O_2 \text{ transport} = CO \times Ca_{O_2} \qquad (1)$$

   2. With the development of ARDS, oxygen transport normally decreases because of the decrease in Ca_{O_2}.
   3. As PEEP is applied and Ca_{O_2} is increased, oxygen transport improves.
   4. With excessive application of PEEP, oxygen transport may decrease because of the effect of PEEP on cardiac output. If

this occurs, fluid therapy, pharmacologic support, or decreasing PEEP is indicated.

K. Effects of PEEP on closing volume

1. Closing volume is that point in a forced vital capacity maneuver at which gravity-dependent airways close.

2. The point at which gravity-dependent airways close may become a larger percentage of the FVC and possibly exceed FRC in anesthetized individuals, postoperative patients, and obese patients.

3. PEEP therapy may have the effect of decreasing closing volume and improving oxygenation in the patients defined; however, no conclusive data supporting this are available.

L. Effect on extravascular lung water

1. There is no evidence that PEEP therapy decreases extravascular lung water.

2. It appears that PEEP therapy actually maintains or increases extravascular lung water.

M. Effect on intracranial pressure

1. Since PEEP impedes venous return, it can be expected to increase intracranial pressure by causing blood to pool in the cranium.

2. If PEEP therapy is required in patients with an increased intracranial pressure, elevation of the head of the patient's bed a distance equal to the amount of PEEP applied can minimize the effects of PEEP on intracranial pressure.

N. Barotrauma and PEEP

1. Any time positive pressure is applied to the lung, the likelihood of barotrauma is increased.

2. However, barotrauma normally occurs when patients simulate coughs, fight the ventilator, or engage in any activity that markedly increases intrapulmonary pressure.

3. When high levels of PEEP are applied, careful monitoring for barotrauma must be maintained. This is necessary because the lung requiring high levels of PEEP is significantly diseased and any increase in airway pressure may result in barotrauma.

O. The effects of PEEP therapy on renal, gastrointestinal, and endocrine function are the same as those of all forms of positive pressure (see Chap. 32).

III. Indications for PEEP Therapy

A. The primary indication for PEEP therapy is ARDS.

    1. PEEP is truly indicated only in patients with a generalized diffuse acute restrictive disease process characterized by:
      a. Decreased pulmonary compliance
      b. Decreased FRC
      c. Refractory hypoxemia
      d. Increased intrapulmonary shunting
    2. PEEP does not correct the refractory hypoxemia associated with a localized disease process such as:
      a. Pneumonia
      b. Pleural effusion
      c. Localized atelectasis
  B. Other indications for PEEP include the treatment of noncardiogenic pulmonary edema or early ARDS. The capillary endothelial changes associated with the early phase are:
    1. Diffuse
    2. Generalized
    3. Cause a decrease in FRC; however, this decrease is minimal
    4. Hypoxemia, which is normally somewhat responsive to oxygen therapy
  C. PEEP therapy has also been recommended for the following pathophysiologic conditions. However, data establishing its efficacy are questionable.
    1. Chest trauma
    2. Cardiogenic pulmonary edema
    3. Following open heart surgery
IV. Physiologic PEEP
  A. The application of 3–5 cm H_2O PEEP to replace the glottic mechanism.
  B. The placement of a foreign body between the vocal cord results in a reflexive decrease in FRC.
  C. This occurs in all individuals but has only been demonstrated to be clinically significant in two populations.
    1. Neonatal/pediatric patients. *This group should not have a short-term artificial airway in place without 3–5 cm H_2O PEEP.* If extubation is indicated they are extubated from 3–5 cm H_2O PEEP rather than from atmospheric pressure.
    2. Patients with severe COPD. Again, establishment of an artificial airway under acute conditions results in a significant decrease in the FRC causing hypoxemia. It is advisable to maintain 5 cm H_2O PEEP in these patients until extubation.
    3. PEEP of 3–5 cm H_2O is often used in the average patient requiring a short-term artificial airway. The efficacy of such

treatment has not been established, nor have any adverse reactions been documented.

V. Prophylactic PEEP

    A. PEEP has been used to prevent ARDS or postoperative pulmonary complications.

    B. No definitive data for or against this application of PEEP are available.

VI. Clinical Goals of PEEP Therapy

    A. The end point of PEEP therapy is defined by:

        1. Adequate arterial oxygenation.

        2. Minimal $F_{I_{O_2}}$.

        3. Adequate cardiovascular function.

    B. Adequate arterial oxygenation:

        1. Defined as a P_{O_2} greater than 60 mm Hg. This normally results in a 90% HbO_2% saturation if there is no significant shift in the oxyhemoglobin dissociation curve (Fig 33–5).

        2. Normal hemoglobin content.

    C. Minimal $F_{I_{O_2}}$

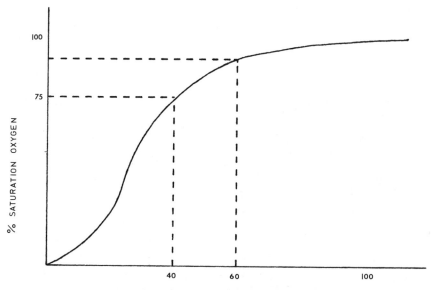

PARTIAL PRESSURE OXYGEN

Fig 33–5.—At a Pa_{O_2} of 60 mm Hg the hemoglobin is approximately 90% saturated with oxygen. Because the curve is relatively flat beyond the 90% saturation level, the Pa_{O_2} must be significantly increased in order to effect a significant change in hemoglobin saturation, whereas increasing the Pa_{O_2} from 40 mm Hg to 60 mm Hg increases the hemoglobin saturation by about 15%.

1. The specific $F_{I_{O_2}}$ that is "safe" to inspire over a period of time has not been determined.
2. Most suspect that an $F_{I_{O_2}}$ greater than 0.50 may cause pulmonary epithelial damage.
3. PEEP therapy should be titrated until an $F_{I_{O_2}}$ less than 0.50 is necessary. Maintaining the $F_{I_{O_2}}$ below 0.40 is ideal.

D. Adequate cardiovascular function
  1. Entails maintaining appropriate cardiac index and cardiac output for the particular patient.
  2. Entails maintaining adequate tissue perfusion.
    a. Normal skin temperature
    b. Normal urinary output
    c. Intact sensorium
    d. Normal $P\bar{v}_{O_2}$
    e. Normal $a - \bar{v}DO_2$

VII. Monitoring PEEP Therapy
A. With the application of PEEP or the alteration of PEEP levels, extensive monitoring of the patient's cardiopulmonary status must be performed.
B. Monitoring should be done 10–20 minutes after each PEEP adjustment and periodically thereafter.
C. Monitoring gas exchange.
  1. Arterial blood gases
  2. Intrapulmonary shunt if accessible
D. Monitoring pulmonary mechanics.
  1. Evaluation of tidal volume, respiratory rate, and work of breathing, if appropriate
  2. Effective static compliance if patient is in control mode or not spontaneously ventilating
E. Monitoring cardiovascular function.
  1. Pulse and blood pressure
  2. Skin color
  3. Skin turgor
  4. Skin temperature
  5. Urinary output
  6. Sensorium
  7. Cardiac output
  8. Cardiac index
  9. $\overline{PAP}$
  10. CVP
  11. PWP
  12. $P\bar{v}_{O_2}$

        13. $a - \bar{v}DO_2$

        14. Oxygen transport

    F. When PEEP level exceeds 15 cm H_2O it is advisable to insert a pulmonary artery catheter for proper evaluation of cardiovascular function.

VIII. Periodic Discontinuation of PEEP

    A. The periodic discontinuation of PEEP should be avoided. This is particularly true when higher levels of PEEP are employed.

    B. Discontinuation of PEEP on a periodic basis results in:

        1. Significant decreases in Pa_{O_2}.

        2. Increase in intrapulmonary shunt.

        3. Possible increased venous return.

        4. Decreased FRC.

        5. Decreased pulmonary compliance.

        6. A complete reversal of the changes accomplished with the application of PEEP.

    C. Once PEEP levels reach or exceed 15 cm H_2O, PEEP should be maintained on the manual ventilators used during suctioning, transport, and chest physiotherapy.

    D. PEEP *should not* be discontinued when hemodynamic monitoring is being performed.

IX. Clinical Application of PEEP

    A. Regardless of the severity of the disease process, all adult patients should be started on 5 cm H_2O PEEP. Pediatric and neonatal patients should be started on 2–3 cm H_2O PEEP.

    B. PEEP levels should be increased in 5 cm H_2O increments in adults, in 2–3 cm H_2O increments in neonatal and pediatric patients, followed by complete monitoring of the effects of PEEP.

    C. If an increase in PEEP results in adverse cardiovascular effects, fluid therapy and/or pharmacologic support should be used to stabilize cardiovascular function before the PEEP level is again increased.

    D. As PEEP is applied, a significant increase in Pa_{O_2} should be noted. If a 20–40 mm Hg increase in Pa_{O_2} is not seen, the "optimal" level of PEEP for that patient may not have been attained.

    E. Once the Pa_{O_2} has shown a reasonable increase and the patient is stabilized cardiovascularly, attempt to decrease the FI_{O_2}.

        1. If the FI_{O_2} is above 0.5, a 0.05 to 0.2 decrease in FI_{O_2} followed by arterial blood gas measurement is indicated.

        2. If the FI_{O_2} is at or below 0.5, decrease the FI_{O_2} by 0.05, followed by arterial blood gas measurement.

   F. The above sequence is used in patients with severe ARDS. If
      the patient has noncardiogenic pulmonary edema or early
      ARDS, 5–15 cm H_2O may be sufficient to maintain Pa_{O_2} at a low
      (<0.5) FI_{O_2}. *Since no significant intrapulmonary shunting from*
      atelectasis normally exists, a marked increase (20–40 mm Hg) in
      the Pa_{O_2} may not be noted.
 X. Technical Application of PEEP
   A. Devices used to apply PEEP are classified as three types:
      1. Orificial resistors: These devices generate PEEP by devel-
         oping a resistance to gas flow (Fig 33–6)
         a. Ohm's law or the law of flow describes how PEEP is
            developed:

$$\text{Resistance (R)} = \frac{\text{pressure (P)}}{\text{flow (\.V)}} \qquad (2)$$

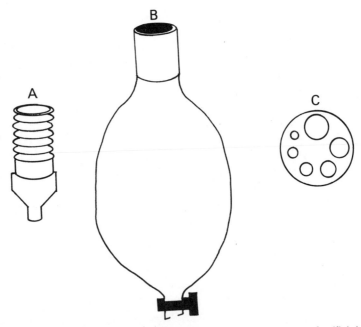

Fig 33–6.—Schematic representation of three common types of orificial resistors. *A,* endotracheal tube adapter attached to flex tube; *B,* screw clamp and
reservoir bag; *C,* variable orificial plate. (From Kacmarek R.M., Dimas S., Reynolds J., et al.: Technical aspects of positive end-expiratory pressure (PEEP):
Part I. Physics of PEEP devices. *Respir. Care* 27:1478–1488, 1982. Reproduced
by permission.)

If equation 2 is solved for pressure, the relationship becomes:

$$pressure = resistance \times flow \qquad (3)$$

   b. Thus, with a fixed resistance, the level of PEEP generated is dependent on the flow through the system.
     (1) Higher flow creates more PEEP.
     (2) Lower flow creates less PEEP.
   c. The major problem with orificial resistors is that PEEP levels are altered if flow through the system changes.
   d. In adults, inadvertently high levels of PEEP can develop if orificial resistors are used.
   e. These PEEP devices are only used in pediatric and neonatal patients, in whom expiratory flows are minimal.
2. Threshold resistors: Devices capable of maintaining a constant predictable and quantifiable PEEP level.
   a. All commonly used adult PEEP devices are normally listed as threshold resistors.
   b. However, all threshold resistors have some orificial properties. If the area across which exhalation occurs is less than the cross-sectional area of the large bore tubing leading to the device, gas flow resistance develops.
   c. It appears that the Emerson water column (Fig 33–7) offers the least resistance to gas flow.
   d. The most commonly used threshold resistor is the balloon-type exhalation valve on ventilator circuits (Fig 33–8).
     (1) Many of the disposable circuits utilizing this type of valve offer significant resistance to gas flow.
     (2) Frequent increases in expiratory pressure are noted with forced exhalation.
     (3) Many produce an expiratory retard with or without PEEP.
   e. Other commonly used threshold resistors with significant orificial properties are
     (1) Weighted ball valves.
     (2) Spring-loaded valves.
     (3) Magnetic valves.
   f. In spite of their limitations, threshold resistors are the devices of choice in the adult. However, care must be taken to evaluate the appropriate function of each of these valves.

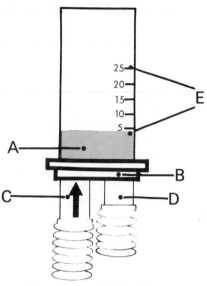

Fig 33–7.—Emerson water column PEEP device. *A*, water reservoir; *B*, flexible diaphragm; *C*, entrance port; *D*, exit port to atmosphere; *E*, calibrated scale in cm H_2O. (From Kacmarek R.M., Dimas S., Reynolds J., et al.: Technical aspects of positive end-expiratory pressure (PEEP): Part I. Physics of PEEP devices. *Respir. Care.* 27:1478–1488, 1982. Reproduced by permission.)

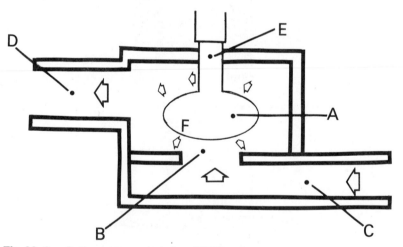

Fig 33–8.—Balloon-type exhalation PEEP valve. *Arrows* represent gas flow. *A*, balloon valve; *B*, outlet orifice; *C*, inlet port; *D*, exit port to atmosphere; *E*, gas nipple; *F*, inferior surface of balloon valve that may occlude outlet orifice. (From Kacmarek R.M., Dimas S., Reynolds J., et al.: Technical aspects of positive end-expiratory pressure (PEEP): Part I. Physics of PEEP devices. *Respir. Care* 27:1478–1488, 1982. Reproduced by permission.)

3. Opposing flow devices: Devices similar to threshold resistors in their ability to maintain a constant, predictable, and quantifiable PEEP level by directing a flow of gas opposing patient exhalation (Figs 33–9 and 33–10).

   a. Minimal orificial resistance is noted with these devices.

   b. These devices are either used in pediatrics/neonatology or for short-term therapy in adults.

B. PEEP applied during positive pressure ventilation.

   1. All of the threshold devices discussed can be easily applied to the expiratory limb of positive pressure ventilators.

   2. The most commonly and easily used of these devices is the balloon-type exhalation valve in the ventilator circuit.

   3. However, the most reliable of these devices appears to be the Emerson water column.

   4. Figures 33–11 and 33–12 illustrate approaches to the application of PEEP to manual ventilators.

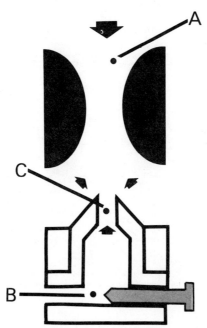

Fig 33–9.—Bourns opposing-flow exhalation PEEP valve. *A,* exhalation outlet; *B,* venturi jet source gas; *C,* venturi jet. Thumb screw adjusts venturi source gas flow. *Small arrows* represents gas entrainment; *large arrows* indicate patient's exhalation. (From Kacmarek R.M., Dimas S., Reynolds J., et al.: Technical aspects of positive end-expiratory pressure (PEEP): Part I. Physics of PEEP devices. *Respir. Care* 27:1478–1488, 1982. Reproduced by permission.)

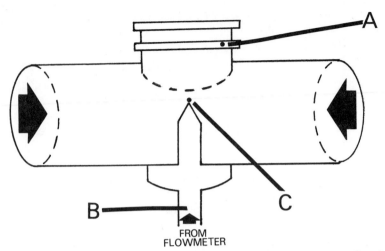

FROM
FLOWMETER

Fig 33–10.—Glazener PEEP device, used in adults for transport or for short-term therapy. *Arrows* represent gas entrainment *A,* exhalation outlet; *B,* venturi jet source gas; *C,* venturi jet. (From Kacmarek R.M., Dimas S., Reynolds J., et al.: Technical aspects of positive end-expiratory pressure (PEEP): Part I. Physics of PEEP devices. *Respir. Care* 27:1478–1488, 1982. Reproduced by permission.)

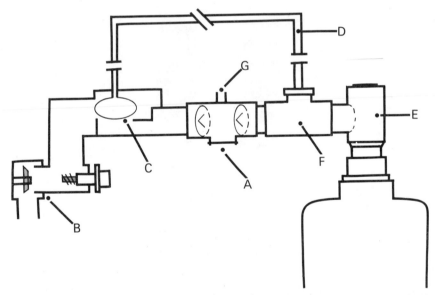

Fig 33–11.—Schematic representation of Universal PEEP system for manual ventilators. *A,* patient T piece with one-way valves; *B,* threshold-resistor PEEP device; *C,* balloon-type exhalation valve; *D,* pressure line to exhalation valve; *E,* manual ventilator gas-collecting head; *F,* T piece with pressure-line tap off; *G,* manometer nipple. (From Kacmarek R.M., Dimas S., Reynolds J., et al.: Technical aspects of positive end-expiratory pressure (PEEP): Part II. PEEP with positive-pressure ventilation. *Respir. Care* 27:1490–1504, 1982. Reproduced by permission.)

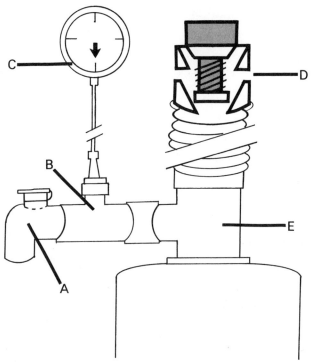

C D

B

A

E

Fig 33–12.—PEEP system for manual ventilators with single exit port gas-collecting head. *A,* patient connection; *B,* T piece with manometer Tap-off; *C,* manometer; *D,* threshold resistor PEEP device; *E,* single exit port gas-collecting head. (From Kacmarek R.M., Dimas S., Reynolds J., et al.: Technical aspects of positive end-expiratory pressure (PEEP): Part II. PEEP with positive-pressure ventilation. *Respir. Care* 27:1490–1504, 1982. Reproduced by permission).

    C. PEEP applied to the spontaneously breathing patient (Fig 33–13).
        1. Patient tolerance of a CPAP system is most directly related to system flow.
            a. System flow must be high enough to meet the patient's peak inspiratory demands (30 to 90 L/min).
            b. At least 4 times the patient's measured minute volume should enter the system.
            c. Flow should leave the system at all times, even at peak inspiration.
            d. A 3- to 5-L anesthesia bag, used as a reservoir, is included on the inspiratory limb. For patients who have very high peak inspiratory flows, two reservoir bags may be included.

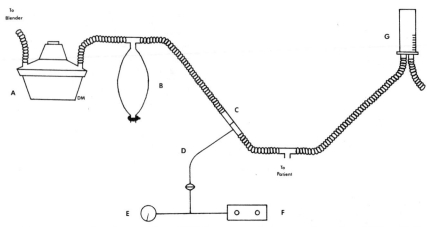

Fig 33–13.—Continuous flow CPAP system. *A,* large volume humidifier; *B,* 5-L reservoir bag; *C,* attachment of high/low pressure alarm and manometer to inspiratory limb; *D,* small bore tubing to alarm and manometer; *E,* pressure manometer; *F,* high/low pressure alarm; *G,* water column PEEP device.

    e. A high/low pressure alarm and a pressure manometer are included in the system to monitor pressure changes.

    f. A properly set up and functioning system should demonstrate no more than a ± 2 cm H_2O fluctuation in pressure about PEEP level.

    g. A screw clamp is attached to the open tail of the reservoir bag to allow pressure relief if the system becomes obstructed.

2. A typical EPAP system is depicted in Figure 33–14.

    a. This system is *not* a constant flow system.

    b. The patient must reduce system pressure to below atmospheric in order to inspire.

    c. The work of breathing with this system is 4 times as great as the work of breathing with a CPAP system.

    d. The use of EPAP systems to deliver PEEP to the spontaneously breathing patient is discouraged secondary to the excessive work of breathing involved.

3. Mask versus artificial airway for the application of CPAP.

    a. Mask CPAP can be used for short-term application of PEEP therapy if PEEP levels do not exceed about 10 cm H_2O.

    b. Patients in whom mask CPAP is used must:

       (1) Be alert, oriented, and cooperative.

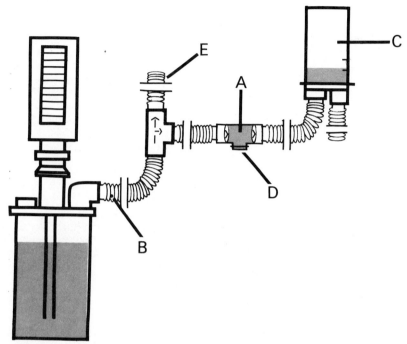

Fig 33–14.—EPAP system. *A,* volume requiring decompression; *B,* constant flow aerosol system; *C,* threshold resistor PEEP device; *D,* patient T piece with one-way valves; *E,* aerosol system reservoir. (From Kacmarek R.M., Dimas S., Reynolds J., et al.: Technical aspects of positive end-expiratory pressure (PEEP): Part III. PEEP with spontaneous ventilation. *Respir. Care* 27:1505–1518, 1982. Reproduced by permission.)

    (2) Have good control of their airway.

  c. A nasogastric tube should be placed to prevent abdominal distention.

  d. Mask CPAP is useful in patients with noncardiogenic pulmonary edema or early ARDS for periods of about 12–36 hours.

  e. The vast majority of patients requiring CPAP also require an artificial airway.

BIBLIOGRAPHY

Annest S.J., Gottlieb M., Paloski W.H., et al.: Detrimental effects of removing end-expiratory pressure prior to intubation. *Ann. Surg.* 191:539–546, 1980.

Bourns Inc. Life Systems Division: *Instruction manual: Bourns infant ventilator model LS-104-105 and Model BP 200.* Riverside, Calif., Bourns Medical Systems.

Bredenberg C.E., Kazui T., Webb W.R.: Experimental pulmonary edema: The effect of positive end-expiratory pressure on lung water. *Ann. Thorac. Surg.* 26:62–70, 1978.

Chapin J.C., Downs J.B., Douglas M.E., et al.: Lung expansion and airway pressure transmission with positive end-expiratory pressure. *Arch.. Surg.* 114:1193–1197, 1979.

Civetta J.M., Barnes T.A., Smith L.O.: "Optimal PEEP" and intermittent mandatory ventilation in the treatment of acute respiratory failure. *Respir. Care* 20:551–557, 1975.

Craig D.B., McCarthy D.S.: Airway closure and lung volumes during breathing with maintained airway positive measures. *Anesthesiology* 36:540–546, 1972.

Demling R.H., Staub N.C., Edmonds L.H.: Effect of end-expiratory airway pressure on accumulation of extravascular lung water. *J. Appl. Physiol.* 38:907–915, 1975.

Douglas M.E., Downs J.B.: Cardiopulmonary effects of PEEP and CPAP, letter. *Anesth. Analg.* 57:347–350, 1978.

Emerson postoperative ventilator operating instructions. Cambridge, Mass., J.H. Emerson Co.

Falke K.J.: Do changes in lung compliance allow the determination of "Optimal PEEP"? *Anesthetist* 29:165–169, 1980.

Gallagher T.J., Civetta J.M.: Goal-directed therapy of acute respiratory failure. *Anesth. Analg.* 59:831–836, 1980.

Fields A., Sterling D.: Open-system IMV with PEEP, letter. *Respir. Care* 24:394–398, 1979.

Garg G.P., Hill G.E.: The use of spontaneous continuous positive pressure (CPAP) for reduction of intrapulmonary shunting in adults with acute respiratory failure. *Can. Anaesth. Soc. J.* 22:284–290, 1975.

Gherini S., Peters R.M., Virgilio R.W.: Mechanical work on the lungs and work of breathing with positive end-expiratory pressure and continuous positive airway pressure. *Chest* 76:251–256, 1979.

Gregory G.A., Kitterman J.A., Phibbs R.H., et al.: Treatment of the idiopathic respiratory distress syndrome with continuous positive airway pressure. *N. Engl. J. Med.* 284:1333–1340, 1971.

Hall J.R., Rendleman D.C., Downs J.B.: PEEP devices: Flow dependent increases in airway pressure, abstract. *Crit. Care Med.* 6:100, 1978.

Hobelmann C.F., Smith D.E., Virgilio R.W., et al.: Left atrial and pulmonary artery wedge pressure differences with positive end-expiratory pressure: The contribution of the pulmonary vasculature. *J. Trauma* 15:951–957, 1975.

Hobelmann C.F., Smith D.E., Virgilio R.W., et al.: Mechanics of ventilation with positive end-expiratory pressure. *Ann. Thorac. Surg.* 24:68–74, 1977.

Hopewell P.C., Murray J.F.: Effect of continuous positive pressure ventilation in experimental edema. *J. Appl. Physiol.* 40:568–570, 1976.

Jardin F., Farcot J., Boisante L., et al.: Influence of positive end-expiratory pressure on left ventricular performance. *N. Engl. J. Med.* 304:387–392, 1981.

Kacmarek R.M., Dimas S., Reynolds J., et al.: Technical aspects of positive end-expiratory pressure: Parts 1–3. *Respir. Care* 27:1478–1518, 1982.

Katz J.A., Ozanne G.H., Zinn S.E., et al.: Time course and mechanisms of lung volume increases with PEEP in acute pulmonary failure. *Anesthesiology* 59:9–14, 1981.

Kirby R.R., Downs J.B., Civetta J.M., et al.: High level positive end-expiratory pressure (PEEP) in acute respiratory insufficiency. *Chest* 67:156–161, 1975.

Liebman P.R., Patten M.T., Manny J., et al.: Humorally medicated alterations in cardiac performance as a consequence of positive end-expiratory pressure (PEEP). *Surgery* 83:594–599, 1978.

Lutch J.S., Murray J.F.: Continuous positive-pressure ventilation: Effects of systemic oxygen transport and tissue oxygenation. *Ann. Intern. Med.* 76:193–201, 1972.

Manny J., Justice R., Hechtman H.B.: Abnormalities in organ blood flow and its distribution during positive end-expiratory pressure. *Surgery* 85:425–431, 1979.

Marotta J., Greenbaum D.M.: PEEP attachment for puritan manual resuscitator. *Respir. Care* 21:862–864, 1976.

McCarthy G.S., Hedenstierna G.: Arterial oxygenation during artificial ventilation: The effect of airway closure and its prevention by positive end-expiratory pressure. *Acta Anaesthesiol. Scand.* 22:563–571, 1978.

Mitzner W., Batra G., Goldberg H.: Lung inflation and extracellular fluid accumulation. *Circulation* 54(suppl. II):14–19, 1976.

Nunn J.F.: *Applied Respiratory Physiology*, ed. 2. London, Butterworth Publishing Co., 1977.

Pepe P.E., Stager M.A., Maunder R.J., et al.: Early application of PEEP in patients at risk for ARDS, abstract. *Am. Rev. Respir. Dis.* 127(suppl.):97, 1983.

Perel A., Eimerl D., Grossberg M.: A PEEP device for a manual bag ventilator. *Anesth. Analg.* 55:745, 1976.

Petty T.L., Nett L.M., Ashbaugh D.G.: Improvement in oxygenation in the adult respiratory distress syndrome by positive end-expiratory pressure (PEEP). *Respir. Care* 16:173–176, 1976.

Quist J., Pontoppidan H., Wilson R.S., et al.: Hemodynamic responses to mechanical ventilation with PEEP. *Anesthesiology* 42:45–52, 1975.

Rose D.M., Downs J.B., Heenan T.J.: Temporal responses of functional residual capacity and oxygen tension to changes in positive end-expiratory pressure. *Crit. Care Med.* 9:79–82, 1981.

Shoemaker W.C., Thompson L. (eds.): *Critical Care: State of the Art.* Fullerton, Calif., Society of Critical Care Medicine, 1981, vol. 2.

Smith R.A., Kirby R.R., Gooding D.O., et al.: Continuous positive airway pressure (CPAP) by face mask. *Crit. Care Med.* 8:483–485, 1980.

Spearman C.B., Sheldon R.L., Egan D.E.: *Egan's Fundamentals of Respiratory Therapy*, ed. 4. St. Louis, C.V. Mosby Co., 1982.

Sturgeon C.I., Douglas M.E., Downs J.B., et al.: PEEP and CPAP: Cardiopulmonary effects during spontaneous ventilation. *Anesth. Analg.* 56:633–639, 1977.

Suter P.M., Fairley H.B., Isenberg M.D.: Optimum end-expiratory airway pressure in patients with acute pulmonary failure. *N. Engl. J. Med.* 292:284–290, 1975.

Shapiro B.A., Harrison R.A., Kacmarek R.M., et al.: *Clinical Application of Respiratory Care*, ed. 3. Chicago, Year Book Medical Publishers, Inc., 1985.

Shapiro B.A., Cane R.D., Harrison R.A.: Positive end-expiratory pressure therapy in adults with special reference to acute lung injury: A review of the literature and suggested clinical correlations. *Crit. Care Med.* 12:127–141, 1984.

Shapiro B.A., Cane R.D., Harrison R.A.: Positive end-expiratory pressure in acute lung injury. *Chest* 83:558–563, 1983.

Toung T.J.K., Saharia P., Mitzner W.A., et al.: The beneficial and harmful effects of positive end-expiratory pressure. *Surg. Gynecol. Obstet.* 147:518–523, 1978.

Venous B., Jacobs H.K., Lim L.: Treatment of the adult respiratory distress syndrome with continuous positive airway pressure. *Chest* 76:257–261, 1979.

Walkinshaw M., Shoemaker W.C.: Use of volume loading to obtain preferred levels of PEEP: A preliminary study. *Crit. Care Med.* 8:81–86, 1980.

Wiegett J.A., Mitchell R.A., Snyder W.H. III: Early positive end-expiratory pressure in the adult respiratory distress syndrome. *Arch. Surg.* 114:497, 1979.

Zamost B.G., Alfery D.D., Johanson I., et al.: Description and clinical evaluation of a new continuous positive airway pressure device. *Crit. Care Med.* 9:109–113, 1981.

Zarins C.K., Virgilio R.W., Smith D.E., et al.: The effect of vascular volume on positive end-expiratory pressure induced cardiac output depression and left atrial wedge pressure discrepancy. *Surg. Res.* 23:348–355, 1977.

34 / Pharmacology

I. General Information
  A. Definitions
    1. General
      a. Drug: Any chemical compound that may be administered to or used in an individual to aid in the diagnosis, treatment, or prevention of disease; to relieve pain; or to control or improve any physiologic disorder or pathologic condition.
      b. LD_{50}: The dosage of a drug that would be lethal to 50% of a test population.
      c. ED_{50}: The dosage of a drug that would have therapeutic effects for 50% of a test population.
      d. TI: Therapeutic index. The numerical ratio of the LD_{50} to the ED_{50} (LD_{50}/ED_{50}). This ratio shows how close the lethal and therapeutic doses of a drug are for a test population. Low indexes mean the therapeutic and lethal doses are similar and the drug has a high potential for overdose or toxic side effects (Fig 34–1).
      e. Potency: The activity of a drug per unit weight. A potent drug has a large biologic activity at a small unit dose (Fig 34–2).
      f. Efficacy: The maximum effect produced by a drug regardless of dose (Fig 34–3).
    2. Drug interactions
      a. Additive: Two drugs, when given together, produce an effect equal to the sum of their individual effects.
      b. Potentiation: Potentiation occurs when a drug active at a specific receptor site is given with a drug inactive at that receptor site, and the resulting effect is greater than that of the active drug alone ($1 + 0 = 3$).
      c. Synergism: Two drugs active at a receptor site, when given together, cause an effect greater than the sum of their individual effects ($1 + 2 = 6$).
      d. Antagonist: A drug whose effects are directly opposite those of another drug.

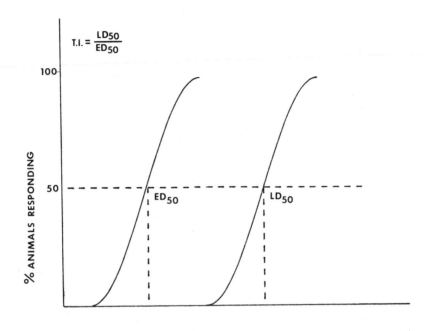

Fig 34–1.—Log-dose response curve demonstrating therapeutic index *(TI)* determination.

(1) Competitive: An antagonist whose effects are directly related to dosage. A competitive antagonist decreases potency but does not affect efficacy of the other drug.

(2) Noncompetitive: An antagonist whose effects are not dose related. Both potency and efficacy of the other drug are decreased.

e. Cumulation: A gradual rise in the body's total drug level that occurs when the administration rate of the drug is greater than the body's rate of removal.

f. Tolerance: The body's ability to increase its metabolism of a drug. Increasing amounts of the drug are required to produce the same effect.

g. Tachyphylaxis: The rapid development of tolerance.

B. Pharmacologic nomenclature

1. Chemical name: Name illustrative of chemical structural formula of the drug.

2. Generic name: Officially adopted name of the drug in the United States; name used in *United States Pharmacopeia.*

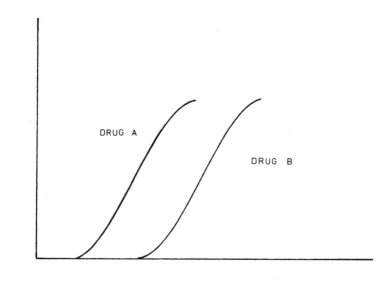

LOG DOSE

Fig 34–2.—Log-dose response curve comparing the potency of two drugs. The potency of drug *A* is greater than that of drug *B*.

       3. Trade or proprietary name: Patented name given a particular drug by the manufacturer that introduced it.

C. Absorption: The specific physical and chemical characteristics of a drug determine the rate of absorption. Routes of administration are listed in order of speed in attaining blood levels after administration.

    Note: Not all drugs may be administered by all routes listed, and the speed of absorption by route may also vary.

       1. Intravenous injection (IV)
       2. Via lung (aerosol)
       3. Intramuscular injection (IM)
       4. Subcutaneous injection (Sub. Q.)
       5. Sublingual and rectal absorption
       6. Oral
       7. Topical

D. Distribution: Movement of the drug to area of desired pharmacologic activity.

       1. Primary mechanism for distribution: Circulatory system.
       2. Topical administration for effect on skin or mucous membrane decreases likelihood of further, undesired distribution.

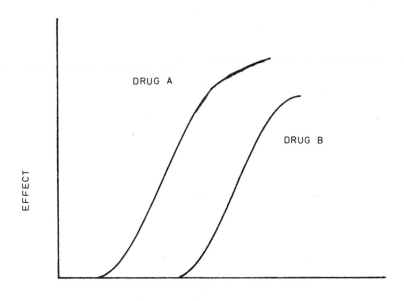

LOG DOSE

Fig 34–3.—Log-dose response curve comparing the efficacy of two drugs. A greater effect is caused by drug *A* than drug *B*. In addition, drug *A* is more potent than drug *B*.

    E. Metabolism: Actual inactivation of the drug by the body.
        1. Primary organ for detoxification: Liver.
        2. Secondary organs for detoxification: Kidney and gastrointestinal tract.
        3. Many drugs may be inactivated by the body's cells or plasma proteins.
    F. Excretion: Mechanism for elimination of the drug from the body.
        1. Primary organ for excretion: Kidney.
        2. Secondary excretion sites:
           a. Gastrointestinal tract
           b. Respiratory tract
           c. All exocrine glands
    G. Side effect: Any physiologic response other than that for which the drug was administered.
  II. Wetting Agents/Diluents
    A. Isotonic solution: A solution equivalent to a 0.9% W/V solution of NaCl. Isotonic solutions are used in respiratory therapy primarily in small-volume nebulizers.

B. Hypertonic solution: A solution with a concentration greater than a 0.9% W/V solution of NaCl. Hypertonic solutions are used in respiratory therapy primarily for sputum induction.
C. Hypotonic solution: A solution with a concentration of less than a 0.9% W/V solution of NaCl. Hypotonic solutions are most commonly used in respiratory therapy in large-volume aerosol generators and seem to have less effect on increasing airway resistance than normal saline or water.
D. Distilled water: Used in respiratory therapy in all types of humidifiers.
III. Mucolytics
  A. Trade name: Mucomyst.
  B. Generic name: Acetylcysteine (N-acetyl-L-cysteine).
  C. Mechanism of action: Lyses disulfide bonds holding mucoproteins together, thus increasing fluidity of mucoid sputum.
  D. Concentration: 20% W/V or 10% W/V solution.
  E. Dosage
    1. Standard dosage: 4 ml of 10% W/V or 20% W/V solution.
    2. Maximum dosage: None specified.
  F. Indications: Thick, retained mucoid or mucopurulent secretions.
  G. Contraindications: Hypersensitivity.
  H. Side effects/hazards
    1. Bronchospasm
    2. Excessive liquefaction of dried, retained secretions
    3. Stomatitis
    4. Hypersensitivity
    5. Nausea
    6. Rhinorrhea
  I. Comments
    1. Highly recommended that drug be administered in conjunction with bronchodilator.
    2. Should be refrigerated after opening.
    3. Should be used within 96 hours after opening.
    4. Reacts with rubber, some plastics, and iron.
    5. Foul smelling.
    6. Should be administered in glass, plastic, or nontarnishable metal container.
    7. Minimal effectiveness on predominantly purulent secretions.
    8. Supplied in 4-ml, 10-ml, and 30-ml vials.
IV. Prophylactic Antiasthmatics
  A. Trade name: Aarane or Intal.

B. Generic name: Cromolyn sodium.
C. Mechanism of action
   1. Inhibits release of histamine and slow-reacting substance of anaphylaxis (SRS-A) during allergic, IgE-mediated responses on pulmonary mast cells.
   2. Suppresses response of mast cell to antigen-antibody reaction.
D. Concentration: 20-mg capsules or 20 mg/2 ml H_2O ampules.
E. Standard dosage: 20 mg three or four times daily.
F. Maximum dosage: 20 mg three or four times daily.
G. Primary indications: Prophylactic maintenance in patients with severe bronchial asthma.
H. Secondary indications: Result of the effect of cromolyn sodium on all mast cells.
   1. Allergic rhinitis
   2. Diarrhea in systemic mastocytosis
   3. Ulcers of the oral mucosa
   4. Nonspecific inflammatory bowel disease
I. Contraindications: Hypersensitivity.
J. Side effects/hazards
   1. Local irritation
   2. Bronchospasm
   3. Maculopapular rash
   4. Urticaria
K. Comments
   1. Ineffective in acute asthmatic attack.
   2. Maximum effect seen after 4 weeks of continuous use.
   3. Sometimes effective in controlling exercise-induced asthma.

V. Detergent
   A. Trade name: Alevaire.
   B. Generic name: Active agent superinone (trade name, Tyloxapol); also contains sodium bicarbonate and glycerine.
   C. Mechanism of action
      1. Tyloxapol reduces the surface tension of mucoid secretions, thereby increasing fluidity.
      2. Sodium bicarbonate increases the pH of secretions, causing polysaccharides in sputum to lyse.
      3. Glycerine has hydroscopic effect for stabilization of aerosol.
   D. Concentration
      1. Tyloxapol: 0.125% W/V
      2. Sodium bicarbonate: 2% W/V
      3. Glycerine: 5% W/V

E. Dosage
  1. Standard dosage
    a. Intermittent use: 4–10 ml undiluted.
    b. May be used continuously.
  2. Maximum dosage: None specified.
F. Indications: Thick, retained secretions, primarily of mucoid type.
G. Side effects/hazards
  1. May cause bronchospasm in asthmatic patients.
H. Comments
  1. Should be refrigerated after opening.
  2. Should be discarded 72 hours after opening.
  3. Should be kept from direct light.
  4. Supplied in 60-ml and 500-ml bottles.

VI. Surface-Active Agent
A. Trade name: Ethyl alcohol, ethanol.
B. Generic name: Ethyl alcohol, ethanol.
C. Mechanism of action
  1. Has direct surfactant-like effect on surface tension of frothy, serum-like fluid developed in acute pulmonary edema.
  2. Breaking up of frothy secretions allows them to occupy a much smaller volume, improving distribution of ventilation.
D. Concentration: 20%–80% solution.
E. Dosage
  1. Standard
    a. Intermittent: 4–10 ml of 50% solution.
    b. Continuous: 500 ml of 50% solution over 24-hour period.
F. Indication: Acute pulmonary edema.
G. Contraindications: Hypersensitivity.
H. Side effects/hazards
  1. Airway irritation
  2. Bronchospasm
  3. Local dehydration
I. Comments: Should not be administered in heated aerosol or ultrasonic nebulizer.

VII. Sympathomimetics: General Considerations
A. General classification
  1. Alpha effect: Constriction of vascular smooth muscle.
  2. Beta effect: Peripheral relaxation of vascular smooth muscle (minimal).

      a. *Beta one:* Positive inotropic and chronotropic cardiac effects.

      b. *Beta two:* Relaxation of nonvascular smooth muscle (bronchodilation).

B. Mechanism of action (Fig 34–4)

   1. Alpha effect: Inhibits membrane-bound adenylcyclase from converting ATP to cyclic 3′5′-AMP.

   2. Beta effect: Stimulates release of membrane-bound adenylcyclase, which increases formation of cyclic 3′5′-AMP (adenosine monophosphate) from ATP (adenosine triphosphate).

D. General therapeutic uses of sympathomimetics

   1. Treatment of generalized bronchoconstriction

   2. Treatment of mucosal congestion

   3. Treatment of allergic disorders

   4. Control of hemorrhage

   5. Treatment of hypotension

   6. Cardiac stimulation

   7. Treatment of heart block

   8. Treatment of CNS disorders

E. Contraindications

   1. Hyperthyroidism

   2. Hypertension

   3. Tachycardia

F. Side effects/hazards

   1. Palpitations

   2. Tachycardia

   3. Hypertension

   4. Restlessness

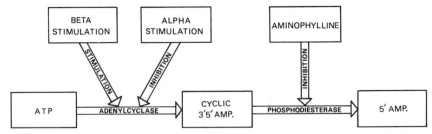

Fig 34–4.—Increased cyclic 3′5′-AMP levels result in bronchodilation. Beta stimulation increases cyclic 3′5′-AMP levels by release of adenylcyclase, whereas aminophylline increases cyclic 3′5′-AMP levels by inhibiting its metabolism by phosphodiesterase. Alpha stimulation inhibits adenylcylase release and therefore decreases cyclic 3′5′-AMP levels.

      5. Fear
      6. Anxiety
      7. Tension
      8. Tremor
      9. Weakness
     10. Dizziness
     11. Pallor
  G. Comments
      1. Tolerance is frequently observed (tachyphylaxis).
      2. Synergistic effects may be seen.
      3. Maximally administered every 2–3 hours.
      4. Normal duration of action is short, up to 3 hours, and may be as short as 1–1½ hours.
VIII. Specific Sympathomimetics (Table 34–1)

TABLE 34–1.—COMPARISON OF AEROSOLIZED SYMPATHOMIMETICS

GENERIC NAME	DRUG	EFFECTS	CONCENTRATION	DOSAGE
Isoproterenol HCl	Isuprel	α 0 β_1 + + + β_2 + + +	1:100; 1:200	0.5 ml 1:200 in 4 ml NS
Racemic epinephrine	Vaponephrine, Micronephrine	α + + β_1 + β_2 + +	2.25% W/V	0.5 ml in 4 ml NS
Isoetharine	Bronkosol, Dilabron	α 0 β_1 + β_2 + +	1% W/V	0.5 ml in 4 ml NS
Epinephrine HCl	Adrenalin	α + + + β_1 + + + β_2 + +	1:100	0.2 ml in 4 ml NS .05 ml of 1:000, SC
Phenylephrine	Neo-Synephrine	α + + + β_1 0 β_2 0	0.25% W/V	0.2 ml in 4 ml NS
Metaproterenol sulfate	Alupent	α 0 β_1 ½+ β_2 + + +	5% W/V .65% spray	0.3 ml in 4 ml NS 2 sprays q 6 hours
Albuteral	Ventolin	α 0 β_1 0 β_2 + + +	0.1 mg spray	2 sprays q 6 hours
Terbutaline sulfate	Bricanyl	α 0 β_1 + β_2 + +	0.2% W/V	0.25–0.5 ml in 4 ml NS

0 none
 + weak
 + + medium
 + + + strong
α alpha
β_1 beta one
β_2 beta two
NS normal saline

A. Isoproterenol HCl
1. Trade name: Isuprel
2. Generic name: Isoproterenol HCl
3. Concentration: 1:100 or 1:200 solution
4. Effects
   a. Alpha: None (0)
   b. Beta one: Strong (+ + +)
   c. Beta two: Strong (+ + +)
5. Dosage by aerosol
   a. Standard
      (1) 0.5 ml of 1:200 solution in 4 ml of normal saline.
      (2) 0.25 ml of 1:100 solution in 4 ml of normal saline.
   b. Maximum
      (1) 1 ml of 1:200 solution in 4 ml of normal saline.
      (2) 0.5 ml of 1:100 solution in 4 ml of normal saline.
B. Racemic epinephrine
1. Trade name: Vaponephrine, Micronephrine
2. Generic name: Racemic epinephrine
3. Concentration: 2.25% W/V solution
4. Effects
   a. Alpha: Medium (+ +)
   b. Beta one: Weak (+)
   c. Beta two: Medium (+ +)
5. Dosage
   a. Standard: 0.5 ml of 2.25% W/V solution of 4 ml of normal saline.
   b. Maximum: 1 ml of 2.25% W/V solution in 4 ml of normal saline.
C. Isoetharine
1. Trade name: Bronkosol, Dilabron
2. Generic name: Isoetharine
3. Concentration: 1% W/V solution
4. Effects
   a. Alpha: None (0)
   b. Beta one: Weak (+)
   c. Beta two: Medium (+ +)
5. Dosage (aerosol)
   a. Standard: 0.5 ml in 4 ml of normal saline.
   b. Maximum: 1 ml in 4 ml of normal saline.
D. Epinephrine HCl
1. Trade name: Adrenalin
2. Generic name: Epinephrine HCl

3. Concentraton: 1:100
4. Effects
    a. Alpha: Strong (+ + +)
    b. Beta one: Strong (+ + +)
    c. Beta two: Medium (+ +)
5. Dosage
    a. Aerosol
        (1) Standard: 0.25 ml in 4 ml of normal saline.
        (2) Maximum: 0.50 ml in 4 ml of normal saline.
    b. Subcutaneous: 0.3–0.5 ml of a 1:1000 solution.

E. Phenylephrine
    1. Trade name: Neo-Synephrine
    2. Generic name: Phenylephrine
    3. Concentration: 0.25% W/V
    4. Effects
        a. Alpha: Strong (+ + +)
        b. Beta one: None (0)
        c. Beta two: None (0)
    5. Dosage
        a. Standard: 0.2 ml in 4 ml of normal saline.
        b. Maximum: 0.5 ml in 4 ml of normal saline.
    6. Comment: Normally administered only as nasal decongestant by spray or drops.

F. Metaproterenol sulfate
    1. Trade name: Alupent, Metaprel
    2. Generic name: Metaproterenol sulfate
    3. Concentration
        a. 10 and 20 mg tablet (oral dosage)
        b. Metered mist: 0.65 mg/spray
        c. Liquid: 5% W/V solution
    4. Effects
        a. Alpha: None (0)
        b. Beta one: Very weak (+)
        c. Beta two: Medium (+ + +)
    5. Dosage
        a. Standard
            (1) One tablet four times daily.
            (2) Two sprays every 4–6 hours.
            (3) 0.3 ml in 4 ml of normal saline via aerosol.
        b. Maximum
            (1) 0.6 ml in 4 ml of normal saline via aerosol.
    6. Comment: Duration of effect up to 6 hours.

G. Albuteral
  1. Trade name: Ventolin, Proventil
  2. Generic name: Albuteral
  3. Concentration: Metered mist: 90 mg per spray, 2-mg and 4-mg tablets
  4. Effects
     a. Alpha: None (0)
     b. Beta one: None (0)
     c. Beta two: Strong (+ + +)
  5. Dosage
     a. Standard: 2 sprays tid or qid; 2 or 4 mg tid or qid.
     b. Maximum: None specified.
  6. Comment: Duration of effect up to 6 hours.
H. Terbutaline sulfate
  1. Trade name: Bricanyl, Brethine
  2. Generic name: Terbutaline sulfate
  3. Concentration: 0.1% W/V; 2.5- and 5-mg tablets
  4. Effects
     a. Alpha: None (0)
     b. Beta one: Weak (+)
     c. Beta two: Medium (+ +)
  5. Dosage
     a. 0.25–1.0 mg subcutaneously.
     b. 0.25–0.5 ml in 4 ml of normal saline solution via aerosol.
     c. 2.5- or 5.0-mg tablets tid.
IX. Sympathomimetics Utilized for Their Effects on the Cardiovascular System
  A. Norepinephrine
    1. Trade name: Levophed, Noradrenalin
    2. Generic name: Norepinephrine
    3. Effects
       a. Alpha: Strong (+ + +)
       b. Beta one: Weak (+)
       c. Beta two: None (0)
    4. Indications: Hypotension
    5. Administration: IV only
  B. Dopamine HCl
    1. Trade name: Intropin, Dopastat
    2. Generic name: Dopamine HCl
    3. Effects: Dose dependent
       a. Low dosages

        (1) Increased renal blood flow

        (2) Mild increase in cardiac output

    b. Moderate dosages

        (1) Increased renal blood flow

        (2) Increased cardiac output

    c. High dosages: Systemic vasoconstriction

  4. Indications

    a. Hypotension

    b. Shock

    c. Renal failure

    d. Myocardial infarction

    e. Other hemodynamic problems

  5. Administration: IV only in appropriate dilution of nonalkaline solutions.

  6. Side effects/hazards

    a. QRS interval widening

    b. Angina

    c. Conduction disturbances

    d. Tachycardia

C. Dobutamine

  1. Trade name: Dobutrex

  2. Generic: Dobutamine

  3. Effects

    a. Alpha: None (0)

    b. Beta one: Moderate (+ +)

    c. Beta two: None (0)

  4. Indications:

    a. Congestive heart failure

    b. Hemodynamic abnormalities

  5. Administration: IV only

  6. Side effects/hazards

    a. Premature ventricular contractions

    b. Anginal pain

    c. Ischemic injury

  7. Comments

    a. Has inotropic selectivity (less increase in heart rate than other drugs).

    b. Decreases systemic vascular resistance.

    c. No increase in pulmonary or systemic blood pressure noted with administration.

X. Noncatecholamines Affecting the Sympathetic Nervous System

  A. Ephedrine

1. Trade name: Ephedrine
2. Generic name: Ephedrine
3. Mechanism of action: Causes release of epinephrine and norepinephrine stored throughout the body
4. Effects (lasting up to 6 hours)
   a. Bronchodilation
   b. Mild cardiac stimulation
   c. Peripheral vasoconstriction
   d. Mild CNS stimulation
5. Indications
   a. Nonemergency allergic reactions
   b. Chronic asthma
   c. Nasal congestion
6. Administration: Oral, intramuscular, or subcutaneous

B. Theophylline
   1. Trade name: Aminophylline
   2. Generic name: Theophylline
   3. Mechanism of action: Inhibits phosphodiesterase (see Fig 34–4) from converting cyclic $3'5'$-AMP to inactive $5'$-AMP.
   4. Effects
      a. Bronchodilation
      b. Cardiac stimulation
      c. Coronary artery dilation
      d. Skeletal muscle stimulation
      e. Diuresis
      f. CNS stimulation
   5. Indications
      a. Acute and chronic asthma
      b. Abnormal respiratory patterns (e.g., Cheyne-Stokes)
      c. Sleep apnea (neonates)
   6. Comments
      a. Administered orally, IM, IV, or by suppository.
      b. Causes gastrointestinal discomfort.

XI. Parasympathomimetics
   A. Action: Enhance effects of parasympathetic nervous system.
   B. Classification of effects
      1. *Muscarinic:* Effect on parasympathetic postganglionic fibers, thus stimulating only the parasympathetic nervous system.
      2. *Nicotinic:* Effect on other sites where acetylcholine is the transmitter substance, thus stimulating sites outside the parasympathetic nervous system.

      a. Voluntary muscle

      b. Sympathetic nervous system

      c. CNS

      d. Adrenal medulla

C. Classification of drug groups

   1. Choline esters (drugs with structure similar to acetylcholine):

      a. Primary effects: Muscarinic with limited nicotinic effects

      b. Primary indications

         (1) Paroxysmal supraventricular tachycardia

         (2) Gastrointestinal disorders

         (3) Urinary bladder disorders

         (4) Bronchial provocation testing

      c. Representative drugs

         (1) Methacholine (generic), Mecholyl (trade)

         (2) Bethanechol (generic), Urecholine (trade)

   2. Naturally occurring alkaloids

      a. Primary effect: Almost exclusively at muscarinic sites

      b. Primary indication: Glaucoma

      c. Representative drug: Pilocarpine (generic and trade)

   3. Cholinesterase inhibitors

      a. Mechanism of action: Competitive inhibition of cholinesterase.

      b. Primary Effect: Strong stimulation at both nicotinic and muscarinic sites.

      c. Therapeutic uses

         (1) Paralytic ileus

         (2) Atony of urinary bladder

         (3) Glaucoma

         (4) Myasthenia gravis (symptomatic)

         (5) Atropine intoxication

         (6) Reversal of nondepolarizing neuromuscular blocking agents

   4. Representative drugs

      a. Neostigmine (generic), Prostigmine (trade)

      b. Pyridostigmine (generic), Mestinon (trade)

      c. Ambenonium (generic), Mytelase (trade)

      d. Edrophonium (generic), Tensilon (trade)

D. Side effects associated with excessive stimulation of parasympathetic nervous system

   1. Gastrointestinal disorders

       2. Cardiovascular problems

       3. Excessive secretion by exocrine glands, (e.g., mucous, salivary)

XII. Parasympatholytics

   A. Action: Inhibition of parasympathetic nervous system.

   B. Mechanism of action: Competitive inhibition of acetylcholine at muscarinic sites only.

   C. Therapeutic uses

       1. CNS disorders

       2. Preanesthesia medication

       3. Ophthalmologic (pupil dilation)

       4. Upper airway allergies

       5. Gastrointestinal disorders

       6. Genitourinary tract disorders

       7. Common cold

       8. Over-the-counter sleeping pills

       9. Motion sickness, nausea and vomiting

     10. Cardiovascular problems

     11. Used with parasympathomimetics for reversal of neuromuscular blocking agents

     12. Bronchodilation

   D. Side effects

       1. Dry mouth

       2. Blurred vision

       3. Urinary retention

       4. Lightheadedness

       5. Fatigue

   E. Representative drugs

       1. Atropa belladonna, atropine (generic)

       2. Hyoscine (generic), Scopolamine (trade)

XIII. Sympatholytics

   A. Action: Inhibition of the sympathetic nervous system.

   B. Alpha-adrenergic blocking agents

       1. Mechanism of action: Direct inhibitory affect at alpha-adrenergic receptor site.

       2. Effects

          a. Prevent excitatory responses of smooth muscle and exocrine glands.

          b. Can cause postural hypotension.

          c. Cause an increase in cardiac output and decrease in total peripheral resistance in normal recumbent subjects.

       3. Therapeutic uses

      a. Hypertension
      b. Peripheral vascular disease
    4. Representative drugs
      a. Phentolamine (generic), Regitine (trade)
      b. Azapetine (generic), Ilidar (trade)
      c. Phenoxybenzamine (generic), Dibenzyline (trade)
  C. Beta-adrenergic blocking agents
    1. Action: Decrease beta one and beta two effects.
    2. Mechanism of action: Competitive inhibition at receptor site.
    3. Effects
      a. Negative inotropic and chronotropic effect on heart.
      b. Slight bronchoconstriction (contraindicated in asthmatics).
      c. May have partial agonist effect.
    4. Therapeutic uses
      a. Cardiac arrhythmias
      b. Angina pectoris
      c. Hypertension
      d. Migraine prophylaxis
      e. Glaucoma
    5. Side effects/hazards
      a. Pulmonary edema
      b. Hypotension
      c. Heart block
    6. Representative drugs
      a. Propranolol (generic), Inderal (trade)
      b. Metaprolol (generic), Lopressor (trade)
      c. Timolol (generic), Bleocardin, Timolide (trade)
      d. Nadolol (generic), Corgard (trade)
      e. Atenolol (generic), Tenormin (trade)
      f. Pindolol (generic), Visken (trade)
XIV. Neuromuscular Blocking Agents
  A. Major action: Interruption of transmission of nerve impulse at skeletal neuromuscular junction, resulting in paralysis.
  B. Categories
    1. *Nondepolarizing* agents
      a. Mechanism of action: Competitive inhibition of acetylcholine at muscle postsynaptic receptor sites. The muscle tissue itself remains sensitive to external stimulation.
      b. Effects

(1) Maximal effects are seen in about 3–4 minutes and persist 20–40 minutes.

(2) Hypotension as a result of histamine release seen occasionally with d-Tubocurarine.

(3) Bradycardia occasionally is seen with pancuronium.

(4) Effects of this group of drugs may be reversed by cholinesterase-inhibiting agents (e.g., neostigmine).

  c. Representative drugs

(1) Tubocurarine (generic), d-Tubocurarine (trade)

(2) Pancuronium (generic), Pavulon (trade)

2. *Depolarizing* agents

  a. Mechanism of action

(1) Causes persistent depolarization of muscle motor end-plates.

(2) As this wave of depolarization proceeds, a rippling of voluntary muscles occurs (muscle fasciculation), usually from the head downward. Since these agents are chemically similar to acetylcholine, they cause continual stimulation of the motor end-plate.

(3) This continual stimulation does not allow time for repolarization; therefore the muscle develops a flaccid paralysis.

(4) With time, the depolarizing agent is metabolized by pseudocholinesterase.

  b. The muscle fiber itself is still sensitive to external stimulation.

(1) Effects seen in about 30–40 seconds and persist 3–5 minutes.

(2) Irreversible.

  c. Representative drugs

(1) Succinylcholine (generic), Anectine (trade)

(2) Decamethonium (generic), Syncurine (trade)

XV. Steroids

  A. Adrenocorticotropic hormone (ACTH) and adrenocorticosteroids

1. Adrenocorticotropic hormone (corticotropin) is produced and released from the adrenohypophysis (anterior pituitary).

2. Physiology of steroid regulation

  a. Release of ACTH into the blood causes the adrenal cortex to release its steroids into the bloodstream.

b. Release of ACTH is affected directly by corticotropin-releasing factor (CRF), which is secreted by the hypothalamus.

c. Blood level of CRF is indirectly affected by blood steroid levels.

d. Thus, there is a cyclic relation between ACTH, CRF and steroid levels (Fig 34–5).

e. An increase in steroid levels causes a decrease in CRF levels, which causes a decrease in ACTH levels. This results in a decrease in steroid levels, which causes an increase in CRF levels, etc., thus maintaining a normal equilibrium.

3. Actions

a. Stimulate glucose formation (i.e., increase blood sugar levels).

b. Diminish glucose utilization.

c. Promote storage of glucose in liver.

d. Regulate rate of synthesis of proteins.

e. Control distribution of body fat.

f. Regulate lipid metabolism.

g. Regulate reabsorption of sodium ions from kidney tubules.

h. Increase urinary excretion of both K^+ and H^+.

i. Maintain normal function of skeletal muscles.

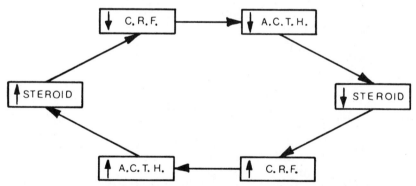

Fig 34–5.—There is a cyclic relationship of corticotropin-releasing factor (CRF), adrenocorticotropic hormone (ACTH), and steroid levels. Normal steroid levels are maintained by this interrelationship. CRF and ACTH levels are directly related; ACTH and steroid levels are also directly related; steroid and CRF levels are indirectly related.

      j. Increase hemoglobin and red cell content of blood.

      k. Maintain normal lymphoid tissue.

      l. Prevent or suppress inflammatory responses caused by hypersensitivity.

   4. Mechanisms of action

      a. Anti-inflammatory: Presumably causes the stabilization of the cellular lysosomal membranes.

      b. Allergic disorders: Has a catabolic effect on lymphoid tissue.

      c. Edema: Decreases capillary permeability by an unknown mechanism.

   5. Therapeutic uses

      a. Allergic asthma

      b. Acute and chronic adrenal insufficiency

      c. Suppression of immune response in organ transplant patients

      d. Congenital adrenal hyperplasia

      e. Adrenal insufficiency secondary to anterior pituitary insufficiency

      f. Arthritis

      g. Rheumatic carditis

      h. Osteoarthritis

      i. Acute inflammatory diseases

   6. Side effects

      a. Cushing's disease

        (1) Moon face

        (2) Hirsutism

        (3) Muscle wasting

        (4) Variable hypernatremia

        (5) Hypokalemia

      b. Hypertension

      c. Aggravation of diabetes mellitus

      d. Necrotizing arteritis in rheumatoid patients

      e. Aggravation of peptic ulcer

      f. Psychotic manifestations

      g. Adrenal atrophy

   7. Representative drugs

      a. Dexamethasone (Decadron)

        (1) Packaged in 10-ml vial with 4 mg per ml (0.4% W/V).

        (2) Administered by aerosol following extubation to diminish inflammation of larynx and trachea.

(3) Dosage: 1 ml of dexamethasone, 0.5 mg of 2.25% racemic epinephrine, and 3 ml normal saline.

  b. Beclomethasone dipropionate (Vanceril)

    (1) Supplied as metered mist of 50 μg per inhalation.

    (2) Used for chronic treatment of bronchial asthma in patients in whom a corticosteroid is indicated.

    (3) Side effects

      (a) Localized (mouth, pharynx, larynx) infection with *Candida albicans* and *Aspergillus niger*.

      (b) Occasional deaths have resulted from ACTH suppression when beclomethasone has been used to replace previous therapies involving corticosteroids with strong systemic activity.

    (4) Dosage:

      (a) Standard: 2 inhalations 3 or 4 times daily.

      (b) Maximum: 22 inhalations per day.

XVI. Diuretics

  A. Action: Increase rate of urine formation.

  B. Effects

    1. Most increase Na^+ excretion.

    2. Most cause an increased loss of K^+.

    3. Most are not affected by acid-base imbalances.

    4. Most can be administered in tablet form.

  C. Therapeutic uses

    1. Pulmonary edema

    2. Congestive heart failure

    3. Chronic or acute renal failure

    4. Systemic fluid overload

  D. Types

    1. Osmotic diuretics

      a. Mechanism of action

        (1) Cause osmotic gradient in urine tubular system, preventing reabsorption of fluid into bloodstream.

        (2) Cause osmotic movement of fluid from tissues into plasma.

      b. Characteristics

        (1) Filterable at the glomerulus.

        (2) Poorly reabsorbed by the renal tubule.

        (3) Pharmacologically inert.

      c. Representative drugs

        (1) Mannitol

(2) Urea

2. Mercurial diuretics
   a. Mechanism of action:
      (1) Prevent reabsorption of Na^+ and Cl^- in proximal convoluted tubule, thereby decreasing the volume of water reabsorbed.
      (2) Promote loss of K^+ and H^+ in distal convoluted tubules.
   b. Characteristics
      (1) May cause metabolic alkalosis with extended use.
      (2) Are ineffective in the presence of systemic metabolic alkalosis.
      (3) Are potentiated in the presence of metabolic acidosis.
   c. Contraindications
      (1) Renal insufficiency
      (2) Acute nephritis
   d. Characteristic drugs
      (1) Mercaptomerin sodium (generic), Thiomerin (trade)
      (2) Meralluride (generic), Mercuhydrin (trade)
      (3) Mersalyl (generic), Salygran (trade)

3. Carbonic anhydrase inhibitors
   a. Mechanism of action: Inhibit effects of carbonic anhydrase in proximal convoluted tubule, thereby increasing the amount of HCO_3^- and the volume of urine excreted.
   b. Representative drugs
      (1) Acetazolamide (generic), Diamox (trade)
      (2) Dichlorphenamide (generic), Daranide (trade)

4. Thiazides
   a. Mechanism of action: Inhibits reabsorption of 5%–10% of Na^+ and Cl^- at distal convoluted tubules.
   b. Characteristics
      (1) Cause an excessive loss of K^+.
      (2) Not affected by acid-base imbalances.
      (3) Can be administered in tablet form.
   c. Representative drugs
      (1) Chlorothiazide (generic), Diuril (trade)
      (2) Hydrochlorothiazide (generic), Hydro-Diuril (trade)
      (3) Hydroflumethiazide (generic), Saluron (trade)
      (4) Methyclorothiazide (generic), Enduron (trade)

5. Loop of Henle diuretics

    a. Mechanism of action: Inhibit reabsorption of Na^+ and Cl^-, primarily at distal and proximal convoluted tubules, thereby increasing the volume of fluid passed as urine.

    b. Characteristics

       (1) Function independently of acid-base status.

       (2) Considered the most potent of all diuretics.

    c. Side effects/hazards

       (1) Loss of K^+ due to increased excretion.

       (2) Development of metabolic alkalosis.

       (3) Aggravation of diabetes mellitus due to impaired glucose tolerance.

    d. Representative drugs

       (1) Ethacrynic acid (generic), Edecrin (trade)

       (2) Furosemide (generic), Lasix (trade)

XVII. Narcotics

  A. Primary use: Analgesia

  B. Mechanism of action: Unclear, but these drugs affect neurotransmission at specific CNS sites, affect autonomic nervous system transmission, and cause some histamine release.

  C. General pharmacologic effects

    1. Analgesic

      a. Alters the perception of pain.

      b. Interferes with the continuance of pain impulses in the spinal cord.

      c. Alters the body's response to the pain stimulus.

      d. May elevate the pain threshold.

    2. Euphoric: Seen at therapeutic dosages.

    3. Hypnotic: With increasing dosages, more subjective CNS depression.

    4. Metabolic: Transient hyperglycemia.

    5. Endocrine: Stimulates the release of antidiuretic hormone.

    6. Pupil size: Miosis.

    7. Gastrointestinal tract: Constipation because of decreased overall activity.

    8. Nausea and vomiting: Direct stimulation of medullary control center.

    9. Cardiovascular system

      a. If patient is well oxygenated and in normal acid-base balance, there are no significant effects.

      b. Cardiac arrhythmias may be seen with acid-base abnormalities.

           c. Hypotension may result due to direct effect on venous smooth muscle and release of histamine.

      10. Respiratory system

           a. Direct depression of medullary respiratory center response to carbon dioxide changes.

           b. Significant decrease in respiratory rate, tidal volume, and minute volume is seen with large dosages.

      11. Cough reflex: Decreased as a result of direct depression of medullary cough center.

  D. Therapeutic uses

    1. Analgesia

    2. Cough control

    3. Emetic

    4. Antidiarrhetic

    5. Pulmonary edema

    6. Control of patients on ventilators

  E. Representative drugs

    1. High potency

      a. Morphine (generic and trade)

      b. Oxymorphone (generic), Numorphan (trade)

      c. Heroin

      d. Levorphanol (generic), Levo-Dromoran (trade)

      e. Methadone (generic), Dolophine (trade)

      f. Phenazocine (generic), Prinadol (trade)

    2. Intermediate potency

      a. Meperidine (generic), Demerol (trade)

      b. Alphaprodine (generic), Nisentil (trade)

      c. Pentazocine (generic), Talwin (trade)

      d. Anileridine (generic), Leritine (trade)

      e. Oxycodone (generic), Percodan (trade)

    3. Low potency

      a. Codeine (generic and trade)

      b. Diphenoxylate (generic), Lomotil (trade)

XVIII. Narcotic Antagonists

  A. Sole use: To reverse effects of narcotics.

  B. Mechanism of action: Competitive displacement of agonist from receptor site.

  C. Partial antagonists

    1. Cause narcotic-like effects in absence of a narcotic.

    2. Cause increased respiratory depression if administered in a nonnarcotic overdose (e.g., barbiturates).

    3. Representative drugs

       a. Nalorphine (generic), Nalline (trade)

       b. Levallorphan (generic), Lorfan (trade)

  D. Pure antagonists: Have only narcotic antagonist properties.

     1. Will not increase respiratory depression in a nonnarcotic overdose.

     2. Representative drug: Naloxone (generic), Narcan (trade)

  E. Duration of effect

     1. 45–60 minutes (*careful monitoring of overdosed patient must be maintained*).

     2. Narcotic's effect may significantly outlast that of the narcotic antagonist.

XIX. Sedative/Hypnotics

  A. Solid or liquid substances that cause a longer generalized depression of the CNS than do anesthetic gases.

  B. Mechanism of action: Selective depression of ascending reticular activating system at either the cellular or synaptic level, resulting in loss of consciousness.

  C. Physiologic effects

     1. Increased dosages cause behavioral changes.

       a. Sedation: Generalized decreased responsiveness.

       b. Disinhibition: Impaired judgment and loss of self-control.

       c. Relief of anxiety.

       d. Ataxia and nystagmus.

       e. Sleep (hypnosis).

       f. Anesthesia.

     2. EEG pattern changes consistent with generalized CNS depression.

     3. Poor analgesia.

     4. Anticonvulsant: (phenobarbital the most effective).

     5. Withdrawal state with repeated long-term use and abrupt discontinuance.

     6. Habit forming.

     7. Voluntary muscle relaxation from spinal cord depression.

     8. Depression of respiratory medullary center with larger doses.

     9. Profound vasomotor depression and shock with larger doses.

    10. No direct effect on myocardium.

  D. Therapeutic uses

     1. Sleep induction

     2. Relief of anxiety (sedation)

       3. Treatment of neurotic anxiety
       4. Relief of depression
       5. Voluntary muscle relaxation
       6. Anticonvulsant
   E. Side effects
       1. Drowsiness
       2. Impaired performance and judgment
       3. Hangover
       4. Drug abuse
       5. Withdrawal state
       6. Overdose
   F. Contraindications
       1. Hypothyroidism
       2. Hypoadrenalism
   G. Types
       1. Barbiturates
          a. Ultra-short acting: Anesthetic agents
             (1) Hexobarbital (generic), Sombucaps (trade)
             (2) Thiopental (generic), Pentothal (trade)
          b. Short acting: Primarily for sleep induction
             (1) Pentobarbital (generic), Nembutal (trade)
             (2) Secobarbital (generic), Seconal (trade)
          c. Intermediate acting: Relief of anxiety
             (1) Amobarbital (generic), Amytal (trade)
          d. Long acting: Anticonvulsant
             (1) Phenobarbital (generic and trade)
       2. Nonbarbiturate sedatives: Hypnotics
          a. Short acting
             (1) Methaqualone (generic), Quaalude (trade)
             (2) Paraldehyde (generic and trade)
             (3) Chloral hydrate (generic)
             (4) Flurazepam (generic), Dalmane (trade)
          b. Intermediate acting
             (1) Meprobamate (generic), Miltown, Equanil (trade)
             (2) Glutethimide (generic), Doriden (trade)
             (3) Diazepam (generic), Valium (trade)
          c. Long acting: Chlordiazepoxide (generic), Librium (trade)
 XX. Antipsychotic Tranquilizers
   A. Action: Alter psychotic state without inducing sedation or hypnosis.
   B. Mechanism of action

      1. Decrease nervous input into the reticular activating system, thereby decreasing reticular activity.

      2. Enhance the breakdown of catecholamines.

      3. Indirectly decrease the formation of norepinephrine.

  C. Characteristics

      1. General effects are subjectively unpleasant.

      2. Non-habit forming.

      3. Causes generalized increased electric activity (evidenced on EEG).

      4. Increasing dosages cause indifference, apathy, motor retardation, and convulsions.

      5. Patient remains arousable.

  D. Therapeutic uses

      1. Schizophrenia

      2. Mania

      3. Anxiety

      4. Anorexia

      5. Amphetamine intoxication

      6. Control of vomiting

  E. Representative drugs

      1. Chlorpromazine (generic), Thorazine (trade)

      2. Promazine (generic), Sparine (trade)

      3. Triflupromazine (generic), Vesprin (trade)

      4. Prochlorperazine (generic), Compazine (trade)

      5. Haloperidol (generic), Haldol (trade)

XXI. Antimicrobial Drugs

  A. These drugs possess *selective toxicity*—the property of being far more toxic for the parasite than for the host cell.

  B. Mechanism of action and representative drug groups

      1. Inhibition of growth by competitive inhibition of metabolism of microbe's proteins

        a. Sulfonamides (Gantrisin)

        b. *P*-aminosalicylic acid (PAS)

      2. Inhibition of cell wall synthesis

        a. Penicillin, ampicillin

        b. Cephalosporins (Keflin, Loridine, Keflex)

        c. Polymyxins

      3. Inhibition of protein synthesis

        a. Chloramphenicol

        b. Tetracycline

        c. Erythromycin

        d. Streptomycin

      e. Kanamycin

      f. Neomycin

      g. Gentamicin

    4. Inhibition of nucleic acid synthesis

      a. Actinomycin

      b. Mitomycin

  C. General principles of antibiotic therapy

    1. Clinical indications of infection should be present.

    2. The specific etiologic diagnosis must be formulated before antibiotic therapy is ordered.

    3. A specimen must be obtained for laboratory culture and sensitivity before therapy is begun.

    4. The most indicated antibiotic should be administered.

    5. The antibiotic should be correlated with the results of culture and sensitivity study.

    6. Patient must take full course of antibiotic therapy.

    7. Antibiotics in general, are not effective against viruses.

XXII. Miscellaneous Drugs Affecting the Cardiovascular System

  A. Cardiac glycosides (digitalis)

    1. Action

      a. Exhibit a positive inotropic effect on the myocardium.

      b. Normally cause increased cardiac output.

      c. Indirectly cause increased renal blood flow and have a diuretic effect.

      d. Slow impulse conduction through the atrioventricular (AV) node and bundle of His.

      e. Exert a direct depressant effect on the sinoatrial (SA) node, causing decreased heart rate.

      f. Increase the refractory period of the AV node.

    2. Mechanism of action: Actions are mediated by vagal and extravagal means. One theory postulates that the drug may cause an increase in intracellular sodium that precipitates increased calcium mobilization. This leads to stronger myocardial contractions.

    3. Therapeutic use

      a. Primarily used in the treatment of congestive heart failure

      b. Atrial fibrillation

      c. Atrial flutter

      d. Paroxysmal atrial tachycardia

      e. Ventricular tachycardia

    4. Side effects/hazards

a. Toxicity (therapeutic dose is one third of the lethal dose)
b. AV block
c. Premature ventricular contractions
5. Representative drugs
    a. Digitoxin (generic), Crystodigin, Purodigin (trade)
    b. Digoxin (generic), Lanoxin (trade)
    c. Lanatoside C (generic), Cedilanid (trade)
    d. Ouabain (generic)
B. Quinidine
  1. Action
    a. Acts as a depressant to myocardium.
    b. Slows depolarization by increasing time necessary to reach action potential.
    c. Alters cardiac muscle permeability to sodium.
    d. Decreases velocity of electric impulse conduction throughout myocardium.
    e. Has curare-like side effect on skeletal muscle.
  2. Mechanism of action: Attaches to lipoproteins present in the myocardial cell membrane, altering cell membrane permeability to positive ions such as sodium, potassium, and calcium. Causes depression of conduction velocity and contractility.
  3. Therapeutic uses
    a. Primary use is treatment of atrial arrhythmias
    b. Premature ventricular contractions
  4. Side effects/hazards
    a. Ventricular tachycardia
    b. Premature ventricular contractions
    c. Ventricular fibrillation
    d. Hypotension
    e. Asystole
    f. Atrial embolism
    g. Respiratory arrest in hypersensitive patients
  5. Representative drugs
    a. Quinidine gluconate
    b. Quinidene sulfate
C. Procainamide (generic), Pronestyl (trade)
  1. Action
    a. Depresses myocardial excitability.
    b. Slows conduction in the atria, bundle of His, and ventricles.

2. Mechanism of action: Attaches to lipoproteins present in the myocardial cell membrane, altering the cell membrane's permeability to positive ions such as sodium, potassium, and calcium.
3. Effects: Causes depression of conduction velocity and contractility.
4. Therapeutic uses
   a. Premature ventricular contractions
   b. Ventricular tachycardia
   c. Atrial fibrillation
   d. Paroxysmal atrial tachycardia
5. Side effects/hazards
   a. AV block
   b. Ventricular extrasystoles (possibly progressing to ventricular fibrillation)

D. Lidocaine (generic), Xylocaine (trade)
   1. Action: Increases the threshold for electrical stimulation of the ventricle.
   2. Mechanism: Appears to act on myocardial tissue in the same manner as quinidine or procainamide.
   3. Therapeutic uses
      a. Cardiac arrhythmias, especially ventricular arrhythmias or those that appear after myocardial infarction
      b. Arrhythmias that may occur during cardiac surgery
   4. Side effects/hazards
      a. Hypotension
      b. Bradycardia
      c. Cardiovascular collapse and cardiac arrest
      d. Seizures

E. Calcium-channel blocking agents
   1. Action: Decreases the inward current of the cardiac action potential.
   2. Mechanism of action: Prevents the influx of calcium ions into cells (primarily myocardial and vascular smooth muscle) at specific membrane sites, thus inhibiting muscle contraction by decreasing the availability of calcium for actin-myosin interaction.
   3. Effects
      a. Decrease myocardial contractility and metabolism.
      b. Decrease blood pressure.
      c. Decrease smooth muscle activity.
      d. General negative inotropic effect.

4. Therapeutic uses
   a. Antiarrhythmic (paroxysmal supraventricular tachycardia, atrial flutter, atrial fibrillation)
   b. Anti-anginal
   c. Improve hemodynamics in cardiomyopathy
   d. Antihypertensive
5. Side effects/hazards
   a. Headache
   b. Nausea
   c. Transient hypotension
   d. Bradycardia   } when used with Beta blocker
   e. Ventricular asystole
6. Representative drug: Verapamil (generic), Calan, Isoptin (trade)

BIBLIOGRAPHY

DeKornfeld T.J.: *Pharmacology for Respiratory Therapy.* Sarasota, Glenn Educational Medical Services, Inc., 1976.

DiPalma J.R.: *Basic Pharmacology in Medicine.* New York, McGraw-Hill Book Co., Inc., 1976.

Egan D.F.: *Fundamentals of Respiratory Therapy,* ed. 3. St. Louis, C.V. Mosby Co., 1977.

Evaluations of Drug Interactions, ed. 2. Washington, D.C., American Pharmaceutical Association, 1976.

Flaum S.F., Zelis R.: *Calcium Blockers.* Baltimore, Urban & Schwarzenberg, Inc., 1982.

Goodman L.S., Gilman A. (eds.): *The Pharmacological Basis of Therapeutics,* ed. 6. Macmillan Publishing Co., Inc., 1980.

Goth A.: *Medical Pharmacology,* ed. 9. St. Louis, C.V. Mosby Co., 1978.

Leonard R.G., Talbot R.L.: Calcium channel blocking agents. *Clin. Pharmacol.* Jan.–Feb., 34:189, 1982.

Mathewson H.S.: *Pharmacology for Respiratory Therapists,* ed. 2. St. Louis, C.V. Mosby Co., 1981.

Meyers F.H., Jawetz E., Goldfine A.: *Review of Medical Pharmacology,* ed. 4. Los Altos, Calif., Lange Medical Publications, 1974.

Product Information. New York, Breon Laboratories, Inc.

Rau J.L.: Autonomic airway pharmacology. *Respir. Care* 22:263, 1977.

Rau J.L.: *Respiratory Therapy Pharmacology.* Chicago, Year Book Medical Publishers, Inc., 1978.

Year Book of Critical Care Medicine 1983. Chicago, Year Book Medical Publishers, Inc., 1983.

Young J.A., Crocker D.: *Principles and Practice of Respiratory Therapy,* ed. 2. Chicago, Year Book Medical Publishers, Inc., 1976.

35 / Microbiology

I. Classification of Microorganisms by Cell Type
  A. Eukaryotic (Protista)
    1. Algae (except blue-green)
    2. Protozoa
    3. Fungi
    4. Slime molds
  B. Prokaryotic (lower Protista)
    1. Blue-green algae
    2. Bacteria
    3. Rickettsiae
    4. Mycoplasmas
II. Eukaryotic Cell Structure (Fig 35–1)
  A. Surface layers
    1. Cell membrane: complex lipoprotein structure.
    2. Cell wall: rigid to moderately rigid polysaccharide structure.
  B. Nucleus
    1. Well-defined nucleus surrounded by nuclear membrane.
    2. Control center for cell growth and development.
      a. Contains chromosomes
      b. Contains RNA
      c. Nuclear membrane continuous with endoplasmic reticulum
  C. Cytoplasmic structures.
    1. Endoplasmic reticulum (ER): system of large sacs and smaller tubules responsible for macromolecular transport.
      a. Smooth ER (without attached ribosomes): involved in lipid and steroid synthesis.
      b. Rough ER (with attached ribosomes): involved in protein synthesis.
    2. Mitochondria: responsible for production of ATP and aerobic metabolism (Kreb's cycle and electron transport chain). Seen in animal cells.
    3. Chloroplasts: contain pigments, starches, and enzymes used in photosynthesis.

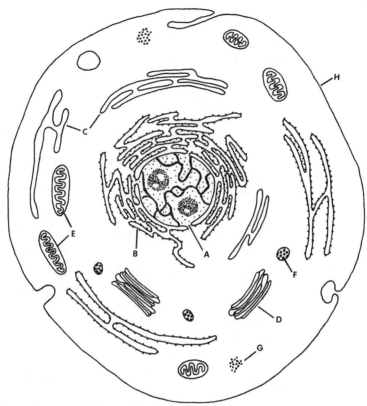

Fig 35–1.—Eukaryotic cell: *A,* nucleus; *B,* rough endoplasmic reticulum; *C,* smooth endoplasmic reticulum; *D,* Golgi body; *E,* mitochondria; *F,* lysosome; *G,* free ribosomes; *H,* cell membrane.

      4. Ribosomes: free or attached to endoplasmic reticulum; responsible for protein synthesis.

      5. Lysosomes: contain proteolytic enzymes for metabolism of ingested organic material.

  D. Motility organelles

      1. Cilia

         a. Numerous on cell exterior.

         b. Move in coordinated waves.

      2. Flagella

         a. Singular or present in small numbers.

         b. Move in undulating motion.

         c. Longer than cilia.

III. Prokaryotic Cell Structure (Fig 35–2)
    A. Surface layers
        1. Cell membrane: lipoprotein structure.
        2. Cell wall: moderately rigid to very rigid structure.
            a. Gram-positive bacteria
                (1) High lipid content
                (2) Murein network: peptide chains attached to larger polysaccharide chains
            b. Gram-negative bacteria: three-layer membrane
                (1) Inner: mucopeptide
                (2) Middle: lipopolysaccharide
                (3) Outer: lipoprotein
    B. Nucleus
        1. No distinct nucleus: no separation from cytoplasm.
        2. Cell may contain one or more regions of nuclear material called nucleoids.
        3. No mitotic apparatus.
        4. Free existence of chromosomes in cytoplasm; may be circular or attached to cell membrane.
    C. Cytoplasmic structures
        1. No ER present.
        2. No mitochondria present. Aerobic metabolic enzymes are present in the form of multienzyme complexes; they are attached to the cell membrane or other internal membranes.
        3. No chloroplasts present. Photosynthetic enzymes and pigments are present in special arrangements; these are not separated from the cytoplasm by a membrane.
        4. Ribosomes: slightly smaller than eukaryotic ribosomes; exist freely in cytoplasm.
        5. Mesosome: found in cell membrane; allow for attachment of DNA in cell division. Found chiefly in gram-positive forms.
        6. No lysosomes present.
        7. Cell nutrients stored by cytoplasmic granules.
    D. Motility organelles
        1. Flagella
            a. Different from eukaryotic flagella.
            b. One or many per cell.
            c. Move in rotary motion.
        2. Pili
            a. Short, fine filaments.

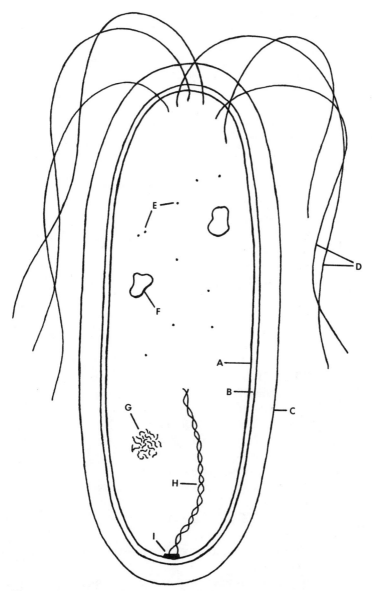

Fig 35–2.—Prokaryotic cell: *A,* cell membrane; *B,* cell wall; *C,* capsule; *D,* flagella; *E,* ribosomes; *F,* storage granule; *G,* nucleoid; *H,* DNA; *I,* mesosome.

        b. Function not known; may function in specialized bacterial sexual reproduction.

IV. Necessary Growth Conditions
    A. Growth medium: requirements vary with bacteria.
        1. Sugar concentration.
        2. Nutrients and minerals: water, carbon, hydrogen, nitrogen, sulfur, phosphorus, amino acids.
    B. Atmosphere
        1. Aerobic: require oxygen for survival.
        2. Anaerobic: cannot grow in presence of oxygen.
        3. Facultative anaerobes: can survive with or without oxygen.
    C. Temperature
        1. Optimal temperature for most bacteria is 30°–40° C.
    D. Osmotic pressure and pH
        1. Osmotic requirement (salt concentration of environment) varies with each bacteria species; most require 0.9% saline.
        2. Optimal pH between 6.0 and 8.0.
    E. Moisture
    Water is essential for all bacterial growth.
    F. Light
        1. Most bacteria prefer darkness.
        2. Ultraviolet and blue light are destructive to bacteria.

V. Microbial Reproduction
    A. Asexual (binary fission)
        1. Most common form of reproduction.
        2. Two identical daughter cells result from single parent cell.
        3. Normal chromosome replication.
    B. Sexual (conjugation)
        1. Present in a few bacterial species.
        2. DNA is transferred from one bacterium to another.

VI. Growth Pattern
    (A new culture of bacteria will develop similar to growth curve seen in Figure 35–3.)
    A. Lag phase: Adaptation to new environment; little reproduction.
    B. Exponential phase: Stage of rapid cell growth.
    C. Stationary phase: Equal death and growth rates.
    D. Death phase: Depletion of culture nutrients and buildup of toxic waste. Death rate exceeds growth rate.

VII. Measurement of Growth
    A. Cell concentration: Expressed as number of viable cells.
    B. Cell density: Expressed as dry weights.

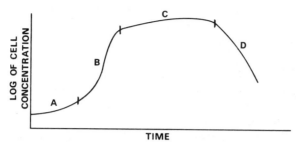

Fig 35–3.—Growth pattern of a new closed culture: *A,* lag phase; *B,* exponential phase; *C,* stationary phase; *D,* death phase.

VIII. Microbial Relationships
    A. Autotroph: Organism capable of using simple inorganic matter as nutrients (nonpathogenic).
    B. Heterotroph: Organism capable of using organic matter to survive (pathogenic).
        1. Saprophyte: Organism that lives on dead organic matter.
        2. Parasite: Organism that lives on or in another organism and that benefits from but does not benefit the host organism.
        3. Symbiosis: Two dissimilar organisms existing together.
            a. Commensalism: Two species existing together: one benefiting, the other not affected.
            b. Antibiosis: Association between two dissimilar organisms that is harmful to one or both.
            c. Ammensalism: Two dissimilar organisms existing together with no effect on each other.
            d. Synnecrosis: Two dissimilar organisms existing together to the detriment of both.
            e. Mutualism: Two dissimilar organisms existing together, each benefiting from the association and unable to survive without it.
IX. Capsule
    A. Layer surrounding outside of cell produced by the cell itself. Common in pathogenic organisms.
    B. Functions
        1. Prevents phagocytosis
        2. Prevents virus attachment
        3. External nutrient storage
    C. Causative factors
        1. High sugar concentration
        2. Presence of blood serum in culture

3. Microorganism living in a host organism
D. Composition: mucilaginous
   1. Polypeptides
   2. Dextran
   3. Polysaccharides
   4. Cellulose
X. Spore
  A. Intermediate form of the organism that develops in response to adverse environmental conditions; will regenerate to vegetative cell when environmental conditions improve.
  B. Protective coat around nucleic material that may remain inside cell (endospore) or extend beyond the width of the cell (exospore).
  C. Metabolically active; contains necessary enzymes for Kreb's cycle.
  D. Resistant to:
   1. Heat
   2. Drying
   3. Lack of nutrients
   4. Toxic chemicals
  E. Spore-forming genera
   1. *Bacillus*
   2. *Clostridium*
   3. *Sporosarcina*
XI. Microbial Shapes (Fig 35–4)
  A. Spherical: coccus
  B. Rod: bacillus
  C. Spiral: spirillum, spirochete
  D. Comma-shaped: vibrios
  E. Spindle-shaped: fusiform
XII. Staining
  Used to identify and categorize bacteria on the basis of cell components.
  A. Gram staining
   1. All bacteria can be separated into two general categories (gram-positive or gram-negative) by virtue of their staining properties. Variation in staining is determined by cell wall construction.
   2. Staining sequence
    a. Basic dye: Crystal violet
    b. Gram's iodine
    c. Alcohol wash
    d. Counterstain: Red dye safranin

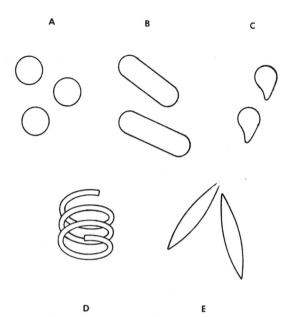

Fig 35–4.—Bacterial shapes: *A,* cocci; *B,* bacilli; *C,* vibrios; *D,* spirillum, spirochette; *E,* fusiform.

   3. Gram-positive bacteria: Stain blue or violet
   4. Gram-negative bacteria: Stain red or pink
  B. Acid-fast (Ziehl-Neelsen's) stain
   1. Identifies bacteria of genus *Mycobacterium*
   2. Acid-fast bacteria: stain red
   3. Staining sequence
    a. Carbol-fuchsin (red)
    b. Hydrochloric acid in alcohol wash
    c. Water wash
    d. Counterstain: Methyl blue
XIII. Definitions
  A. Inflammation: Specific tissue response to stress by living agents or to electric, chemical, or mechanical trauma, evidenced by vascular dilatation, fluid exudation, accumulation of leukocytes, or any combination of the three.
  B. Contamination: Presence of a microorganism in otherwise sterile environment.
  C. Infection: Inflammation caused by multiplication of pathogenic microorganisms.
  D. Pathogen: Any disease-producing microorganism.

E. Virulence: Heightened ability of an organism to produce infection in its host.

F. Immunity: Level of resistance of a body to effects of a deleterious agent (e.g., pathogenic microorganism).

G. Superinfection: Infection developed primarily in the debilitated or immunosuppressed patient previously treated with antibiotics.

H. Pyrogenic: Fever-inducing inflammatory process.

I. Nosocomial infection: Hospital-acquired infection.

J. Aerobic: Growing only in presence of oxygen.

K. Anaerobic: Growing only in absence of oxygen.

L. Toxins: Poisonous substances produced by bacteria
1. Exotoxin
   a. Primarily produced by gram-positive bacteria.
   b. Is protein and normally is diffused by bacteria into surrounding media.
   c. Some are extremely lethal.
2. Endotoxin
   a. Primarily produced by gram-negative bacteria.
   b. Is a lipopolysaccharide and normally is released when the bacterial cell is destroyed.

M. Vegetative cell: Metabolically active form of a bacterium in which reproduction can occur.

XIV. Frequently Encountered Pathogenic Genera (Table 35–1)
A. *Bacillus*
1. Genus characteristics
   a. Gram-positive.
   b. Large rod, aerobic.
   c. Arranged in chains.
   d. Spore forming.
   e. Secretes exotoxin.
2. Species
   Bacillus anthracis
   a. Diseases (primarily animal; less common in man):
      (1) Skin infections
      (2) Septicemia
      (3) Pneumonia (woolsorters' disease)
      (4) Enteritis
      (5) Meningitis
      (6) Anthrax
   b. Found in soil.
   c. Transmitted via injured skin or inhalation.

TABLE 35-1.—Commonly Encountered Bacterial Genera

GENERA	GRAM STAIN	SHAPE/CONFIGURATION	AEROBIC/ANAEROBIC	SPECIES	ANTIBIOTIC SUSCEPTIBILITY
Bacillus	Positive	Rod, chain	Aerobic	Anthracis	Penicillin
Clostridium	Positive	Rod, separate, chain, pairs, palisade	Anaerobic	Tetani, Botulinum perfringens	Penicillin
Corynebacterium	Positive	Rod, palisade	Aerobic	Diphtheriae	Penicillin Erythromycin
Diplococcus	Positive	Coccus, encapsulated pairs	Aerobic	Pneumoniae	Penicillin
Staphylococcus	Positive	Coccus, clusters	Aerobic	Aureus	Penicillin Tetracycline
Streptococcus	Positive	Coccus, chain	Aerobic	Groups A, B, C, & D	Penicillin
Mycobacterium	Positive	Rod, separate or "cords"	Aerobic	Tuberculosis, leprae	Isoniazid Rifampin Ethambutol Streptomycin
Neisseria	Positive	Coccus, pairs	Aerobic	Meningitidis	Penicillin
Proteus	Negative	Rod, separate	Aerobic	Mirabilis, Vulgaris	Penicillin Ampicillin Gentamicin
Pseudomonas	Negative	Rod, separate	Aerobic	Aeruginosa	Streptomycin Carbenicillin Gentamicin Polymixins Chloramphenicol
Serratia	Negative	Rod, separate	Aerobic	Marcescens	Gentamicin
Escherichia	Negative	Rod, separate	Aerobic, facultatively anaerobic	Coli	Gentamicin Sulfonamides Cephalosporin
Klebsiella	Negative	Rod, separate	Aerobic	Pneumoniae	Gentamicin
Haemophilus	Negative	Rod, separate	Aerobic	Influenzae, Haemolyticus, Parainfluenzae	Ampicillin Chloramphenicol
Salmonella	Negative	Rod, separate	Aerobic, facultatively anaerobic	Typhi, Enteritidis	Ampicillin Chloramphenicol

        d. Treatment: penicillin.

B. *Clostridium*

  1. Genus characteristics

    a. Gram-positive.

    b. Rod, aerobic.

    c. Found singly, in pairs, in parallel groups (palisade), or in short chains.

    d. Spore forming.

    e. Secretes exotoxins.

  2. Species

    Clostridium botulinum

    a. Causes botulism.

    b. Found in poorly canned or preserved foods.

    c. Transmitted via ingestion of infected foods.

    d. Treatment: antitoxins.

    Clostridium perfringens

    a. Causes gas gangrene.

    b. Found as normal intestinal flora; found in animal manure and soil.

    c. Transmitted via deep wounds.

    d. Treatment:

      (1) Surgical debridement

      (2) Hyperbaric oxygen

      (3) Penicillin

      (4) Antitoxins

    Clostridium tetani

    a. Produces tetanus.

    b. Found in soil.

    c. Transmitted via deep wounds.

    d. Treatment:

      (1) Surgical debridement

      (2) Antitoxins

      (3) Penicillin

C. *Corynebacterium*

  1. Genus characteristics

    a. Gram-positive.

    b. Rod (often club-shaped), aerobic.

    c. Often arranged in a palisade pattern.

    d. Secrete exotoxin.

  2. Species

    Corynebacterium diphtheriae

       a. Causes diphtheria.

       b. Transmitted through contact with contaminated individuals.

       c. Treatment:

         (1) Antitoxin (most effective)

         (2) Penicillin

         (3) Erythromycin

D. *Diplococcus* (also called *Pneumococcus*)

   1. Genus characteristics

     a. Gram-positive.

     b. Coccus, aerobic.

     c. Found in encapsulated pairs.

   2. Species

     Diplococcus pneumoniae

     a. Diseases:

       (1) Most common pathogen causing bacterial, lobar pneumonia; characteristic "rusty" sputum

       (2) Sinusitis

       (3) Meningitis

       (4) Endocarditis

       (5) Bacteremia

       (6) Septic arthritis

       (7) Osteomyelitis

     b. Found as normal flora of the upper respiratory tract in 30%–70% of the population (especially hospital personnel).

     c. Transmitted by inhalation, injured skin.

     d. Treatment: penicillin.

E. *Staphylococcus*

   1. Genus characteristics

     a. Gram-positive.

     b. Coccus, aerobic, and facultatively anaerobic.

     c. Arranged in irregular clusters.

     d. Produces an exotoxin and enterotoxin.

   2. Species

     Staphylococcus aureus

     a. Diseases:

       (1) Normally produces pimples, abscesses, or boils

       (2) Pneumonia

       (3) Empyema

       (4) Wound infection

(5) Septicemia

    b. Found as normal flora of skin and respiratory and gastrointestinal tracts (especially in hospital personnel).

    c. Transmitted by body contact, contact with contaminated articles, and blood and lymphatics from localized infections.

    d. Treatment:

       (1) Penicillin

       (2) Tetracycline

F. *Streptococcus*

  1. Genus characteristics

    a. Gram-positive.

    b. Coccus, aerobic.

    c. Arranged in chains.

    d. May produce capsules.

  2. Classifications

    a. Group A, beta-hemolytic streptococci: Septicemia, tonsillitis, scarlet fever, pneumonia, nasopharyngitis, middle ear infections, rheumatic fever, endocarditis, glomerulonephritis.

    b. Group B, beta-hemolytic streptococci: Female genital tract infections; may cause endocarditis, meningitis, neonatal sepsis.

    c. Group C, beta-hemolytic streptococci erysipelas: Throat infections and opportunistic infections.

    d. Group D, beta-hemolytic streptococci: Urinary tract infections and endocarditis.

    e. Found commonly in man, animals, and plants.

    f. Transmitted by contact with other individuals.

    g. Treatment: penicillin.

G. *Mycobacterium*

  1. Genus characteristics

    a. Gram-positive.

    b. Rod, aerobic.

    c. Inert forms found singly: Virulent strains are found in "cords"—two chains in a side-by-side, parallel arrangement.

  2. Species

  Mycobacterium tuberculosis

    a. Diseases:

       (1) Pulmonary tuberculosis

       (2) Spinal tuberculosis

(3) Urinary tract tuberculosis
b. Pulmonary tuberculosis transmitted via inhalation of droplet nuclei.
c. Treatment:
    (1) Isoniazid (INH)
    (2) Ethambutol
    (3) Rifampin
    (4) Streptomycin

Mycobacterium leprae (Hanson's bacillus)
a. Causes leprosy.
b. A true parasite—found only in host.
c. Transmitted via intimate contact.
d. Treatment:
    (1) Isoniazid (INH)
    (2) Ethambutol
    (3) Rifampin
    (4) Streptomycin

H. *Neisseria*
  1. Genus characteristics
    a. Gram-positive.
    b. Coccus, aerobic.
    c. Found as diplococci with their adjacent sides flattened.
  2. Species
    Neisseria meningitidis
    a. Diseases:
       (1) Meningococcal meningitis
       (2) Bacteremia
       (3) Pneumonia
    b. Nasopharyngeal normal flora.
    c. Transmitted via lymph canal in predisposed individuals; method of transmission of virulent strains is still unknown.
    d. Treatment: penicillin.

I. *Proteus*
  1. Genus characteristics
    a. Gram-negative.
    b. Rod, aerobic, and facultatively anaerobic.
    c. Found as a single organism.
  2. Species
    Proteus mirabilis, Proteus vulgaris
    a. Diseases (usually opportunistic):
       (1) Chronic urinary tract infections

        (2) Pneumonia

        (3) Gastroenteritis

        (4) Bacteremia

    b. Found as normal fecal flora.

    c. Transmitted by contact.

    d. Treatment:

        (1) Gentamicin

        (2) Penicillin

        (3) Ampicillin

        (4) Streptomycin

J. *Pseudomonas*

  1. Genus characteristics

    a. Gram-negative.

    b. Rod, aerobic, and facultatively anaerobic.

    c. Found as a single organism.

  2. Species

    Pseudomonas aeruginosa

    a. Diseases opportunistic; cause up to 10% of all hospital-acquired infections.

        (1) Pneumonia (characteristic green, odiforous sputum)

        (2) Wound infection

        (3) Urinary tract infection

        (4) Empyema

        (5) Meningitis

        (6) Septicemia

    b. Found in soil and water; frequently cultured from nebulizers.

    c. Transmitted via person-to-person contact.

    d. Treatment:

        (1) Carbenicillin

        (2) Gentamicin

        (3) Polymixins

        (4) Chloramphenicol

K. *Serratia*

  1. Genus characteristics

    a. Gram-negative.

    b. Rod, aerobic.

    c. Found as a single organism.

  2. Species

    Serratia marcescens

    a. Diseases:

        (1) Empyema

        (2) Septicemia

        (3) Wound infections

        (4) Hospital epidemics

     b. Widely distributed in nature.

     c. Treatment: gentamicin.

L. *Escherichia*

  1. Genus characteristics

     a. Gram-negative.

     b. Rod, aerobic, and facultatively anaerobic.

     c. Found as a single organism.

  2. Species

    Escherichia coli

     a. Disease (45% of all hospital-acquired infections):

        (1) Necrotizing pneumonia

        (2) Septicemia

        (3) Endocarditis

        (4) Meningitis

        (5) Wound infections

        (6) Urinary tract infections

     b. Found as normal flora of the gastrointestinal tract.

     c. Transmitted via person-to-person contact.

     d. Treatment:

        (1) Gentamicin

        (2) Sulfonamides

        (3) Cephalosporin

M. *Klebsiella*

  1. Genus characteristics

     a. Gram-negative.

     b. Short rod, aerobic, and facultatively anaerobic.

     c. Found as a single organism.

     d. Produce capsules.

  2. Species

    Klebsiella pneumoniae (Friedlander's bacillus)

     a. Diseases:

        (1) Necrotizing pneumonia (characteristic "red currant jelly" sputum)

        (2) Lung abscesses

        (3) Endocarditis

        (4) Septicemia

     b. Found as normal flora in the nose, mouth, and intestines.

     c. Treatment: gentamicin.

N. *Haemophilus*

  1. Genus characteristics

        a. Gram-negative.

        b. Minute rod, aerobic, and facultatively anaerobic.

        c. Found as a single organism.

    2. Species

     Haemophilus influenzae (Pfeiffer's bacillus)

        a. Diseases:

            (1) Most common cause of epiglottitis in children

            (2) Meningitis

            (3) Laryngitis

            (4) Croup

            (5) Subacute bacterial endocarditis

        b. Found as normal flora in the upper respiratory tract.

        c. Treatment:

            (1) Chloramphenicol

            (2) Ampicillin

     Haemophilus haemolyticus

        a. Causes pharyngitis.

        b. Found as normal flora in the upper respiratory tract.

        c. Treatment.

            (1) Chloramphenicol

            (2) Ampicillin

     Haemophilus parainfluenzae

        a. Causes bacterial endocarditis.

        b. Found as normal flora in the upper respiratory tract.

        c. Treatment:

            (1) Chloramphenicol

            (2) Ampicillin

  O. *Salmonella*

    1. Genus characteristics

        a. Gram-negative.

        b. Rod, aerobic, and facultatively anaerobic.

        c. Found as single organism.

        d. Forms exotoxin.

        e. Resistant to freezing.

    2. Species

     Salmonella typhi

        a. Causes typhus.

        b. Found in sewage.

        c. Transmitted through contaminated water, less frequently contaminated food.

        d. Treatment:

            (1) Chloramphenicol

            (2) Ampicillin

Salmonella enteritidis
 a. Diseases:
  (1) Enteritis
  (2) Enteric fever that may progress to meningitis, en-
      cephalitis, endocarditis, or nephritis
  (3) Gastroenteritis
 b. Found in animals, particularly shellfish, swine, and
    fowl.
 c. Transmitted orally via contaminated milk, turtles, and
    eggs; and undercooked chicken, fish, clams, and pork.
 d. Treatment:
  (1) Chloramphenicol, ampicillin
  (2) Strict liquid diet
XV. *Mycoplasma*
  A. Structure
   1. Surface layer
    a. Three-layer membrane.
    b. No cell wall.
   2. Nucleus
    a. No distinct nucleus.
    b. Circular DNA.
   3. Cytoplasmic structures
    a. Ribosomes—randomly distributed; occasionally seen in
       helical formation.
    b. Granules—contain various enzymes.
   4. Motility organelles: None present.
  B. Genus characteristics
   1. Gram-negative.
   2. Highly pleomorphic, aerobic.
   3. Present as singular organisms.
  C. Species
   Mycoplasma hominis
   1. Diseases:
    a. Pharyngitis
    b. Tonsillitis
    c. Pelvic inflammatory disease
   2. Found as normal flora in the upper respiratory and genito-
      urinary tracts.
   3. Transmitted via person-to-person contact.
   4. Treatment:
    a. Tetracycline
    b. Erythromycin
    c. Body may produce antibodies to the organisms

Mycoplasma pneumoniae (Eaton agent, primary atypical pneumonia, pleuropneumonia-like organism [PPLO])
  1. Causes a self-limiting respiratory syndrome that may have generalized symptoms or be asymptomatic.
  2. Found as normal flora of the upper respiratory tract.
  3. Transmitted via person-to-person contact
  4. Treatment:
     a. Tetracycline
     b. Erythromycin
XVI. *Rickettsiae*
   A. Considered a true bacterium
      1. Contains DNA and RNA.
      2. Multiplies by binary fission.
      3. Has metabolic enzymes.
      4. Can be killed or controlled by antibiotics.
   B. Characteristics
      1. Gram-positive, requires special staining techniques for identification.
      2. Pleomorphic rod or coccus.
      3. Occurs singly, paired, chained, or in filaments.
      4. Diseases have clinical findings of fever, headaches, malaise, and rash.
         a. Typhoid fever
         b. Rocky Mountain spotted fever
         c. Q fever
         d. Trench fever
      5. Normally inhabits arthropods as an obligate intracellular parasite.
      6. Transmitted via bite of infected organism.
      7. Treatment
         a. Para-amino benzoic acid
         b. Chloramphenicol
         c. Tetracycline
XVII. Viruses
   A. Structure
      1. Surface layers:
         a. Simple virus: protein coat
         b. Complex virus: protein coat with some polysaccharides and lipids present (lipoprotein membrane)
      2. Nucleus: No nucleus: single strand of DNA or RNA present.
      3. Cytoplasmic structure:

   a. No organelles present
   b. Contain no metabolic enzymes
   4. Motility organelles: None present.
 B. Characteristics
   1. Do not stain by conventional means.
   2. Come in a variety of shapes and forms, all of which are
      very small (maximum diameters 0.1–0.3 mµ).
   3. Obligate intracellular parasite.
   4. Replication by diverting host metabolism to produce new
      viruses.
   5. No antibiotic susceptibility.
 C. Species
   1. Respiratory syncytial virus (RSV)
      Single most important agent causing infantile bronchio-
      litis and pneumonia.
   2. Influenza virus
      Causes an acute respiratory tract infection characterized
      by chills, malaise, fever, muscular aches, prostration,
      cough, and sputum production.
   3. Parainfluenza virus
      *Primary cause of croup in children and also may cause
      other upper respiratory problems.*
   4. Adenovirus
      Commonly causes both upper and lower respiratory in-
      fections, pharyngitis, rhinitis, otitis, and laryngitis.
   5. Rhinovirus
      Primary agent causing the common cold.
XVIII. Fungi
 A. Structure
   1. Single cells: yeasts.
   2. Tubular strands of single cells: more complex forms. Hy-
      phae, or series of branching filaments, that form myce-
      lium.
      a. Vegetative mycelium: part of fungus feeding and grow-
         ing in medium.
      b. Aerial mycelium: part of fungus protruding from me-
         dium.
 B. Reproduction
   1. Sexual sporulation.
   2. Asexual sporulation.
 C. Types
   1. Saprophytic fungi: *Aspergillus fumigatus*

      a. Found in immunosuppressed patients, patients with leukemia, and patients receiving corticosteroid therapy.

      b. Enters respiratory system, causing a severe pneumonia that may lead to hemorrhagic pulmonary infarction or granulomas.

  2. Superficial and cutaneous fungi

      a. Tinea pedis (athlete's foot).

      b. Tinea corpens (ringworm).

      c. Tinea capitis (ringworm of scalp).

  3. Mucous membrane invader—*Candida albicans*

      a. Normal flora of respiratory, gastrointestinal, and female genital tracts.

      b. Found in immunosuppressed or debilitated patients and in individuals on excessive antibiotic therapy.

      c. May cause septicemia, thrombophlebitis, endocarditis.

  4. Subcutaneous fungi: cause sporotrichosis

  5. Systemic fungi

      a. Histoplasmosis

      b. Coccidiomycosis

XIX. Normal Flora

  A. Skin

    1. Staphylococci

    2. Streptococci

    3. Coliform bacteria

    4. Enterococci

    5. Diphtheroids (aerobic and anaerobic)

    6. *Proteus* species

    7. *Pseudomonas* species

    8. *Bacillus* species

    9. Fungi (lipophilic)

  B. Respiratory tract

    1. Staphylococci

    2. Streptococci

    3. *Klebsiella*

    4. *Neisseria* species

    5. *Haemophilus* species

    6. Diplococci (pneumococci)

    7. *Mycoplasma*

    8. *Candida albicans* and other fungi

  C. Gastrointestinal tract

    1. Coliform bacteria

2. Enterococci
3. *Clostridium* species
4. *Proteus* species
5. Yeasts
6. *Penicillium* species
7. Enteroviruses
8. *Pseudomonas aeruginosa*
9. Streptococci
10. Staphylococci
11. *Alcaligenes faecalis*
12. *Bacteroides* species
13. *Lactobacillus* species

BIBLIOGRAPHY

Brock T.D.: *Biology of Microorganisms.* Englewood Cliffs, N.J., Prentice-Hall, Inc., 1970.

DeLaat N.C.D.: *Microbiology for the Allied Health Professions,* ed. 2. Philadelphia, Lea & Febiger, 1979.

Griggs B.M., Reinhardt D.T.: *Fundamentals of Nosocomial Infections Associated with Respiratory Therapy.* New York, Projects in Health, Inc., 1975.

Jawetz E., Melinick J.L., Adelberg E.A.: *Review of Medical Microbiology,* ed. 12. Los Altos, Calif., Lange Medical Publications, 1976.

Mikat D.M., Mikat K.W.: *A Clinician's Guide to Bacteria,* ed. 2. Indianapolis, Eli Lilly and Co., 1975.

Novikoff A.B., Holtzman E.: *Cells and Organelles,* ed. 2. New York, Holt, Rinehart and Winston, 1976.

Shapiro B.A., Harrison R.A., Trout C.A.: *Clinical Application of Respiratory Care.* Chicago, Year Book Medical Publishers, Inc., 1975.

Smith L.A.: *Principles of Microbiology,* ed. 7. St. Louis, C.V. Mosby Co., 1973.

Swanson C.D., Webster D.L.: *The Cell,* ed. 4. Englewood Cliffs, N.J., Prentice-Hall, Inc., 1977.

Walton J.R., et al.: Serratia bacteremia from mean arterial pressure monitors. *Anesthesiology* 43:113, 1975.

36 / Sterilization

I. Definitions
  A. *Sterilization:* Complete destruction of all types of microorganisms.
  B. *Germicide:* Chemical or physical agent used to destroy all types of microorganisms.
  C. *Disinfectant: Germicidal agent used on inanimate objects.*
  D. *Bactericide:* Chemical or physical agent used to destroy bacteria in non-spore-forming states.
  E. *Sporicide:* Chemical or physical agent used to destroy spores.
  F. *Bacteriostatic:* Chemical or physical agent used to inhibit bacterial growth.
  G. *Antiseptic:* Chemical agent used to destroy or inhibit the growth of microorganisms on living tissue.
  H. *Asepsis:* Removal of microorganisms and/or prevention of recontamination with microorganisms.
  I. *Decontamination:* Process of removing a contaminant by chemical or physical means.
  J. *Sanitization:* Any process that reduces total bacterial contamination to a level consistent with safety.
II. Preparation for Sterilization
  A. Equipment must be washed clean of all organic matter.
    1. Use an alkaline soap to prevent formation of curds on the equipment.
    2. Hand wash small items with a brush.
    3. Ultrasonic washers may be used for large items.
  B. Rinsing should be complete.
  C. Air-dry
  D. Package appropriately for the sterilization process to be used.
III. Mechanisms of Action of Various Agents
  A. Denaturation and coagulation of protein
    1. Denaturation: Chemical alteration of a protein's structure, causing it to lose some or all of its unique or specific characteristics.
    2. Coagulation: Solidification of protoplasmal protein into a gelatinous mass.

580

    B. Surface tension alteration
       1. Lowering aqueous plasma surface tension increases plasma membrane permeability, allowing an influx of fluid.
       2. The increased permeability causes cellular lysis.
    C. Interference with intracellular metabolic pathways: Normally either the cell is destroyed or multiplication is inhibited.
IV. Sterilization by Heat
    A. The mechanism of action is denaturation and coagulation.
    B. Efficiency of heat sterilization is determined by the heat capacity of the gas involved in the sterilization process.
    C. Heat capacity of water at any temperature significantly exceeds the heat capacity of air.
    D. Steam has a heat capacity many times greater than that of water at the same temperature due to the latent heat of varporization of water molecules.
    E. Heat capacity of steam increases logarithmically with increasing pressure.
    F. Order of efficiency of sterilization by heat
       1. Steam under pressure (autoclave)
       2. Steam at atmospheric pressure
       3. Boiling water
       4. Dry heat under pressure
       5. Dry heat at atmospheric pressure
       6. Water below its boiling point (pasteurization)
    G. Autoclaving
       1. Steam and pressure are used to produce the most efficient method of sterilization.
       2. Sterilization occurs as a result of heat transfer from the condensation and evaporation of steam on the surface of the substance being sterilized.
       3. Equipment is packaged in material that allows steam to enter but prevents microorganisms from entering.
         a. Muslin
         b. Linen cloth
         c. Kraft paper
         d. Nylon
         e. Brown paper
         f. Crepe paper
         g. Vegetable parchment
       4. Variables involved in proper autoclaving
         a. Temperature
         b. Pressure

    c. Concentration of steam

5. Holding time is the minimum amount of time necessary to kill spores at a specific pressure.
6. The actual sterilization time is one and one half times the holding time.
7. Examples of autoclaving cycles:
    a. 121° C at 15 psi for 15 minutes
    b. 126° C at 20 psi for 10 minutes
    c. 134° C at 29.4 psi for 3 minutes
8. Heat-sensitive indicators are applied to all equipment to be autoclaved.
    a. These indicate that the equipment has been exposed to conditions necessary for sterilization.
    b. *They do not indicate sterilization.*
9. Biologic indicators are used to ensure that actual sterilization has been accomplished.
    a. *Bacillus stearothermophilus* spores are normally used because of their high heat resistance.
    b. Capsules containing 10^6 spores should be placed in at least one load per day and inspected for viable cells.

H. Dry heat
1. Efficiency is considerably lower than steam heat.
2. In general, dry heat should be used only on materials in which moist heat would be deleterious or unable to permeate the product being sterilized.
3. Temperature-time relationships
    a. 170° C: 60 minutes
    b. 160° C: 120 minutes
    c. 150° C: 150 minutes
    d. 140° C: 180 minutes
    e. 121° C: Overnight

I. Pasteurization
1. The submergence of equipment in medium hot water for a specified period of time.
2. Pasteurization is effective only in the destruction of vegetative cells.
3. Equipment is immersed in water at a temperature of 75° C for 10 minutes.
4. When the equipment is removed from the pasteurization unit, it must be dried and packaged.

V. Ethylene Oxide Sterilization (ETO; $[CH_2]_2O$)
  A. Characteristics of ETO

1. A gas at room temperature but liquefies readily under moderate pressure.
2. Has a pleasant ethereal odor.
3. Causes irritation of tissues, especially the mucous membranes.
4. ETO is flammable and explosive at certain concentrations and temperatures.
5. Normally used in 10%–12% mixtures with carbon dioxide or halogenated hydrocarbons (e.g., dichlorodifluoromethane [Freon 12], which act as a damping agent) making up the remainder of the gas mixture. These mixtures are nonflammable at temperatures up to 55° C.

B. Mechanism of action
1. Alkylation occurs at specific enzyme sites and interrupts normal metabolism and reproduction.
2. Coordination of the following factors is necessary for proper sterilization:
   a. Gas concentration
   b. Humidity
   c. Temperature
   d. Time
3. The addition of H_2O vapor increases sensitivity of both vegetative cells and spores to ETO.
4. Sterilization proceeds most rapidly at relative humidities of 30% and slows progressively below or above that level.
5. Other factors being equal, the effectiveness of ETO doubles for each 10° C rise in temperature up to 60° C.
6. System pressure for carbon dioxide mixtures is between 20 and 30 psi, and for hydrocarbon mixtures, between 5 and 7 psi.
7. Typical systems
   a. Temperature 54.4° C, relative humidity 30%–60%, and pressure 5–7 psi with 450 mg of $(CH_2)_2O$ per liter of air for 6 hours results in sterilization.
   b. If the concentration of $(CH_2)_2O$ is raised to 850 mg/L, sterilization occurs in 3 hours.
8. The packaging material used should be permeable to humidity and $(CH_2)_2O$, but not to microorganisms.
   a. Wrapping paper
   b. Cloth
   c. Muslin
   d. Polyethylene

    e. Nylon film

  9. The use of indicator tape identifies exposure to ETO but does not guarantee sterility of equipment.

  10. A biologic indicator is used to ensure that conditions necessary for sterility have been achieved. Cultures of *Bacillus subtilis* var. globigii should be used daily.

  11. Aeration time

    a. Most materials require at least a 24-hour aeration time in a well-ventilated area (aeration chambers can significantly decrease this time).

    b. Substances made of neoprene rubber or polyvinyl chloride require extended aeration times: up to 7 days, depending on thickness: because of their tendency to absorb $(CH_2)_2O$.

  12. ETO residues

    a. Substances that have been previously gamma irradiated, especially polyvinyl chloride, react with $(CH_2)_2O$ to form ethylene chlorhydrin, which is very irritating to tissue.

    b. If the material to be sterilized is not dry, the water on it reacts with $(CH_2)_2O$ to form ethylene glycol (this usually results in a very sticky residue on the material).

VI. Gamma Irradiation

  A. Gamma waves are very short wavelength light waves possessing extremely high energy and having the ability to ionize a substance.

  B. Ionization of water molecules inactivates DNA molecules by increasing the rate of reaction of DNA with hydrogen and hydroxyl ions.

  C. Advantages

    1. High efficiency.

    2. Negligible temperature change.

    3. Equipment may be prepackaged and sealed.

  D. Disadvantages

    1. Sterilization time prolonged 48–72 hours.

    2. Polyvinyl chloride may release chlorine gas.

    3. Feasible only on a large-scale industrial level.

VII. Liquid Disinfectants

  A. Alcohol

    1. Ethyl alcohol: 50%–70% most efficient.

    2. Isopropyl alcohol: 75%–100% most efficient.

    3. Effective against vegetative cells.

    4. Ineffective against viruses and spores.

B. Acetic acid
1. A 1:1 mixture of vinegar with tap water is bacteriostatic.
2. Used to disinfect equipment in the home.
3. Minimal toxicity to tissue.
C. Formaldehyde
1. Formaldehyde: Formalin in a 37% solution.
2. It is used in disinfectant solutions.
3. Formalin is very effective when used in combination with isopropyl alcohol or hexachlorophene.
4. It is sporicidal with prolonged exposures of 6–12 hours.
5. It is toxic to tissues and has a pungent, penetrating, irritating odor.
D. Phenol and related compounds
1. Considerable variation in concentration.
2. Some preparations virucidal.
3. No sporicidal properties.
4. Irritating to tissue.
E. Iodine and related compounds
1. Concentrations variable.
2. Efficient bactericidal activity.
3. No sporicidal activity.
F. Mercurial compounds
1. Concentrations variable.
2. Poor germicides.
3. Normally considered bacteriostatic only.
4. Rapidly inactivated by organic substances.
G. Quaternary ammonium compounds
1. Selective bactericidal activity.
2. Not destructive to tuberculosis bacillus spores or enteroviruses.
3. Rapid loss of potency, especially in the presence of protein.
H. Glutaraldehyde (Table 36–1)
1. Cidex (activated alkaline glutaraldehyde, pH 7.5–8.5)
   a. The equipment should be completely washed and partially dried.
   b. Cidex is effective in the presence of protein material if immersion is complete.
   c. A 10-minute exposure is germicidal.
   d. A 10-hour exposure is sporicidal.
   e. Cidex is toxic to tissue.
   f. Equipment must be rinsed completely after exposure, left to air dry, and packaged in a sterile manner.

TABLE 36–1.—COMPARISON OF CIDEX AND SONACIDE

PROPERTY	CIDEX	SONACIDE
pH	7.5–8.5	2.7–3.7
Germicidal time	10 min	20 min
Sporicidal time and temperature	10 hr at room temperature	1 hr at 60° C
Toxicity	Toxic	Extremely toxic
Solution life	28 days	28 days

  g. Maximum solution life is 28 days.
 2. Sonacide (acid glutaraldehyde, pH 2.7–3.7)
  a. The equipment should be completely washed and partially dried.
  b. A 10-minute exposure is germicidal except for *Mycobacterium*.
  c. A 20-minute exposure is completely germicidal.
  d. Heated sonacide (60° C) is sporicidal after 1 hour.
  e. It is extremely toxic to tissue.
  f. Equipment must be rinsed completely after exposure, left to air dry, and packaged in a sterile manner.
  g. Maximum solution life is 28 days.
VIII. Filtration
 A. Sterilization or disinfection of gases and liquids is particularly difficult.
 B. High-efficiency particulate air filters are the most effective filters available.
  1. They remove particles as small as 0.3 μ with a 99.97% efficiency.
  2. Used primarily in laminar flow rooms and hoods.
 C. Membrane filters are used on most respiratory therapy equipment.
  1. They are composed of thin sheets of cellulose esters or other polymeric material folded many times to ensure a large surface area.
  2. Most may be autoclaved for reuse; however, some are disposable.
  3. Some are effective against viruses.

BIBLIOGRAPHY
American Hospital Association Advisory Committee on Infections: *Infection Control in the Hospital*, ed. 4. Chicago, American Hospital Association, 1979.
AMA Z–79, Subcommittee on Ethylene Oxide Sterilization: Ethylene oxide sterilization: A guide for hospital personnel. *Respir. Care* 22:12, 1977.

Bageant R.A., et al.: In-use testing of four glutaraldehyde disinfectants in the cidematic washer. *Respir. Care* 26:1255–1261, 1981.

Becker K.O.: Decontamination area for inhalation therapy. *J. Am. Hosp. Assoc.* 45:68, 1971.

Becker K.O.: Inhalation therapy department chooses ETO. *J. Am. Hosp. Assoc.* 45:681, 1971.

Block S.S.: *Disinfection, Sterilization and Preservation,* ed. 2. Philadelphia, Lea & Febiger, 1977.

Boyd R.F., Hoerl B.G.: *Basic Medical Microbiology,* ed. 2. Boston, Little, Brown & Co., 1981.

Haselhuhn D.H., Brason F.W., Borick P.M.: In-use study of buffered glutaraldehyde for cold sterilization of anesthesia equipment. *Anesth. Analg.* 46:468, 1967.

Leach E.D.: A new synergized glutaraldehyde-phenate sterilizing solution and concentrated disinfectant. *Infect. Control* 1:26–31, 1981.

McLaughlin A.J.: *Manual of Infection Control in Respiratory Care.* Boston, Little, Brown & Co., 1983.

Masferrer R., Marguez R.: Comparison of two activated glutaraldehyde solutions: Cidex solution and Sonacide. *Respir. Care* 22:257, 1977.

Nelson E.J.: Respiratory therapy equipment contamination surveillance program: Part I. Techniques of infection control in respiratory therapy and anesthesia. Seattle, Olympic Medical Corp., Series 5, 1977.

Perkins J.J.: *Principles and Methods of Sterilization in Health Sciences,* Springfield, Ill., Charles C Thomas, Publisher, 1969.

Rendell-Baker L., Roberts R.B.: Safe use of ethylene oxide sterilization in hospitals. *Anesth. Analg.* 51:658, 1972.

Rubbo S.D., Gardner J.F.: *A Review of Sterilization and Disinfection.* Chicago, Year Book Medical Publishers, Inc., 1965.

Starkey D.H., Himmelsbach C.K.: On the avoidance of failures in sterilization. *Hospitals* 48:143, 1974.

Sykes G.: *Disinfection and Sterilization.* London, E. and E.N. Spon. Ltd., 1958.

Sykes M.K.: Sterilization of ventilators. *Int. Anesthesiol. Clin.* 10:131, 1972.

Synder J.E.: Infection control. *Hospitals* 44:80, 1970.

Synder R.W., Cheatle E.L.: Alkaline glutaraldehyde, an effective disinfectant. *Am. J. Hosp. Pharm.* 22:321, 1965.

Technical Standards and Safety Committee, AART: Recommendations for respiratory therapy equipment: Processing, handling and surveillance. *Respir. Care* 22:928, 1977.

Wilson R.D., et al.: An evaluation of the acidemic decontamination system for anesthesia equipment. *Anesth. Analg.* 51:658, 1972.

Index

Adrenomedullary hormones
circulation and
pulmonary, 121
systemic, 120
heart rate and, 129
myocardial contractility and, 136–137
Aerobic, 562, 566
Aerosol
clearance of, 392
definition of, 391
deposition of, 391
optimal, ventilatory pattern for,
391–392
generators (*see* Nebulizer)
oxygen delivery systems, mechanical,
375
penetration of, 391
optimal, ventilatory pattern for,
391-392
stability of, 391
sympathomimetics in COPD, 304
therapy, 391-396
goals of, 393
hazards of, 393
indications for, 392-393
in pneumonia, 324
Afterload, 133-135, 231
PEEP and, 503
Air
bubbles contaminating blood gases,
212
compressed, cylinders, calculation of
duration of flow from, 360
entrainment, 427
fractional distillation of, 368
pollutants, 300
trapping, 301
increased, due to IPPB, 409
Airway
artificial, 381
obstruction, acute, management
of, 388
after smoke inhalation, 332
care, 381–390
cuffs, 386–388
deflation technique, 388
high-volume, low-pressure, 387
inflation techniques, 387–388
Kamen-Wilkinson, 387
Lanz, 387
pressures, monitoring of, 388

lower, 47–61
maneuvers
expiratory, 440
inspiratory, 440
nasopharyngeal, 381
obstruction, 381
aerosol therapy and, 393
partial, 82
partial, congenital, 349
oropharyngeal, 381
pressure
mean, 477
mean, effect of positive pressure
on, 462
peak, 481, 482, 483
positive, continuous (*see* CPAP)
positive, expiratory (*see* EPAP)
resistance, 42, 76, 80–82, 293
increased, due to IPPB, 410
mechanical ventilation and, 483
suctioning, 388–389
technique, 389
upper, 38–47
reflexes, 89
Alarm systems: ventilator, 440, 484
Albuteral, 538
Alcohol
as disinfectant, 584–585
ethyl, 533
Aldosterone, 160–161
Alevaire, 532–533
Algae, 558
blue-green, 558
Alkalosis, 145
metabolic
compensated, 94
myocardial contractility and, 136
primary causes of, 210
respiratory, 202
compensated, 93–94
myocardial contractility and, 136
in pulmonary disease, obstructive,
303
in pulmonary disease, restrictive,
314
in pulmonary embolism, 326
Alkylation, 583
Allergen inhalation tests, 287
Allergies, 300
asthma and, 310
Alpha$_1$ antitrypsin deficiency, 305

Heart *(cont.)*
  septal defect causing, ventricular, 341
  failure, and thoracoskeletal restrictive lung disease, 327
  fibroskeleton, 259
  glycosides, 554–555
  index, 239
    monitoring after PEEP, 514
  output, 127–137, 138, 140, 141
    arteriovenous oxygen content difference and, 509, 510
    capillary, 217
    decreased, due to IPPB, 409–410
    effect of positive pressure on, 463, 464
    kidney and, 157
    measurement techniques, 236–239
    monitoring after PEEP, 514
    PEEP and, 503, 504, 505
    shunted, 217
  rate, 127
    control of, 128–130
    ECG interpretation, 262
  rhythm *(see* Rhythm)
  sound, first, 124
  valves *(see* Valve)
Heat
  (See also Thermal)
  dry, sterilization by, 582
  latent *(see* Latent heat)
  specific, 16
  sterilization by, 581–582
  units of, 16
Helium, 358
  dilution study, 275
Hematocrit, 97
Hemes, 183
Hemodynamic
  effects of PEEP, 505–507
  monitoring, 229–241
    during mechanical ventilation, 484
  values, neonatal, 174
Hemoglobin, 97
  abnormal, 188
  buffering system, 201
  carrying capacity, 183–185
  content, 219
  fetal, 188
  reduced, 421
  structure, 183–185

Hemoptysis, 309
  IPPB causing, 410
  in pulmonary embolism, 325
Hemothorax, 317
Henderson-Hasselbalch equation, 196–197
Henry's law, 26
Heparin: as blood gas contaminant, 211–212
Hering-Breuer reflex, 90
Hernia: diaphragmatic, 330, 349
Heroin, 550
Heterotroph, 563
Hexobarbital, 552
Hilum, 63
His bundle, 257, 258, 259
Histamine, 532, 550
  inhalation test, 285–286
Histoplasmosis, 578
Histotoxic hypoxia, 370
H_2O *(see* Water)
H_2O_2, 373
Hook's law, 27–28
Hormone
  adrenocorticotropic, 544–547
    in myasthenia gravis, 329
  adrenomedullary *(see* Adrenomedullary hormones)
  antidiuretic, 160, 549
HPO_4^{-2}, 161, 163
Huffing, 403
Humidifier oxygen delivery systems: cascade-type, 375–377
Humidity, 21–22
  absolute, 21
    maximum, 21
  aerosols and, 391
  effect on Dalton's law, 22–23
  relative, 21–22
Hyaline membrane, 374
Hydrochloride acid administration: dilute, calculation of, 211
Hydrochlorothiazide, 548
Hydro-Diuril, 548
Hydroflumethiazide, 548
Hydrogen
  bonding, 15
  ion, 91, 94, 161
    concentration, expressions of, 10–11
  peroxide, 373

Streptokinase: in pulmonary embolism, 326
Streptomycin, 553
  for *Mycobacterium*
    leprae, 571
    tuberculosis, 571
  for *Proteus*, 572
Stress: generalized increased, and ventilator commitment, 467
Stridor: congenital laryngeal, 349
Stroke volume, 125, 127, 134, 137, 229, 230
  control of, 130–137
Subaortic stenosis, 342
Subatmospheric pressure, 72
Subcutaneous
  emphysema (*see* Emphysema, subcutaneous)
  injection, 529
Subglottic edema, 386
Sublimation, 17
Sublingual absorption: of drugs, 529
Submucosal glands, 42, 57
  hypertrophy, 307
Succinylcholine, 544
Suction, 381
Suctioning, airway, 388–389
  technique, 389
Sudden infant death syndrome, 355–356
Sulfonamides, 553
  for *Escherichia coli*, 573
Superinfection: definition of, 566
Superoxide
  dismutase, 373, 374
  radical, 373
Supersaturated solution, 4
Supraventricular tachycardia, 269
Surface
  -active agent, 533
  area, body, 239
    neonatal, 180
  tension, 28–29, 76–77
    alteration, 581
    PEEP and, 501
Surfactant, 29, 501
  development, 166–167
  in pulmonary alveolar proteinosis, 326

in respiratory distress syndrome
  adult, 323
  infant, 335
"Sweat test," 353
Symbiosis, 563
Sympathetic
  nerve fibers, 101
  nervous system (*see* Nervous system, sympathetic)
  response in asthma, 311
  stimulation, 121, 122
    cardiac excitatory center and, 139
    vasoconstriction and, 138
    vasodilation and, 138
  tone, 463
Sympatholytics, 542–543
  heart rate and, 129
  myocardial contractility and, 137
Sympathomimetics, 533–539
  alpha effect, 533
  in asthma, 312
  beta effect, 533
  beta one, 534
  beta two, 534
  in bronchospasm, 304
  heart rate and, 129
  in mucosal edema, 304
  myocardial contractility and, 137
Syncurine, 544
Synergism, 527
Synnecrosis, 563
Systemic
  arterial system, 125
  circulation, 118–121
    control of, 119
  hypertension, 134
  pressure
    interstitial colloid osmotic, 246
    PEEP and, 505
  resistance (*see* Resistance, systemic)
Systole, 123
  atrial, 123–124
  ventricular, 124–125, 126
Systolic pressure, 229, 230, 232

T

Tachycardia, 139
  atrial, 265
  sinus, 264